Neural Degeneration and Repair

Edited by
Hans Werner Müller

Related Titles

H. Nothwang, E. Pfeiffer (Eds.)

Proteomics of the Nervous System

2008
ISBN 978-3-527-31716-5

O. von Bohlen und Halbach, R. Dermietzel

Neurotransmitters and Neuromodulators

Handbook of Receptors and Biological Effects

2006
ISBN 978-3-527-31307-5

G. Thiel (Ed.)

Transcription Factors in the Nervous System

Development, Brain Function, and Diseases

2006
ISBN 978-3-527-31285-6

R. Shulman, D. Rothman (Eds.)

Brain Energetics and Neuronal Activity

Applications to fMRI and Medicine

2004
ISBN: 978-0-470-84720-6

Neural Degeneration and Repair

Gene Expression Profiling, Proteomics,
and Systems Biology

Edited by
Hans Werner Müller

WILEY-
VCH

WILEY-VCH Verlag GmbH & Co. KGaA

The Editor

Prof. Dr. Hans Werner Müller
Heinrich-Heine University Düsseldorf
Department of Neurology
Moorenstrasse 5
40225 Düsseldorf
Germany

Cover illustration
The cover picture shows an immunofluorescence
image of sensory neurons (red) in a dorsal root
ganglion expressing gastric inhibitory polypeptide
(green). The neurons respond to peripheral
nerve injury by altered gene expression.
With kind permission of Bettina Buhren and
Hans Werner Müller.

Library of Congress Card No.: applied for

British Library Cataloguing-in-Publication Data
A catalogue record for this book is available from
the British Library

**Bibliographic information published by
the Deutsche Nationalbibliothek**
Die Deutsche Nationalbibliothek lists this publication in the Deutsche Nationalbibliografie; detailed
bibliographic data are available in the Internet at
http://dnb.d-nb.de

Printed in the Federal Republic of Germany
Printed on acid-free paper

Typesetting   Thomson Digital, Noida, India
Printing   Strauss GmbH, Mörlenbach
Binding   Litges & Dopf GmbH, Heppenheim

ISBN: 978-3-527-31707-3

Contents

Neural Degeneration and Repair: Gene Expression Profiling, Proteomics, and Systems Biology
Edited by Hans Werner Müller
Copyright © 2008 WILEY-VCH Verlag GmbH & Co. KGaA, Weinheim
ISBN: 978-3-527-31707-3

Preface

During the past ten years, since the introduction of microarray technology, neuroscientists became aware that highly complex gene expression networks are activated in traumatic nervous system injuries and devastating neurodegenerative disorders such as Alzheimer's disease (AD) and Parkinson's disease (PD). The classical approach of studying single or small sets of genes or proteins has been quite disappointing to dissect the intricate network of molecular reactions and failed to provide a more complete picture of the pathophysiological and degenerative events. Despite a great deal of initial skepticism, the advent of microarray technology that allows the study of changes in gene expression at a (near) genome wide scale has opened a new avenue for a molecular systems approach to neural degeneration and repair. As a step further, proteome analysis, the "analysis of the entire PROTEin complement expressed by a genOME", involves the simultaneous separation, identification and/or quantification of hundreds or thousands of proteins from a single tissue sample.

There is a desperate need for a critical overview of the present state of research in this field that has reached a certain state of maturation and acceptance and is at the edge to be widely and routinely used among neuroscientists all over the world. Thus, it appears to be timely to describe the potential as well as the limitations of the application of these recent technologies to highly relevant neurological disorders such as trauma, neurodegenerative disorders and neural tumors and their transition into clinical applications (diagnosis, prevention, therapy).

This book highlights the state-of-the-art application of microarrays and proteomics in systems neurobiology and translational neuroscience from genome research to clinical application with particular emphasis on peripheral (PNS) and central nervous system (CNS) injury and repair, neuropathic pain, ageing and neurodegenerative diseases such as AD, PD, and neurooncology. Microarray technology will not only be critically compared with previously existing high-throughput gene expression technologies. As outlined in the following chapters, the genomic and proteomic technologies have proven a tremendous impact on elucidating genetic networks and molecular pathways underlying successful axonal plasticity, regeneration and retrograde axonal signaling in the damaged PNS and CNS. Moreover, the potential of pharmacogenomics for future applications in personalized therapies, the

Neural Degeneration and Repair: Gene Expression Profiling, Proteomics, and Systems Biology
Edited by Hans Werner Müller
Copyright © 2008 WILEY-VCH Verlag GmbH & Co. KGaA, Weinheim
ISBN: 978-3-527-31707-3

development of new quantitative proteomics technologies (SILAC, ICAT, iTRAC), and the impact of novel redox proteomics approaches to analyze protein modifications due to oxidative damage in nerve cell cultures and animal models of AD are presented. On the other hand, gene expression profiling of gliomas has opened entirely new perspectives on tumor classification and deciphering tumor heterogeneity, pathway-associated expression signatures, and lineage-specific molecular signatures to localize the origin of a glial tumor.

We hope that this book provides useful information for a wide range of basic researchers and biomedical and clinical scientists from the level of neurobiology/medical students, postdocs to advanced specialists in academics as well as industry.

I am very grateful to all the people who contributed to this book, especially to Dr. Andreas Sendtko and Claudia Grössl from Wiley-VCH.

Düsseldorf, January 2008   *Hans Werner Müller*

List of Contributors

Lan Bao
Chinese Academy of Sciences
Shanghai Institutes for Biological
Sciences
Institute of Biochemistry and
Cell Biology
Laboratory of Molecular Cell Biology
320 Yue Yang Road
200031 Shanghai
P.R. China

Frank Bosse
Heinrich-Heine University
Molecular Neurobiology Laboratory
Department of Neurology and
Biomedical Research Center
Moorenstrasse 5
40225 Düsseldorf
Germany

Nicole Brazda
Heinrich-Heine University
Molecular Neurobiology Laboratory
Department of Neurology and
Biomedical Research Center
Moorenstrasse 5
40225 Düsseldorf
Germany

Peter Buckley
University of Pennsylvania
Department of Pharmacology
36th Hamilton Walk
Philadelphia, PA 19129
USA

D. Allen Butterfield
University of Kentucky
Department of Chemistry
Center of Membrane Sciences, and
Sanders-Brown Center on Aging
121 Chemistry-Physics Bldg.
Lexington, KY 40506-0055
USA

Simone Di Giovanni
University of Tübingen
Laboratory for Neuroregeneration
and Repair
Hertie Institute for Clinical Brain
Research
Otfried-Müller-Strasse 27
72076 Tübingen
Germany

James Eberwine
University of Pennsylvania
Department of Pharmacology
36th Hamilton Walk
Philadelphia, PA 19129
USA

Neural Degeneration and Repair: Gene Expression Profiling, Proteomics, and Systems Biology
Edited by Hans Werner Müller
Copyright © 2008 WILEY-VCH Verlag GmbH & Co. KGaA, Weinheim
ISBN: 978-3-527-31707-3

Mike Fainzilber
Weizmann Institute of Science
Department of Biological Chemistry
76100 Rehovot
Israel

James W. Fawcett
University of Cambridge
Centre for Brain Repair
Department of Clinical Neurosciences
Cambridge
United Kingdom

Daniel H. Geschwind
University of California at Los Angeles
School of Medicine
Department of Neurology
710 Westwood Plaza
Los Angeles, CA 90095-1769
USA

Jeanine Jochems
University of Pennsylvania
Department of Pharmacology
36th Hamilton Walk
Philadelphia, PA 19129
USA

Fabian Kruse
Heinrich-Heine University
Molecular Neurobiology Laboratory
Department of Neurology and
Biomedical Research Center
Moorenstrasse 5
40225 Düsseldorf
Germany

Patrick Küry
Heinrich-Heine University
Molecular Neurobiology Laboratory
Department of Neurology and
Biomedical Research Center
Moorenstrasse 5
40225 Düsseldorf
Germany

Matthew R. Mason
Laboratory for Neuroregeneration
Netherlands Institute for Neuroscience
Amsterdam
The Netherlands

Izhak Michaelevski
Weizmann Institute of Science
Department of Biological Chemistry
76100 Rehovot
Israel

Jeremy A. Miller
University of California at Los Angeles
Department of Neurology
Interdepartmental Program in
Neuroscience
710 Westwood Plaza
Los Angeles, CA 90095-1769
USA

Hans W. Müller
Heinrich-Heine University
Department of Neurology and
Biomedical Research Center
Molecular Neurobiology Laboratory
Moorenstrasse 5
40225 Düsseldorf
Germany

Tanea Reed
University of Kentucky
Department of Chemistry
203 Chemistry-Physics Bldg.
Lexington, KY 40506-0055
USA

Guido Reifenberger
Heinrich-Heine University
Department of Neuropathology
Moorenstrasse 5
40225 Düsseldorf
Germany

Markus J. Riemenschneider
Heinrich-Heine University
Department of Neuropathology
Moorenstrasse 5
40225 Düsseldorf
Germany

August B. Smit
Vrije Universiteit
Department of Molecular and
Cellular Neurobiology
Center for Neurogenomics and
Cognitive Research
1105 AZ Amsterdam
The Netherlands

Floor J. Stam
Vrije Universiteit
Department of Molecular and
Cellular Neurobiology
Center for Neurogenomics and
Cognitive Research
1105 AZ Amsterdam
The Netherlands

Rukhsana Sultana
University of Kentucky
Department of Chemistry
203 Chemistry-Physics Bldg.
Lexington, KY 40506-0055
USA

Joost Verhaagen
Laboratory for Neuroregeneration
Netherlands Institute for Neuroscience
Amsterdam
The Netherlands

Christina F. Vogelaar
University of Cambridge
Centre for Brain Repair
Department of Clinical Neurosciences
Cambridge
United Kingdom

Hua-Sheng Xiao
Chinese Academy of Sciences
Shanghai Institutes for Biological
Sciences
Institute of Neuroscience and
Key Laboratory of Systems Biology
320 Yue Yang Road
200031 Shanghai
P.R. China

Xu Zhang
Chinese Academy of Sciences
Shanghai Institutes for Biological
Sciences
Institute of Neuroscience and
Key Laboratory of Neurobiology
320 Yue Yang Road
200031 Shanghai
P.R. China

1

Microarrays in Systems Neurobiology and Translational Neuroscience – From Genome Research to Clinical Applications

Jeremy A. Miller and Daniel H. Geschwind

1.1
Introduction

Although microarray technology was introduced just 10 years ago, over 20 000 articles have been published using this technology as of 2006, covering areas ranging from soil ecology and yeast genomics to cancer and neurological disorders. In neuroscience, much of this represents publications since 2000, showing a remarkable trajectory as well as reflecting early skepticism that has now given way to acceptance and appreciation (Figure 1.1). Entire transcriptomes can now be assayed on a single chip at a reasonable cost, and technologies are becoming cheaper and more accurate day by day. In basic neuroscience research, microarrays have been used to assess gene expression differences across mouse strains [1], brain areas [2], cell types [3–5], and brain tumor strains [6]. They have also been used to identify genes that play an important role in neural stem cell biology [7,8], mouse models of neurodevelopmental disorders [9], and postmortem assessments of many neurodegenerative diseases such as Alzheimer's disease (AD) [2,10–15], Parkinson's disease (PD) [16], Huntington's disease (HD) [17,18], amyotrophic lateral sclerosis (ALS) [19,20], and schizophrenia [21]. In addition to providing a useful tool for basic neuroscience research, microarrays hold significant promise clinically as patient classifiers in acute and chronic neurological diseases [22].

This chapter summarizes the current state of microarray technology, presenting several clinical applications. In the next section, gene expression technologies leading up to microarray technologies are presented along with alternative high-throughput techniques. Section 1.3 provides a primer on how to design and implement a successful microarray experiment and presents challenges to the field and analytic methods that have been developed to get the most out of expression data. The last section summarizes recent microarray experiments in the field of neuroscience, highlighting key, representative papers documenting state-of-the-art experimental design, clinical uses in brain cancer, and the use of peripheral blood as a substitute for brain tissue in various neuropsychiatric conditions. Finally, genomic DNA microarrays are briefly discussed, along with speculation on the future of clinical microarray applications.

Neural Degeneration and Repair: Gene Expression Profiling, Proteomics, and Systems Biology
Edited by Hans Werner Müller
Copyright © 2008 WILEY-VCH Verlag GmbH & Co. KGaA, Weinheim
ISBN: 978-3-527-31707-3

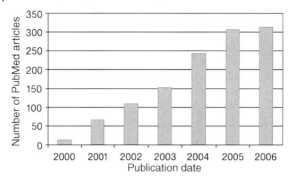

Figure 1.1 Acceptance and use of microarrays in the twenty-first century. Since the year 2000, publications on microarrays have gained popularity in the area of neurosciences, indicating their more widespread acceptance and use as a viable tool. The X-axis indicates publication year, while the Y-axis indicates number of publications turning up in PubMed searches for ''microarray'' and ''brain''.

1.2
Gene Expression Before Microarrays

Since the discovery of DNA in the early 1900s and the subsequent discovery of RNA as the substrate for protein synthesis, gene expression assays have become an essential component of disease research. Gene expression approaches initially took a gene-centric view. A scientist would hypothesize a relationship between a gene and a phenotype, and then test this hypothesis using methods such as Northern blot and *in situ* hybridization. In Northern blot analysis, mRNA is denatured and separated by weight on a gel using agarose gel electrophoresis, transferred onto a membrane, and hybridized with complementary labeled probes [23]. Thus, gene expression correlates with intensity of the labeling. *In situ* hybridization, on the contrary, involves directly applying labeled probes to the tissues of interest to determine where the mRNA is expressed *in situ* [24]. Although still important for studying single genes, these high-resolution techniques are at a disadvantage with regard to the throughput now available using techniques such as RT-PCR, serial analysis of gene expression (SAGE), differential display, and microarrays. As is the case in complex, dynamic tissues such as the brain and nervous system, there is often a trade-off between scale and resolution [25].

1.2.1
High-Throughput Gene Expression Techniques

A paradigm shift occurred in the early 1990s, as technology improved and knowledge of the genome became widely accessible. This challenged scientists to move from a gene-by-gene study to develop methods that took into consideration the entire system of gene expression, moving from the unimolecular to the systems level [26]. One of the earliest methods using high-throughput techniques to identify a large number of genes differentially expressed between two tissues or conditions was differential-display reverse-transcription polymerase chain reaction (DDPCR) [27]. In DDPCR, the 5′ end of mRNA is bound to anchor primers and reverse transcribed. A subset of this cDNA is then PCR amplified near its 3′ end using short arbitrary primers. The resulting amplified cDNAs from two samples are run side by side on a gel, and any differentially displayed bands of interest can be excised from the gel, reamplified, cloned, and sequenced. This method is relatively inexpensive and can test gene expression of all transcripts amplified simultaneously; however, every interesting band has to be sequenced individually, and the completion of the human genome project has rendered such time-consuming sequencing unnecessary.

Representational difference analysis (RDA) represents a more elegant genome-wide subtraction method that, unlike DDPCR, does not require sifting through an entire gel of genes to find some that are different [7,28,29]. In RDA, populations of mRNA from two separate tissues are transcribed into cDNA, digested using restriction enzymes, converted into primers, and PCR amplified. These populations are then cross-hybridized by combining an excess of one population (driver) and using that to remove identical transcripts from the less concentrated population (tester). By iteratively performing this process with each population as the driver and the tester, and then shotgun cloning the subtraction products, libraries for genes enriched in each tissue can be created. We have used this method coupled to microarray screening, which provides a powerful approach to screening genetic subtractions [7,28].

1.2.2
Contemporaneous Alternatives to Microarrays

SAGE [30] is one of the several high-throughput sequencing methods that provide a powerful technique for high-resolution assessment of gene expression in a relatively small number of samples. In SAGE, cDNA is positionally anchored using restriction digestion, and short nucleotide chains around 14 base pair (bp) are removed from specific positions in each molecule, serving as tags, concatenated together into polymers of such tags, many multiples of which can be processed in a single sequencing run. Thus, small tags of each gene are present in proportion to their abundance in the starting mRNA and can be counted by efficient sequencing and bioinformatic identification of the gene from which they originate. The resolution in SAGE is limited only by the cost and time of sequencing, but it typically requires about 2000 sequencing reactions for each SAGE library to identify 50 000 tags. However, often one needs to sequence 1 million or more tags to identify low-abundance species in a complex tissue such as the CNS. To compare two tissues, several such libraries need to be prepared from each tissue, making this a high-resolution but low-throughput approach (relative to sample numbers that can be studied). In theory, this technique is sensitive enough to find any mRNA species and has the advantage over differential display, as each sequencing run determines multiple mRNA species. In practice, however, this technique is too expensive and time consuming for massive parallelization and clinical use.

Massively parallel signature sequencing (MPSS) determines mRNA counts using a principle similar to SAGE [31]. In MPSS, fluorescently labeled cDNAs from the input sample are hybridized to a microbead cDNA library, and hybridized beads are fluorescently sorted and placed on a 2D grid. All beads are then simultaneously decoded and digested 4 bp at a time by binding unique adaptors, which can be read using a charge-coupled device (CCD). MPSS has all the advantages of SAGE and can read many more mRNA species for similar time investment (~250 000), but it requires special equipment and is expensive. Thus, for most, it remains primarily a research tool for in-depth investigation of a few specific samples of interest, although the recent advent of new sequencing technologies will significantly decrease the price of these clone and count techniques.

1.2.3
Microarray Technologies

Microarrays balance sensitivity and throughput to allow efficient study of about 10 000 detected mRNA species in parallel in a large number of samples. This may not allow the maximum depth possible as with MPSS or SAGE but has the advantage of high scalability. The first high-throughput gene expression study, published in 1987, was carried out by Augenlicht *et al.* who used a nylon membrane containing 4000 cDNA sequences to examine gene expression changes in colon cancer [32]. Once solid substrates replaced nylon in the 1990s, this method provided a relatively cheap, quick, and reproducible way for high-throughput gene expression analysis. Owing to the abundant clinical and research applications of this technology, many groups and companies have created their own microarray platforms. Although an entire chapter could be devoted to describing the similarities and differences of these platforms (see [33]), there are two general categories of microarrays: one-color arrays and two-color arrays.

1.2.3.1 One-Color Oligonucleotide Arrays
One-color oligonucleotide (oligo) arrays (or chips) marked the first of the commercial microarray technologies [34–38] and were released by Affymetrix in 1996. These arrays required the development of two novel methodologies. Light directed chemical synthesis allows for the direct application of hundreds of thousands of nucleotides to specific positions on the chip at once, bypassing the need for PCR-amplified cDNA probes. By masking all array positions not associated with the applied nucleotide and repeating this chemical coupling for each nucleotide using multiple masks, gene-specific oligo probes, 25 bp in length, are synthetically created. After synthesis of the array, laser fluorescence microscopy can detect hybridization of fluorescently labeled cDNA (target). Expression values for each gene can then be deduced by averaging over multiple probes and using mismatch probes (where the 13th bp has been purposely changed) to account for nonspecific binding.

1.2.3.2 **Two-Color Arrays**

Contemporaneous with the development of oligonucleotide arrays, a separate yet equally powerful method for running massively parallel gene expression experiments was created [39–43] in which thousands of cDNA probes between 0.2 and 2.5 kb in length were PCR amplified and printed onto poly-L-lysine-coated microscope glass slides using one of two printing techniques. In mechanical microspotting (or passive dispensing) – currently the more popular method – the target is loaded into a dispensing pin using capillary action and placed onto the cDNA microarray by directly contacting the slide. Drop-on-demand (or inkjet) printers use pins with piezoelectric fittings to drop a precise amount of the target onto the slide using an electrical current, without actually having the pins contact the slide. Once synthesized, these cDNA arrays, unlike their one-color counterparts, detect the differential expression between two reference samples, each of which is labeled with separate dyes (typically Cy3-dUTP and Cy5-dUTP). Hybridization fluorescence signals from each dye are detected separately with a dual-wavelength laser scanner and combined into a single pseudocolor image using computer software. Recently, most two-color platforms have shifted from cDNA probes to longer oligonucleotides (30–60 bp), as oligos are generally more customizable, potentially more target specific, and less difficult to amplify and purify than cDNAs. The Agilent platform is an example of a commercial two-color platform based on oligonucleotides [44].

1.2.3.3 **Bead-Based Arrays**

Most current microarray systems, whether one-color (Affymetrix) or two-color (Agilent), are based on oligos attached to a solid substrate, each with a known address. Illumina universal bead arrays [45,46], however, consist of densely packed wells, $\sim 3\,\mu m$ in diameter, which are randomly filled with beads containing 75 bp chimeric oligos. These wells are etched either into bundles of fiber-optic strands or onto specialized chips. Each array has an average coverage of ~ 30 beads per feature, with the exact number variable due to the random filling of wells. For each bead, oligonucleotides consist of a 25 bp bead identifier followed by a 50 bp gene-specific probe, and $\sim 700\,000$ such oligos are attached to each bead. Bead types are decoded by repeated hybridization (and subsequent dehybridization) of fluorescently labeled cDNA sequences complementary to the bead identifiers. Fluorophores are chosen such that each bead has a unique sequence of fluorescent signals (e.g., red-green-none-red-red-none-green-red after eight hybridizations). After decoding, cRNA from one sample is fluorescently labeled and scanned, and the absolute abundance of transcript is determined by averaging the intensities of each bead containing that transcript.

1.3
Designing and Implementing a Microarray Experiment – From Start to Finish

Many articles and guides on the basic design of microarray experiments in the field of neuroscience are available [47–50]. Here, we highlight some of the key issues, starting with the basics.

1.3.1
Choosing the Proper Microarray Platform

Given optimal conditions, all microarray platforms work very well; however, conditions are never optimal, and issues such as experimental assay, local expertise, cost, and gene coverage all play a role in platform selection. A two-color design is most suited for comparative assays, for example, if the experimental goal is to compare multiple tissues from a single subject (tumor versus normal tissue, cerebellum versus cortex, etc.). However, experiments seeking to correlate gene expression with phenotype (such as aging) in a single tissue tend to use one-color arrays; although two-color arrays can be used, by comparing each sample with the same reference sample [41,51]. This choice should be dictated by the statistical design of the analysis, so as to allow optimal power to detect the desired changes.

Another issue to consider is cost versus reproducibility. Laboratory-made spotted oligo arrays cost significantly less than factory-born arrays, whether one-color or two-color, but require more effort to make. All microarrays are prone to batch effects, which can be removed by proper normalization [52,53], but may be more significant in homemade arrays. Thus, in a research-based experiment, custom arrays may be appropriate, whereas biomarker assays would more likely require factory-made arrays since thousands of identical arrays will eventually have to be made quickly. Then, local expertise has also to be taken into account. If all of the current lab personnel were trained using a specific kind of array, then the continued use of those arrays would decrease both experimental time and error. One more advantage of homemade arrays is that they are not vulnerable to changes in designs of manufacturers during the course of a series of experiments, as has been the case with every commercial platform so far.

The final issue to consider when choosing an array platform is customizability versus scalability. Both homemade and Agilent two-color arrays allow for the quick and cheap creation of arrays containing any target of interest. For example, if an experimenter aims to test the expression of multiple splice variants of a gene or to make a biomarker assay for testing the expression of 100 specific genes, such arrays would be appropriate. Nimblegen, which uses a mirror-based masking system, has the maximum synthetic flexibility and offers custom arrays on a commercial platform [54]. A wide variety of configurations are available, but the cost is far higher than homemade spotted arrays. Spotted array technologies do not lag far behind, however, as just about every microarray platform currently has an array to test the expression of every known human transcript. All of these factors have to be taken into account while choosing a proper platform for the experiment at hand.

1.3.2
Preparing the Tissue for Hybridization

After selecting the microarray platform, tissue must be acquired and prepared in such a way to avoid inducing unwanted changes in gene expression. An experiment using postmortem tissue must carefully control for gender, ethnicity, and cause of death to avoid outlier arrays [22,47,55]. Once tissue is acquired it must be properly cared for, as excessive postmortem interval, changes in pH or temperature, or improper tissue handling at any stage can lead to RNA degradation [50]. Nonlinear or excessive PCR can selectively amplify smaller segments of cDNA, leading to increased variability, while improper tissue preservation can make a sample completely unusable. Generally, an experiment should include duplicate spots or arrays to quantitatively assess variability due to human error or choice of array platform, thus, effectively determining the sensitivity of the experiment [50].

The precise steps to be taken between tissue acquisition and target hybridization depend highly on the experiment at hand and generally involve the use of a series of well-characterized procedures and commercially available kits. Generally, mRNA or total RNA samples are extracted from the tissue or cells of interest and converted into their cDNA sequences. In the case of genomic DNA assays, DNA is cut into manageable sizes. When necessary, the cDNA is then amplified. Finally, each sample is fluorescently labeled using one or two dyes, as required.

1.3.3
Single-Cell Assays and Tissue Heterogeneity

Under ideal conditions, microarrays can detect mRNA in relative abundances as low as one part per 500 000 [39,43], allowing for a resolution of 3–10 copies per cell in simple tissues and cell lines. In practice, however, while these species may be detected, their detection may not be reliable enough to ascertain differential expression; so it is safer to assume reliable detection at the 1/100 000 level. In the nervous system and other complex tissues consisting of multiple cell types with uniquely expressed transcripts, resolution of cell type specific species is hampered [50]. To increase resolution, therefore, many microarray experiments now use single-cell assays to filter individual cell types of interest from heterogeneous tissue before assessing changes in gene expression [25], although this also has its costs.

Many cell purification assays, including flow cytometry, microaspiration, and laser-capture microdissection (LCM), have arisen to combat tissue heterogeneity in different situations. Flow cytometry allows thousands of cells per second to be counted, examined, and separated based on any of a number of characteristics of the cells [56]. This method is generally used to quickly obtain large quantities of a single cell type. Several studies have recently demonstrated the use of automated flow sorting [3,4] for purifying neurons from developing and adult brains [4]. In addition, fluorescence can also be applied manually [5], although it is more tedious. The use of automated sorting allows for large-scale purification of thousands of neurons in a single sort. Cells can be labeled by tracer injection [3] or in genetically modified mice [4], which are now available in many forms via the GENSAT project [57]. Microaspiration, on the contrary, involves patching onto individual cells and removing them one at a time [58]. This process is much more painstaking than flow cytometry and provides many fewer cells; however, it can provide much more accurate dissections, and it even allows for dissection of only certain elements of the cell (soma, dendrites, etc. [59]). In LCM, a tissue slice is prepared by labeling cells of interest and placing the slice below a transfer cap on a laser-mounted microscope. Once a labeled cell is located under the microscope, a laser beam can be activated, transferring the cell to the transfer film [60]. Using LCM, several hundred cells can be collected in a relatively short time using a simple assay. Like flow cytometry, LCM allows for assaying a relatively large number of cells, and like microaspiration, it allows for the inspection of cells before acquisition, although cell extraction is not quite as precise.

1.3.4
Microarray Hybridization and Scanning

In two-color assays, equal amounts of differently labeled target from the two samples are combined and cohybridized, while Affymetrix array assays only require hybridization of target from a single sample. In both cases, hybridization lasts overnight, and then arrays are rinsed to remove any nonspecifically bound cDNA. A tunable laser then excites the remaining bound target at the fluorescent frequency of each dye, while a CCD or confocal microscope collects the fluorescence intensities. Most scanners come with their own preprocessing software, although stand-alone programs, such as DNA-Chip Analyzer (dChip) [61] or Imagene [62], can also be used.

1.3.5
Preprocessing

One important issue in microarray studies is how to go from a series of images to a table of expression values for each probe set. While methods differ between platforms, preprocessing can generally be divided into six steps: image analysis, data import, background adjustment, normalization, summarization, and quality assessment [52]. In image analysis, spot detection methods convert pixel intensities to probe intensities, and background levels are stored. Data import methods then take all image analysis files, bring them together, and convert them into a form recognized by the relevant software. Next, probe intensities are background-adjusted to account for nonspecific hybridization and noise in the scanner. All images are then normalized to account for variations among arrays. In some microarray platforms, summarization takes intensities from all spots on an array representing a single probe set and converts them into a single value representing the amount of RNA transcript. Finally, all of the data are assessed for quality, and any measurements falling outside an acceptable range of random noise are omitted.

Custom two-color arrays and Affymetrix chips use very different strategies for preprocessing. Custom two-color arrays use a much more intuitive method; for each sample, a red or a green spot on the array represents each probe set, and the ratio of these values represents the relative abundance of that transcript. In Affymetrix chips, multiple probe pairs consisting of a perfect match and a mismatch oligo represent each probe set on the array. The mismatch probe differs from the perfect match probe only in the 13th nucleotide and is used to account for nonspecific binding. Absolute expression values are then obtained by averaging the difference of intensities between each probe pair for a given gene. Whatever the platform, once preprocessing is complete and a core table of gene expression is obtained, data analysis is ready to begin. Many methods have been used to extract signals from Affymetrix arrays and their utility varies according to the experimental design and conditions [52]. Recent comparisons of these techniques suggest that combining the methods of microarray suite (MAS) background correction, quantile normalization, MAS perfect match probe correction, and median polish expression summary offers clear improvements over the manufacturers software [53]. Additionally, the R package "ProbeFilter" can be used to eliminate many of the nonfunctioning and nonspecific Affymetrix probes to further improve the data quality (http://arrayana-lysis.mbni.med.umich.edu/MBNIUM.html).

1.3.6
Gene Expression Analyses

Standard gene expression analyses involve finding all genes that significantly differ between two categories (Alzheimer's disease versus control hippocampus [12], cortex versus cerebellum [63], tumor 1 versus tumor 2 [6], etc.). The most common method for categorization is to rank each gene by ratio, and then to consider all genes with a ratio greater than X (or less than $1/X$) differentially expressed, where X is chosen on the basis of the level of statistical significance desired (Figure 1.2). A more elegant, higher powered method of analysis is to correlate gene expression in a single tissue with a related phenotype (age [64], neurofibrillary tangle burden [11], body weight [65], etc.). In this method, the Pearson correlation between expression and phenotype is calculated and any significantly correlated genes ($P < 0.05$, typically) are recorded. These analyses produce several to thousands of significant genes, from which a select few are generally investigated. There are many valid analytic approaches and high-quality free software, such as BioConductor (http://www.bio-conductor.org/ [66]) and Multiexperiment Viewer (http://www.tm4.org/mev.html), available for analysis. It is best to consult a statistician to ensure design and analysis are optimally performed.

1.3.7
Analytical Challenges

One major issue in microarray analysis is determining which genes to follow up from the list of significant genes, often numbering in the thousands. A few large-scale efforts, including public efforts such as the Gene Ontology Consortium (GO; http://www.geneontology.org/) and Kyoto Encyclopedia of Genes and Genomes (KEGG; http://www.genome.jp/kegg/), and private efforts like BioCarta (http://www. biocarta.com/genes/index.asp), have gone into categorizing genes into biologically meaningful groups. GO, for instance, provides a hierarchical framework of terms related to biological processes, molecular function, and cellular components.

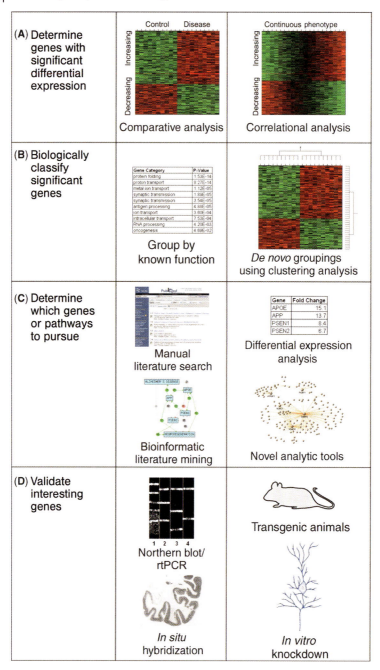

Figure 1.2 (legend see p.11)

As the function of new genes becomes known, they are assigned relevant GO categories, which are then stored in a publicly accessible database. To navigate this database, various programs such as expression analysis systematic explorer (EASE) [67] and gene set enrichment analysis (GSEA) [68] have been created. EASE searches for overexpression of GO terms in a gene list of interest (e.g., all downregulated genes) compared to a reference list (e.g., all genes present on the array). GSEA takes all genes present on the array, ranks them by fold change, and then searches for gene ontology categories with many highly ranked genes, providing power to detect genes not identified with conventional methods. WebGestalt (http://bioinfo.vanderbilt. edu/webgestalt/) allows many of these pathway-related analyses to be performed and stored online in a user-friendly environment, and the web site keeps up-to-date links to many analytic tools [69]. Commercially available programs such as Ingenuity Pathways Analysis (IPA; Ingenuity Systems, www.ingenuity.com), which are highly curated, also help locate genes of interest relative to known pathways.

If many significant genes fall into one or two GO categories, choosing the most significant genes in those categories would be one option. Alternatively, literature-mining tools such as Chilibot [70] allow a user to input a list of terms (genes or phenotypes), return all known relationships between all terms in the list, and suggest hypotheses for new relationships. More focused literature searches can be performed using GeneCards [71], a web site compiling links to everything that it can find about every human gene, including links to primers, RNAi products, knockout mice, and so on. Web sites such as the Allen brain atlas (http://www.brainatlas.org/ aba/) and WebQTL (http://www.genenetwork.org/) provide information about gene expression patterns for thousands of genes in the mouse brain, and in some cases correlate knocking out of various genes with phenotype. A list of other useful web sites for gene expression analysis is included in Table 1.1.

◄───

Figure 1.2 Determining genes of interest from a microarray experiment. (A) After acquiring and preprocessing microarray data, significantly expressed genes are determined using a method depending on the experimental design. In comparative analyses, with two (or more) distinct groups of samples, fold-change measurements determine differential expression, whereas in analyses with a continuous phenotype, differentially expressed genes are those with the highest Pearson correlation with the phenotype of interest. (B) These differentially expressed genes are then biologically classified, both by considering the known function of each gene in a Gene Ontology or KEGG pathway analysis and by looking at *de novo* groupings of genes using hierarchical or *k*-means clustering. (C) Of the tens to thousands of significant genes and pathways typically discovered in microarray analyses, generally only a select few are pursued, and determining relevant genes to pursue is a critical step. Genes essential to significant pathways can be determined by searching the literature either manually using PubMed or GeneCards, or though bioinformatic literature mining tools like Chilibot and IPA. However, relevant genes may be chosen based on expression alone, either by taking genes with the highest differential expression or by using novel analytic tools such as gene coexpression analysis to determine genes with high connectivity. (D) Selected genes are then validated technically using low-throughput methods such as Northern blot and *in situ* hybridization, and genes with confirmed differential expression are then functionally validated using various *in vitro* and *in vivo* genetic manipulations, such as RNAi-mediated knockdown and transgenic knockouts.

Table 1.1 Additional web sites of interest in microarray analysis.

Web site	Description
http://bioinformatics.org/	Bioinformatics tools and information
http://brownlab.stanford.edu/	Information on microarrays at Stanford and links to collaborating labs
http://derisilab.ucsf.edu/	Information on yeast molecular biology and human infectious disease
http://genome.ucsc.edu/	A comprehensive tool for scanning and analyzing the human genome
http://ihome.cuhk.edu.hk/%7Eb400559/	A nearly complete list of web sites related to functional genomics
http://pevsnerlab.kennedykrieger.org/	A comprehensive list of bioinformatic-related tools and databases
http://rana.lbl.gov/	Useful software and web tools for genomic and gene expression analyses
http://www.genenetwork.org/	A set of linked resources for systems genetics in mice
http://www.geneontology.org/	The main gene ontology web site with tools for gene expression analysis
http://www.informatics.jax.org/	A comprehensive mouse genomics resource
http://www.ncbi.nlm.nih.gov/geo/	A repository for thousands of publicly available, MIAME compliant microarray data sets
http://www.ncbi.nlm.nih.gov/gquery/	A list of all major NIH databases
http://www.nervenet.org/	Several useful genetics and gene mapping databases, as well as a mouse brain library

This list represents a comprehensive, but by no means all-inclusive, list of web sites useful for bioinformatic analysis of gene expression data. Many of these web sites have an extensive set of links to numerous other expression-related sites.

Still, moving from the gene list to function remains difficult using conventional methods. We have been very interested in moving to a systems level of understanding of gene expression data and have used the merging of network theory and systems biology, a technique of recent origin, from which extremely powerful methods for quantifying gene coexpression have developed [72–75]. These coexpression methods group genes on the basis of similarity of their expression values to each other and take advantage of three properties of biological systems: (1) gene (and protein) expression networks follow a scale-free topology, meaning that – like airports – a few "hub" genes share similar expression patterns with many other genes, but most connect to only a few other genes; (2) these hub genes are generally more important to cellular function than less connected genes; and (3) groups of genes with similar expression patterns are generally involved in similar biological functions. We have used this approach to identify key targets of human brain evolution [74] and therapeutic targets in cancer [76], thus proving for the first time that these techniques can revolutionize the kind of information obtained from a microarray experiment. Ultimately, a combination of these methods should be used to determine which genes to follow up, and some, if not all, of the chosen genes should be validated using other methods.

1.3.8
Validating Results

Northern blot, *in situ* hybridization, and various forms of PCR are still generally used to quantitatively or qualitatively replicate the most interesting differentially expressed genes. There has been some debate in the literature about whether microarray experiments, when run properly, are more or less accurate than the techniques used to validate them. Low-stringency microarray hybridizations may show higher background, decreasing observed expression differences as compared to single-gene techniques [10]. However, small pipetting errors or incorrect choice of a housekeeping gene for normalization may lead to quantification errors in RT-PCR, which are not found when using microarray platforms [77]. In any case, successful gene expression validation, as generally occurs with highly significant results, provides even more confidence in the ability of microarrays to find phenotype-related expression changes in a highly parallel fashion. More importantly, genes discovered using microarrays and validated using alternative methods generally provide a starting point for determining therapeutic targets in the disorder being studied [47].

1.4
Clinical Applications

Microarray studies generally fall into one of the two main categories. Some studies seek to identify molecular changes in disease or injury, while others aim to identify molecular biomarkers associated with disease (Figure 1.3). Studies identifying molecular changes in disease provide valuable information about pathological changes associated with disease. These studies look at tissues directly affected by disease pathology, which, with the notable exception of cancer tissue or the rare surgical specimen obtained in dementia or epilepsy, generally cannot be obtained while the subjects are alive; as a result such research cannot be directly applied in a clinical setting. However, biomarker identification studies only look at tissue readily accessible with the goal of accurately classifying patients using a simple gene expression assay. This section will focus on clinical uses of microarrays such as biomarker discovery, prognosis, diagnosis, and treatment/response studies. We will begin by presenting a short summary of notable studies in neurological disease research that have advanced the field significantly, suggesting new therapeutic targets for disease and injury treatments.

1.4.1
Neurological Disease-Relevant Research

So many microarray studies have been conducted in the area of basic neuroscience research that an entire review can be written on this topic alone. However, many of them end up with a gene list useful as a database of genes only, as they do not go beyond

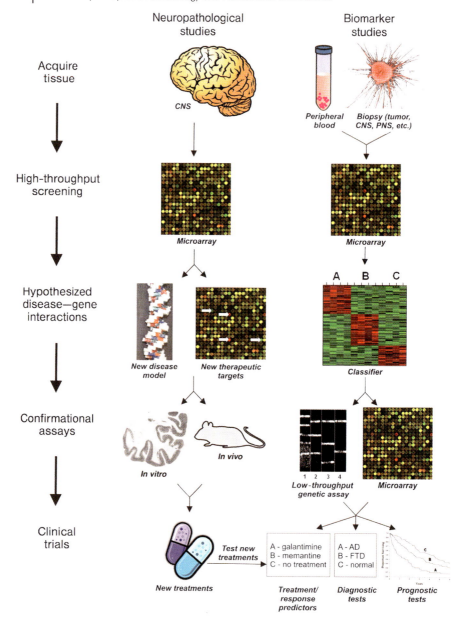

Figure 1.3 Parallel methodologies in neuro-pathological and biomarker studies. Since the tissue is generally acquired postmortem in neuropathological studies (left), these studies seek to answer the question, "What went wrong in this disease and why?" However, biomarker studies (right) use peripheral blood as well as tumor and other biopsy tissues in living patients to answer the question, "How can we classify patients?" In both types of studies, high-throughput screenings are performed on acquired tissue (see Figure 1.2) to determine possible disease–gene interactions. In neuropathological studies, these interactions come in the form of new disease models and therapeutic targets. Treatments for these

that. Here we review a few significant studies because they introduce other key aspects of microarray research or suggest new therapeutic targets for neurological diseases.

1.4.1.1 Incipient Alzheimer's Disease

In the most elegant study on AD published to date, Blalock *et al.* [11] used microarrays to study gene expression changes specific to early stages of Alzheimer's disease and noted which changes were sustained throughout AD progression. To do this, gene expression in samples were correlated to the cognitive status of each individual at death (MiniMental State Examination), as well as to their pathological profile (neurofibrillary tangle burden). Genes were considered AD genes if they were significantly correlated with either NFT burden or MMSE score. They were further considered early AD genes if they were also correlated when the analysis was limited to comparison of control and incipient subjects, finding an upregulation of tumor suppressors and other genes regulating cell proliferation and differentiation, as well as the expected upregulation of apoptosis and downregulation of synaptic transmission pathways.

While many AD microarray studies have been published in the past 5 years [11–15], this study was significant for a few reasons. First, the complexity of AD was taken into consideration when designing the experiment. Instead of designating subjects as either diseased or control, each individual's cognitive ability and Tau pathology were correlated to gene expression as described above. Second, the sample size was large enough to provide decent statistical power ($N = 31$) and allow for significant correlations in early AD using only half the samples. Careful tissue handling and microarray analysis methods resulted in very low false discovery rates for microarray experiments, further increasing statistical power. Additionally, raw data from this experiment were uploaded to the Gene Expression Omnibus (GEO) repository (http://www.ncbi.nlm.nih.gov/geo/) so that other researchers could review these data using other methods. Finally, results from this microarray analysis were used to suggest a new model of incipient AD progression along myelinated axons. None of the results were validated functionally or by alternative methods, however, and no aspects of the model were tested, thereby limiting the possible clinical applications of these results.

◄───────────────────────────────────────

Figure 1.3 (*Continued*)

hypothesized therapeutic targets can then be tested *in vivo* or *in vitro*, either using known interacting compounds or by screening large libraries, with successful treatments then entering clinical trials. Disease–gene interactions in biomarker assays, however, are used to classify patients based on diagnosis, prognosis, response to treatment, or a number of other clinically relevant measures. Any promising classifications are then retested in an independent cohort of individuals using either low- or high-throughput tests, as necessary. New treatments from neuropathological studies of a disease can be tested clinically on patients predicted by biomarker assays to have poor prognosis and no predicted response to available treatments, thus providing patients for the clinical trials and possible new treatments to patients who would otherwise not be treated.

1.4.1.2 Using Animal Models to Study Neurodegeneration

An ideal microarray experiment will make predictions that can be validated *in vitro* and *in vivo*, leading to new results with clinical applications. One early example of this was in multiple sclerosis (MS) [78], where findings in human patients were extended to functional validation in mice. Such studies are few and far between because of the effort needed to validate experiments in animal models. One such study on dementia by our group recently compared gene expression changes in mice expressing the most common FTD-causing human mutation in Tau with wild-type control mice [79]. This study found genes up- or downregulated with Tau mutation in cortex, cerebellum, brain stem, and spinal cord, suggesting that pathologically unaffected areas (like cerebellum) would show upregulation of neuroprotective genes. This hypothesis was tested using multiple *in vitro* and *in vivo* assays, focusing on puromycin-sensitive aminopeptidase (PSA) – a gene which resides very close to tau on chromosome 17, and which was upregulated in cerebellum. For example, in a fly transgenic model of tauopathies, PSA loss of function worsened the rough eye phenotype, and *in vitro*, PSA digested recombinant Tau protein. These results suggest that PSA overexpression may be a viable mechanism for treatment of many neurodegenerative disorders involving tauopathies, and have identified a major new pathway for Tau degradation *in vivo* [79].

Animal models are also useful for determining cell type specific markers. In some situations, multiple morphologically similar cell types will reside in the same cortical areas, making discrimination of these cell types difficult. Corticospinal motor neurons reside in layer V of the cortex along with other projection neurons, for example, and degenerate in upper motor neuron disorders such as ALS. Arlotta and colleagues [3] discovered markers specific to three types of cortical projection neurons in developing mouse cortex by using retrograde labeling of axonal projection fields and fluorescence activated cell sorting (FACS) to separate each cell type, and then ran microarrays on each pure cell line. Using immunohistochemistry and loss of function knockout assays, they found that CTIP2 was specific to corticospinal motor neurons and was required for axonal pathfinding in the spinal cord. While this study cannot be directly applied to adult brain, it provides evidence that functions of specific molecules in specific cell types can be determined using microarray screening and animal models.

1.4.1.3 Determining Gene Pathways Using Meta-Analysis

Meta-analysis of microarrays provides a novel method for extracting groups of genes involved in similar biological pathways. If two genes that may show similar expression patterns in one data set by chance are coexpressed in multiple data sets, it is more likely that the two genes are functionally related. Lee *et al.* [80] looked at gene coexpression across 60 data sets, finding a substantial number of correlated expression patterns (connections) that occurred in multiple studies. Additionally, the probability that two genes were functionally related (as measured in overlapping GO terms) was directly correlated with the number of connections between those two genes. Furthermore, many of the genes could be clustered into groups related to translation, transcription, cell adhesion, electron transport, and many other biologically relevant categories based solely on their multistudy connections. With more microarray data becoming publicly available every day and with computer processor speeds increasing exponentially, such multistudy meta-analyses have the potential to provide high-throughput pathway predictions for genes expressed in the brain and other tissues [74].

1.4.2
Cancer Research

Cancer research represents one of the few fields of microarray study where results from the lab can be directly applied clinically (see [6] for review). Unlike most neurological disorders where diseased tissue can only be acquired from a patient postmortem, tumor samples can be removed from living patients. Tumors can then be classified based on the survival or treatment response of patients in the future. In this section, we will explore various microarray applications in cancer genomics, focusing on applications related to brain tumors.

1.4.2.1 Tumor Classification and Patient Diagnosis
Traditionally, tumors are classified morphologically based on their microscopic resemblance to their CNS cell of origin or developmental progenitor cell [81]. Malignant tumors tend to look more like dedifferentiated precursor cells showing mitotic activity, tumor necrosis, and angiogenesis [6]. Less aggressive tumors, on the contrary, resemble their normal tissue counterparts, often making clinical diagnosis difficult. While this classification scheme works with reasonable accuracy, morphologically identical tumors can exhibit distinct mutational patterns and altered signaling pathways, as well as respond differently to identical drug treatments. An alternative method for categorizing tumor samples is gene expression profiling. In situations where biopsy material cannot be morphologically characterized clearly as either malignant or benign, a clinical test for gene expression patterns characteristic of specific tumor types would be quite useful. By disregarding prior knowledge and grouping tumors entirely on the basis of their transcriptional similarity, unsupervised methods can often uncover morphologically unrecognized tumor subtypes, thereby allowing for a more precise diagnosis of tumor malignancy [51].

Multiple experiments have shown that tumors from different cell types and with different levels of aggressiveness show distinct gene expression patterns [6]. One such example is glioma, where standard morphological categorizations have been useful for predicting survival but not the response to treatment [82]. Shai *et al.* performed unsupervised hierarchical clustering of various gliomas on a panel of 170 genes differentially expressed between tumor types. Glioblastomas, lower grade astrocytomas, and oligodendrogliomas, they concluded, have transcriptional signatures distinct from one another and from normal white matter tissue [82]. Additionally, secondary glioblastomas showed a wide range of expression patterning, suggesting that they constitute a very heterogeneous group. A more recent, large-scale study based on the gene expression profile of a panel of 595 genes [83] found distinct subsets of morphologically identical gliomas, confirming the hypothesis of glioblastoma heterogeneity. More important, these tumor subtypes predicted patient survival better than the standard methods, suggesting that tumor gene expression profiling would be a viable alternative for patient prognostic tests.

1.4.2.2 Determining Patient Prognosis

In addition to classifying tumors for diagnostic purposes, gene expression profiles can be used as biomarkers to predict patient survival. Accurate prognostic tests are useful to determine how aggressive a cancer treatment administered to a patient should be. If a malignant tumor goes untreated, a patient will likely relapse; however, aggressive treatment can lead to severe side effects, including permanent cognitive and psychological deficits [84]. Current clinical methods for risk classification in medulloblastoma fail to identify 20–30% of average-risk patients with resistant disease as well as those patients who might be overtreated [85], suggesting that more accurate methods for risk stratification are necessary. Molecular prognostic markers, as measured by microarray, RT-PCR, or Western blot, provide one such method that, as preliminary results indicate, will be more accurate than traditional methods.

An early cDNA microarray study of 60 medulloblastoma samples found that patient survival could be predicted using as few as eight genes, independent of the clinical variables traditionally used to stratify patients as average versus high risk [86]. These results suggested that not only could gene expression profiles be used as a biomarker for patient survival, but also that such classifiers would be a realistic option for the clinical setting, as so few genes were needed for classification. With the price of microarrays decreasing, repeatability is now becoming more of an issue than small gene number. As mentioned above, a recent microarray study of gliomas found that expression-based tumor classification using a panel of 595 genes is a more powerful predictor of survival than age, pathological type, or grade [83]. A subset of this classifier has been validated on an external data set, and despite the fact that a different microarray platform was used, this classifier significantly outperformed the initial histopathology grading classification. In both the initial and the validation study, samples could be classified to one of the four glioma subtypes that predicted patient survival with high accuracy. Recent experiments have led to similar findings in less common forms of brain cancer, such as ependymal neoplasms [87], suggesting that such prognostic tests may be universally applicable to many forms of brain cancer. These results indicate that a small panel of genes can be used to predict patient survival with high accuracy and to determine whether a patient needs aggressive intervention.

1.4.2.3 Predicting Therapeutic Response to Treatment

Just as prognostic tests could be used to prevent patient overtreatment and minimize side effects, tests predicting therapeutic response would prevent ineffective treatments from being administered, thus allowing a patient to receive proper treatment as quickly as possible. Such screens are important because administration of resistant chemotherapies to a patient can lead to the development of secondary antineoplastic drug resistance, and drugs that at one point would have been useful would no longer be effective [88]. In a proof-of-principle study, Staunton et al. [89] developed gene expression classifiers for sensitivity or resistance of human cancer cell lines to

232 compounds. They measured expression of 6817 genes on a panel of 60 human cancer cell lines, finding classifiers of between 5 and 200 genes whose expression patterns could accurately predict chemosensitivity for approximately one third of the compounds tested. A similar, more focused study published recently tested chemosensitivity of 30 cell lines to 11 anticancer drugs at clinically achieved concentrations [88]. Prediction profiles for each chemotherapy agent were compiled and had an overall accuracy of 86%, once again demonstrating the applicability of microarray technology in drug resistance prediction. Additionally, 67 genes associated with resistance to at least four drugs were found from these profiles. Many of these associations were confirmed using RT-PCR, providing new candidate genes associated with multidrug resistance.

1.4.2.4 Determining Therapeutic Targets for Cancer

Glioblastomas and medulloblastomas represent some of the most common forms of malignant brain tumors in adults and children, respectively. Even with aggressive treatment, patients with glioblastomas have a median survival time of only 15 months after diagnosis [76], and only 50% of children with medulloblastomas survive to adulthood, often with severe psychological and cognitive side effects [84]. Clearly, new treatment approaches for these and other cancers are necessary. One screening approach for novel therapeutic targets for cancer treatment is gene expression based high-throughput screening (GE-HTS) [90]. First, microarrays are used to find a small number of genes that serve as markers for a desired cellular state, such as differentiation. Next, thousands of compounds of interest are individually combined with a cancer cell line in a high-throughput manner. The molecular markers found using microarrays are then measured using RT-PCR for the cell lines with each combined compound to see which ones have been transformed into the desired cellular state. In a study of leukemia cells, Stegmaier *et al.* found that eight of the 1739 compounds tested caused cancer cells to differentiate, leading to growth arrest; after further validation they concluded these to be viable therapeutic targets [90]. Using this method, discovery of new therapeutic targets requires no special assays or reagents and no prior target validation, as the gene expression profiles serve as markers for the state in question.

Coexpression analysis of gene expression data has also been used to discover new molecular targets for glioblastoma treatment. In a significant recent advance, Horvath and colleagues applied a systems biology approach to study 120 patient glioblastoma samples [76]. They built a network in one set of 55 arrays and validated it in an independent group of 65 arrays. This network grouped genes into five modules using coexpression, one of which was significantly enriched in cell growth genes. They identified a set of key hub genes that were driving glioblastoma proliferation in this module, thus providing a proof-of-principle functional validation of the network predictions. By looking at the 10 most connected genes in this module, they found that most genes had already been identified as potential cancer targets, and all but one were associated more with glioblastoma survival than the traditional proliferation markers (Ki67 and PCNA). Additionally, inhibition of ASPM, a novel therapeutic target, was confirmed to inhibit glioblastoma cell growth using siRNA.

Similar results were duplicated using breast cancer samples, suggesting that these results extend across cancer types.

This study presented a new computational technique that can be applied to any cancer microarray experiment and led to insights not observable with standard analysis of differential expression [75]. With the rapidly increasing popularity of microarray and enough studies already published, new therapeutic targets should be discoverable merely by reanalyzing existing data sets using novel computational techniques, such as sophisticated network analyses.

A recent microarray study suggests that new cancer treatments may be found simply by combining old chemotherapies together in novel ways. Cheok *et al.* [91] studied single-agent versus combination therapy in patients with acute lymphocytic leukemia, by comparing gene expression profiles before and after treatment in patients who were treated with methotrexate, mercaptopurine, or both. They found that the combined effect of both chemotherapies was profoundly different from the additive effects of patients taking either drug. Thus, new treatments may be found simply by combining old treatments in novel ways and screening such combinations using microarrays.

1.4.3
Using Peripheral Tissues as a Substitute for Brain Tissue

In most neurological diseases, the affected tissue that holds the key to patient survival cannot be directly assessed in a clinical setting. In these situations, alternative methods must be used for diagnosis and treatment. For example, in many cases damage to the brain can be indirectly assessed using peripheral tissue or blood. Many scientists are rightly skeptical that peripheral, nonneural tissues can provide a window into the CNS. However, as we will discuss, current results indicate that a significant proportion of CNS genes are expressed in peripheral blood or lymphoblasts, and that these tissues can be used to identify biomarkers, if not therapeutic pathways.

1.4.3.1 Gene Expression Profiling of Disease
Unique blood biomarkers have been found for all kinds of neurological disorders, including stroke, hypoxia, multiple sclerosis, depression, Down's syndrome, HD, and seizure, as well as general neurological distress [92–94]. The first study to link transcriptional changes in peripheral blood to brain dysfunction measured gene expression in adult rat blood monocytes, 24 hours postinjury, for a variety of induced injuries [95]. Using several hundred genes as a biomarker, animals with ischemic strokes, hemorrhagic strokes, kainate-induced seizures, hypoxia, and insulin-induced hypoglycemia could be genetically distinguished from controls and each other. Many other genes were similarly regulated in each type of injury, suggesting they are stress related. Similar results were found when the experiment was repeated using rat cortex, confirming the link between peripheral gene expression changes and disease [96]. More recently, studies have compared gene expression in human blood following ischemic stroke [97,98], finding that only a small number of genes were required to distinguish controls from stroke patients. Such studies suggest that a blood test for stroke using either RT-PCR or even microarrays will be very possible in the near future.

One study, probably the most comprehensive to date, relating peripheral blood profiling to disease looked at genes upregulated in subjects with presymptomatic and symptomatic HD and compared age- and sex-matched controls [17]. This study was very well designed, using multiple microarray platforms and quantitative RT-PCR, as well as a test and training set assay, to confirm results. It found that gene expression profiles could separate not only HD subjects from controls, but also presymptomatic from symptomatic subjects, with early presymptomatic subjects having profiles similar to controls and late presymptomatic subjects showing profiles similar to symptomatic HD subjects. Additionally, these upregulated transcripts were less elevated in HD subjects taking the histone deacetylase inhibitor sodium phenylbutyrate, which is a potential experimental therapy. Finally, as with the animal models of acute injury, these genes upregulated in blood were also elevated in the postmortem HD caudate, suggesting that blood mRNA may reflect disease pathways in the brain. Thus, microarrays of peripheral blood can be used not only to diagnose diseases, but also to subcategorize patients with a specific disease, either by specific subphenotype or by treatment response. This provides another key point – biomarkers identified in chronic neurodegenerative diseases such as inherited ataxias and dementia may provide a more proximal and quantitative end point than clinical scales, which may be less sensitive to therapy, especially in the short term. In this manner, biomarkers of disease progression can be used to determine therapeutic efficacy early in a treatment course, increasing the power and reducing the cost of clinical trials.

1.4.3.2 Dividing Complex Phenotypes into Subtypes Using Microarrays

Many other microarray studies in peripheral blood have also found that gene expression profiles alone can subdivide patients with complex diseases. A recent study on Tourette syndrome (TS) found that a subset of patients show overexpression of six cytotoxic T-cell/natural killer cell genes [99]. These results support the hypothesis that pediatric autoimmune neuropsychiatric disorders associated with streptococcal infections (PANDAS) can play a role in the onset of tic disorders and obsessive compulsive disorder (OCD), which is currently unproven [100]. The Sharp lab has also applied this approach to diseases with no obvious blood phenotypes, such as tuberous sclerosis complex 2, neurofibromatosis type 1, and Down's syndrome, finding in all three cases different blood profiles for patients versus controls [101]. Additionally, Down's syndrome patients with congenital heart disease showed different profiles than those without, and tuberous sclerosis patients with autism showed different profiles than those without. These studies suggest that whatever the causes of complex diseases, the resulting phenotypes can be distinguished from one another using blood biomarkers; furthermore, these blood biomarkers may also indicate the underlying mechanisms behind disease phenotypes [93].

In some cases, similar phenotypes may actually show multiple gene expression profiles. For example, a recent study of mRNA expression of leukocytes in patients with major depression disorder revealed 12 genes differentially expressed between depressed patients and controls [94]. Additionally, half of the depressed subjects showed altered expression of many more genes with no corresponding phenotypic manifestation. As depression is a complex neuropsychiatric disease, there may be multiple pathophysiological conditions that trigger it, possibly partially explaining why only a subset of depressed patients respond to treatment. Another equally complicated phenotype is autism. We have recently used microarrays to study autism cases with single-gene etiologies and validate these pathways in idiopathic autism [115]. In this study, we compared mRNA expression between autistic males with a fragile X mental retardation 1 gene (FMR1-RM) mutation, autistic males with a 15q11–q13 duplication (dup(15q)), and controls. In addition to finding distinct gene expression profiles for each autism group, we also found a set of 68 genes commonly dysregulated in both types of autism, including a potential molecular link between the two autistic groups (CYFIP1), which we confirmed *in vitro*. These results suggest that not only can microarrays be used to subdivide complex phenotypes, but they may also be useful for determining the underlying effects of complex disorders.

1.4.3.3 Applying Blood Classification to Treatments
Peripheral blood profiles can also divide patients on the basis of their responses to treatment. These effects can be seen in two ways: (1) patients taking specific drugs show specific profiles, and (2) patients who respond to treatment show different profiles from those who do not. For example, epileptic children treated with carbamazepine or valproic acid each show characteristic gene expression changes compared with controls [101]. Additionally, children who successfully responded to valproic acid had different peripheral blood profiles from those who still had seizures. The most studied disease in this area of research is multiple sclerosis (MS); reviewed in [102]. In short, MS studies of peripheral blood gene expression changes have found notable results: (1) MS patients have a different profile than controls; (2) remitting patients show different expression patterns than relapsing patients; (3) a subset of the MS profile overlaps with systemic lupus erythematosus, suggesting an "autoimmune disease" fingerprint; (4) both interferon-beta and methylprednisolone treatments result in unique molecular signatures; and (5) there were profiles that predicted response to certain MS drugs.

Although most microarray studies require age- and sex-matched controls, some treatment response studies can be self-controlled, removing much of the statistical variability in comparisons. Using this approach, Kalman *et al.* tested the effect of the selective serotonin and noradrenaline reuptake inhibitor, venlafaxine, on gene expression in lymphocytes [103]. Blood was taken from six otherwise healthy, elderly individuals from the same nursing home both before the start of venlafaxine treatment and 4 weeks after the start of treatment. Although this study had a very small sample size, the genetic and environmental factors were both well controlled, since the same individuals were used for both pre- and posttreatment conditions, and since nursing home life placed each subject on the same diet with similar daily routines. Fifty-seven genes related to ionic homeostasis, cell survival, neural plasticity, signal transduction, and metabolism were found to significantly change expression between pre- and posttreatment. These expression changes corresponded to a decrease in clinical levels of depression as measured by the Beck Depression

Inventory. Thus, blood expression profiling has the potential to both help uncover the physiological effects of drugs on the CNS and to separate subjects based on their responses to treatment, thereby preventing the overtreatment of individuals suffering from one of the many neurological disorders.

1.4.3.4 Advantages and Disadvantages of Using Blood Genomics for Brain Disorders

Blood is an ideal substrate for clinical use as it can be acquired inexpensively and easily from any living patient. RNA can be stabilized immediately after extraction using vacutainer tubes (such as PAXgene and TEMPUS), reducing or eliminating many of the factors associated with postmortem tissue [92]. Additionally, unique gene expression profiles for many neurological diseases have been found in blood (as described above). Furthermore, many of the same genes are involved in the disease profiles for both blood and brain [96], with some studies showing significant correlations between gene expression changes in both substrates [17]. Thus, not only can blood provide transcriptional biomarkers for disease, subphenotypes, and treatment response, but it may also provide insight into underlying molecular mechanisms.

Brain disorders are not, however, the only factors determining gene expression in blood. In fact, just about any imaginable variable can have this effect, including, among other things, age, sex, race, diet, time of day, medication, exercise, stress, genetics, glucose levels, and time since last meal [92,94]. Conversely, some genes are expressed exclusively in the brain, and therefore will not be induced in the blood. Furthermore, any changes that do occur in the blood generally are on the order of 1.5–2.0-fold, compared with changes as high as 10-fold in cancer genomics – an issue that can be partially circumvented by using pure cell types [93]. Thus, any successful study must have a large enough sample size to account for all of these factors, with control and disease patients carefully matched. In fact, before clinical trials of any sort can be successful, some standardized method for normalizing disease samples as compared to controls must be developed.

1.4.3.5 Pure Cell Line Assays in Peripheral Blood

As with postmortem tissue, many transcriptional changes in blood that occur in response to neurological disease or injury are cell type specific. For example, most gene expression changes in acute stroke occur in neutrophils and monocytes, while changes in Tourette syndrome occur mostly in natural killer and cytotoxic CD8 T cells, and those in migraine generally occur in platelets [92]. Most MS studies are performed on peripheral blood mononuclear cells, a subset of blood cells involved in immune response [102]. With such small magnitude gene expression changes found in blood relative to brain, pure cell assays are often essential for peripheral blood profiling. Pure cell lines can also help control for unwanted gene expression variations. Lymphoblasts in particular are useful for genetic research as they are easy to acquire and can be cryopreserved and converted into cell lines, providing an inexhaustible supply of genetic material [104]. In fact, many studies have utilized lymphoblastoid cell lines for pharmacogenetic studies. In short, pure cell lines allow for a more precise understanding of transcriptional changes due to illness or injury.

1.4.4
Other Types of Microarrays in Clinical Setting

While this chapter primarily emphasizes mRNA-targeting microarrays, DNA-targeting microarrays also play a significant role in clinical diagnoses in areas such as molecular karyotyping and single nucleotide polymorphism (SNP) genotyping. In general, these arrays include oligos that target specific sequences across the genome. Depending on the specific question asked, current technologies allow the entire genome to be assayed on a single chip at fairly high density.

1.4.4.1 Gene Dose, Molecular Karyotyping, and Chromosomal Abnormalities

High-density DNA arrays have been used since the late 1990s to measure the gene dose effect of specific genomic regions across single chromosomes, as well as the entire genome [105–107]. These arrays allow for mapping of chromosomal copy number, for example, in diseases like Klinefelter's and Down's syndromes. High-throughput assays can simultaneously assess regional duplications, deletions, and amplifications with an average marker spacing of ~25 kb [107]. Such high-density coverage can detect microdeletions associated with developmental disorders, for example, without any need to relate phenotype to genotype [22]. Additionally, by using SNPs as oligonucleotides on microarrays, neutral chromosomal aberrations such as uniparental disomy can also be detected [107,108]. While such abnormalities commonly show no health or developmental effect, imprinting errors in chromosome 15 can lead to Prader–Willi syndrome and Angelman syndrome, and errors in chromosome 11 can lead to Beckwith–Wiedemann syndrome [109]. In short, these increasingly high-throughput arrays overcome many limitations of currently used clinical diagnostic tests, which are often subjective and low throughput, requiring relatively large amounts of DNA.

1.4.4.2 SNP Genotyping and Beyond

As cDNA microarrays can assess the expression of all genes in a single hybridization, whole-genome SNP arrays can assess variability across the entire genome at increasingly high densities. Current arrays from Affymetrix and Illumina can assess over 500 000 SNPs at once, allowing for large-scale association and linkage studies in increasingly short times and at low prices [110,111]. Such studies promote a gradual increase in genome-to-disease associations. Clinical studies have already begun to identify individuals at risk for cardiovascular disease, cancer, diabetes, and deep vein thrombosis, as well as adverse drug reactions [112]. In principle, genomic variation that dictates a drug response or indicates susceptibility to any disease could be optimally assessed using SNP genotyping. Unlike cDNA microarrays in which the readout is scalable, SNP arrays can be designed as binary, where the relevant spot fluoresces or not depending on which nucleotide is present. This binary quality of SNP genotyping results in a low error rate, making such arrays ideal in clinical setting. SNP band hybridization with primer exclusion arrays can also be used for gene resequencing. Affymetrix currently offers over 300 000 bp of resequencing on one array. By measuring signal intensity over a group of adjacent probes, one can simultaneously assess changes in copy number on any of these SNP array platforms. Such copy number variation regions are a significant source of genetic variation, and this approach will likely be important [113,114].

1.4.5
Future Clinical Applications: Pharmacogenomics

Alone and in combination with other systems-level measurements such as neuroimaging, microarray technology provides a valuable tool for optimizing individualized therapies for neurological diseases. In individualized therapy, the patient's genetic and biological makeup is assessed and scanned for potential biomarkers to determine which, if any, treatment is necessary (Figure 1.4) [22]. SNP genotyping can be used to determine susceptibility to various neurological disorders, and then to predict treatment outcome or adverse effects in patients. Transcriptional changes in peripheral blood can be used to diagnose patients and assess the effectiveness of various treatments, both before and after drug administration. Tumors found through imaging and other techniques can be identified and patient prognosis can

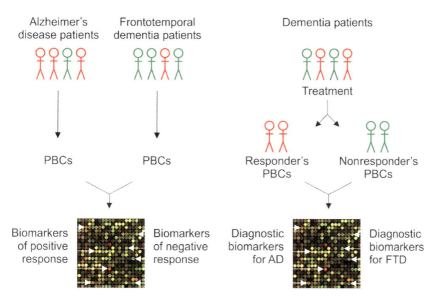

Figure 1.4 Microarray use for individualized medicine. Left: Microarrays may be used to augment current clinical diagnostic protocols. By hybridizing mRNA from peripheral blood cells (PBCs) of dementia patients onto diagnostic microarrays, clinicians could use the expression pattern to determine whether a patient is more likely to have Alzheimer's disease or frontotemporal dementia. Right: Microarrays may be used to determine effective disease treatments. Before beginning a new treatment, gene expression or SNP microarrays may be used to predict treatment response and possible adverse effects in dementia patients. In theory, such diagnostic, prognostic, and treatment-response predictors could be implemented using microarray technology for any disease or injury with a gene expression signature in PBCs or biopsy tissue.

be determined using microarray technologies. In short, standardized microarray chips will start to be available to identify and properly treat most neurological diseases and injuries within the next decade.

Although a few such clinical tests are available and many other pharmacogenomic studies are underway, the goal of large-scale individualized therapies is still far from attained. Before microarrays reach routine clinical use, batch effects need to be decreased by standardizing the methodology and automating as much of the process as possible [112]. Although such assays have improved in quality since their introduction, there is room for additional development. Also, data mining tools need to provide integration of transcriptional and translational data, in addition to imaging, clinical, and histopathological data. With publication of many new large-scale biomarker assays and with constant advances in microarray reliability and data analysis options, individualized medicine is slowly becoming a realistic tool for the clinician.

References

1 Sandberg, R., Yasuda, R., Pankratz, D., Carter, T., Del Rio, J., Wodicka, L., Mayford, M., Lockhart, D. and Barlow, C. (2000) Regional and strain-specific gene expression mapping in the adult mouse brain. *Proceedings of the National Academy of Sciences of the United States of America*, **97** (20), 11038–11043.

2 Brown, V., Ossadtchi, A., Khan, A., Cherry, S., Leahy, R. and Smith, D. (2002) High-throughput imaging of brain gene expression. *Genome Research*, **12** (2), 244–254.

3 Arlotta, P., Molyneaux, B., Chen, J., Inoue, J., Kominami, R. and Macklis, J. (2005) Neuronal subtype-specific genes that control corticospinal motor neuron development *in vivo*. *Neuron*, **45** (2), 207–221.

4 Lobo, M., Karsten, S., Gray, M., Geschwind, D. and Yang, W. (2006) FACS-array profiling of striatal projection neuron subtypes in juvenile and adult mouse brains. *Nature Neuroscience*, **9** (3), 443–452.

5 Sugino, K., Hempel, C., Miller, M., Hattox, A., Shapiro, P., Wu, C., Huang, J. and Nelson, S. (2005) Molecular taxonomy of major neuronal classes in the adult mouse forebrain. *Nature Neuroscience*, **9** (1), 99–107.

6 Mischel, P., Cloughesy, T. and Nelson, S. (2004) DNA-microarray analysis of brain cancer: molecular classification for therapy. *Nature Reviews. Neuroscience*, **5** (10), 782–792.

7 Geschwind, D.H., Ou, J., Easterday, M.C., Dougherty, J.D., Jackson, R.L., Chen, Z., Antoine, H., Terskikh, A., Weissman, I.L., Nelson, S.F. and Kornblum, H.I. (2001) A genetic analysis of neural progenitor differentiation. *Neuron*, **29** (2), 325–339.

8 Phillips, R., Ernst, R., Brunk, B., Ivanova, N., Mahan, M., Deanehan, J., Moore, K., Overton, G. and Lemischka, I. (2000) The genetic program of hematopoietic stem cells. *Science*, **288** (5471), 1635–1640.

9 D'Agata, V., Warren, S., Zhao, W., Torre, E., Alkon, D. and Cavallaro, S. (2002) Gene expression profiles in a transgenic animal model of fragile X syndrome. *Neurobiology of Disease*, **10** (3), 211–218.

10 Ginsberg, S., Hemby, S., Lee, V., Eberwine, J. and Trojanowski, J. (2000) Expression profile of transcripts in Alzheimer's disease tangle-bearing CA1 neurons. *Annals of Neurology*, **48** (1), 77–87.

11 Blalock, E., Geddes, J., Chen, K., Porter, N., Markesbery, W. and Landfield, P.

(2004) Incipient Alzheimer's disease: microarray correlation analyses reveal major transcriptional and tumor suppressor responses. *Proceedings of the National Academy of Sciences of the United States of America*, **101** (7), 2173–2178.

12 Colangelo, V., Schurr, J., Ball, M., Pelaez, R., Bazan, N. and Lukiw, W. (2002) Gene expression profiling of 12633 genes in Alzheimer hippocampal CA1: transcription and neurotrophic factor down-regulation and up-regulation of apoptotic and pro-inflammatory signaling. *Journal of Neuroscience Research*, **70** (3), 462–473.

13 Emilsson, L., Saetre, P. and Jazin, E. (2006) Alzheimer's disease: mRNA expression profiles of multiple patients show alterations of genes involved with calcium signaling. *Neurobiology of Disease*, **21** (3), 618–625.

14 Ricciarelli, R., d'Abramo, C., Massone, S., Marinari, U., Pronzato, M. and Tabaton, M. (2004) Microarray analysis in Alzheimer's disease and normal aging. *IUBMB Life*, **56** (6), 349–354.

15 Loring, J., Wen, X., Lee, J., Seilhamer, J. and Somogyi, R. (2001) A gene expression profile of Alzheimer's disease. *DNA and Cell Biology*, **20** (11), 683–695.

16 Mandel, S., Grunblatt, E., Riederer, P., Amariglio, N., Jacob-Hirsch, J., Rechavi, G. and Youdim, M. (2005) Gene expression profiling of sporadic Parkinson's disease substantia nigra pars compacta reveals impairment of ubiquitin-proteasome subunits SKP1A, aldehyde dehydrogenase, and chaperone HSC-70. *Annals of the New York Academy of Sciences*, **1053**, 356–375.

17 Borovecki, F., Lovrecic, L., Zhou, J., Jeong, H., Then, F., Rosas, H.D., Hersch, S.M., Hogarth, P., Bouzou, B., Jensen, R.V. and Krainc, D. (2005) Genome-wide expression profiling of human blood reveals biomarkers for Huntington's disease. *Proceedings of the*

National Academy of Sciences of the United States of America, **102** (31), 11023–11028.

18 Sugars, K. and Rubinsztein, D. (2003) Transcriptional abnormalities in Huntington disease. *Trends in Genetics*, **19** (5), 233–238.

19 Dangond, F., Hwang, D., Camelo, S., Pasinelli, P., Frosch, M., Stephanopoulos, G., Stephanopoulos, G., Brown, R. and Gullans, S. (2004) Molecular signature of late-stage human ALS revealed by expression profiling of postmortem spinal cord gray matter. *Physiological Genomics*, **16** (2), 229–239.

20 Jiang, Y.M., Yamamoto, M., Kobayashi, Y., Yoshihara, T., Liang, Y., Terao, S., Takeuchi, H., Ishigaki, S., Katsuno, M., Adachi, H., Niwa, J., Tanaka, F., Doyu, M., Yoshida, M., Hashizume, Y. and Sobue, G. (2005) Gene expression profile of spinal motor neurons in sporadic amyotrophic lateral sclerosis. *Annals of Neurology*, **57** (2), 236–251.

21 Mirnics, K., Middleton, F., Marquez, A., Lewis, D. and Levitt, P. (2000) Molecular characterization of schizophrenia viewed by microarray analysis of gene expression in prefrontal cortex. *Neuron*, **28** (1), 53–67.

22 Geschwind, D. (2003) DNA microarrays: translation of the genome from laboratory to clinic. *Lancet Neurology*, **2** (5), 275–282.

23 Alwine, J., Kemp, D. and Stark, G. (1977) Method for detection of specific RNAs in agarose gels by transfer to diazobenzyloxymethyl-paper and hybridization with DNA probes. *Proceedings of the National Academy of Sciences of the United States of America*, **74** (12), 5350–5354.

24 Gall, J. and Pardue, M. (1969) Formation and detection of RNA–DNA hybrid molecules in cytological preparations. *Proceedings of the National Academy of Sciences of the United States of America*, **63** (2), 378–383.

25 Coppola, G. and Geschwind, D.H. (2006) Microarrays and the microscope:

balancing throughput with resolution. *The Journal of Physiology*, **575** (2), 353–359.

26 Geschwind, D. (2000) Mice, microarrays, and the genetic diversity of the brain. *Proceedings of the National Academy of Sciences of the United States of America*, **97** (20), 10676–10678.

27 Liang, P. and Pardee, A. (1992) Differential display of eukaryotic messenger RNA by means of the polymerase chain reaction. *Science*, **257** (5072), 967–971.

28 Dougherty, J. and Geschwind, D. (2002) Subtraction-coupled custom microarray analysis for gene discovery and gene expression studies in the CNS. *Chemical Senses*, **27** (3), 293–298.

29 Hubank, M. and Schatz, D. (1994) Identifying differences in mRNA expression by representational difference analysis of cDNA. *Nucleic Acids Research*, **22** (25), 5640–5648.

30 Velculescu, V., Zhang, L., Vogelstein, B. and Kinzler, K. (1995) Serial analysis of gene expression. *Science*, **270** (5235), 484–487.

31 Brenner, S., Johnson, M., Bridgham, J., Golda, G., Lloyd, D.H., Johnson, D., Luo, S., McCurdy, S., Foy, M., Ewan, M., Roth, R., George, D., Eletr, S., Albrecht, G., Vermaas, E., Williams, S.R., Moon, K., Burcham, T., Pallas, M., DuBridge, R.B., Kirchner, J., Fearon, K., Mao, J. and Corcoran, K. (2000) Gene expression analysis by massively parallel signature sequencing (MPSS) on microbead arrays. *Nature Biotechnology*, **18** (6), 630–634.

32 Augenlicht, L., Wahrman, M., Halsey, H., Anderson, L., Taylor, J. and Lipkin, M. (1987) Expression of cloned sequences in biopsies of human colonic tissue and in colonic carcinoma cells induced to differentiate *in vitro*. *Cancer Research*, **47** (22), 6017–6021.

33 Hardiman, G. (2004) Microarray platforms – comparisons and contrasts. *Pharmacogenomics*, **5** (5), 487–502.

34 Fodor, S., Read, J., Pirrung, M., Stryer, L., Lu, A. and Solas, D. (1991) Light-directed spatially addressable parallel chemical synthesis. *Science*, **251** (4995), 767–773.

35 Fodor, S., Rava, R., Huang, X., Pease, A., Holmes, C. and Adams, C. (1993) Multiplexed biochemical assays with biological chips. *Nature*, **364** (6437), 555–556.

36 Jacobs, J. and Fodor, S. (1994) Combinatorial chemistry – applications of light-directed chemical synthesis. *Trends in Biotechnology*, **12** (1), 19–26.

37 Lockhart, D.J., Dong, H., Byrne, M.C., Follettie, M.T., Gallo, M.V., Chee, M.S., Mittmann, M., Wang, C., Kobayashi, M., Horton, H. and Brown, E.L. (1996) Expression monitoring by hybridization to high-density oligonucleotide arrays. *Nature Biotechnology*, **14** (13), 1675–1680.

38 Lipshutz, R., Fodor, S., Gingeras, T. and Lockhart, D. (1999) High density synthetic oligonucleotide arrays. *Nature Genetics*, **21** (1 Suppl.), 20–24.

39 Schena, M., Shalon, D., Davis, R. and Brown, P. (1995) Quantitative monitoring of gene expression patterns with a complementary DNA microarray. *Science*, **270** (5235), 467–470.

40 Schena, M., Heller, R., Theriault, T., Konrad, K., Lachenmeier, E. and Davis, R. (1998) Microarrays: biotechnology's discovery platform for functional genomics. *Trends in Biotechnology*, **16** (7), 301–306.

41 Iida, K. and Nishimura, I. (2002) Gene expression profiling by DNA microarray technology. *Critical Reviews in Oral Biology and Medicine*, **13** (1), 35–50.

42 Eisen, M. and Brown, P. (1999) DNA arrays for analysis of gene expression. *Methods in Enzymology*, **303**, 179–205.

43 Brown, P. and Botstein, D. (1999) Exploring the new world of the genome with DNA microarrays. *Nature Genetics*, **21** (1 Suppl.), 33–37.

44 Wolber, P., Collins, P., Lucas, A., De Witte, A. and Shannon, K. (2006) The

Agilent *in situ*-synthesized microarray platform. *Methods in Enzymology*, **410**, 28–57.

45 Fan, J., Gunderson, K., Bibikova, M., Yeakley, J., Chen, J., Wickham Garcia, E., Lebruska, L., Laurent, M., Shen, R. and Barker, D. (2006) Illumina universal bead arrays. *Methods in Enzymology*, **410**, 57–73.

46 Gunderson, K.L., Kruglyak, S., Graige, M.S., Garcia, F., Kermani, B.G., Zhao, C., Che, D., Dickinson, T., Wickham, E., Bierle, J., Doucet, D., Milewski, M., Yang, R., Siegmund, C., Haas, J., Zhou, L., Oliphant, A., Fan, J.B., Barnard, S. and Chee, M.S. (2004) Decoding randomly ordered DNA arrays. *Genome Research*, **14** (5), 870–877.

47 Mirnics, K. and Pevsner, J. (2004) Progress in the use of microarray technology to study the neurobiology of disease. *Nature Neuroscience*, **7** (5), 434–439.

48 Karsten, S., Kudo, L. and Geschwind, D. (2004) Microarray platforms: introduction and application to neurobiology. *International Review of Neurobiology*, **60**, 1–23.

49 Lockhart, D. and Barlow, C. (2001) Expressing what's on your mind: DNA arrays and the brain. *Nature Reviews. Neuroscience*, **2** (1), 63–68.

50 Luo, Z. and Geschwind, D. (2001) Microarray applications in neuroscience. *Neurobiology of Disease*, **8** (2), 183–193.

51 Quackenbush, J. (2006) Microarray analysis and tumor classification. *The New England Journal of Medicine*, **354** (23), 2463–2472.

52 Huber, W., Irizarry, R. and Gentleman, R. (2005) *Bioinformatics and Computational Biology Solutions Using R and Bioconductor (Statistics for Biology and Health)*, Springer.

53 Choe, S., Boutros, M., Michelson, A., Church, G. and Halfon, M. (2005) Preferred analysis methods for Affymetrix GeneChips revealed by a wholly defined control dataset. *Genome Biology*, **6** (2), R16.1–R16.16.

54 Nuwaysir, E.F., Huang, W., Albert, T.J., Singh, J., Nuwaysir, K., Pitas, A., Richmond, T., Gorski, T., Berg, J.P., Ballin, J., McCormick, M., Norton, J., Pollock, T., Sumwalt, T., Butcher, L., Porter, D., Molla, M., Hall, C., Blattner, F., Sussman, M.R., Wallace, R.L., Cerrina, F. and Green, R.D. (2002) Gene expression analysis using oligonucleotide arrays produced by maskless photolithography. *Genome Research*, **12** (11), 1749–1755.

55 Vawter, M., Crook, J., Hyde, T., Kleinman, J., Weinberger, D., Becker, K. and Freed, W. (2002) Microarray analysis of gene expression in the prefrontal cortex in schizophrenia: a preliminary study. *Schizophrenia Research*, **58** (1), 11–20.

56 Schwartz, A. and Fernández-Repollet, E. (2001) Quantitative flow cytometry. *Clinics in Laboratory Medicine*, **21** (4), 743–761.

57 Heintz, N. (2004) Gene expression nervous system atlas (GENSAT). *Nature Neuroscience*, **7** (5), 483.

58 Ginsberg, S., Elarova, I., Ruben, M., Tan, F., Counts, S., Eberwine, J., Trojanowski, J., Hemby, S., Mufson, E. and Che, S. (2004) Single-cell gene expression analysis: implications for neuro-degenerative and neuropsychiatric disorders. *Neurochemical Research*, **29** (6), 1053–1064.

59 Kacharmina, J., Crino, P. and Eberwine, J. (1999) Preparation of cDNA from single cells and subcellular regions. *Methods in Enzymology*, **303**, 3–18.

60 Emmert-Buck, M., Bonner, R., Smith, P., Chuaqui, R., Zhuang, Z., Goldstein, S., Weiss, R. and Liotta, L. (1996) Laser capture microdissection. *Science*, **274** (5289), 998–1001.

61 Li, C. and Wong, W. (2001) Model-based analysis of oligonucleotide arrays: model validation design issues and standard error application. *Genome Biology*, **2** (8), 1–11. research0032.0031–research0032.0011.

62 Medigue, C., Rechenmann, F., Danchin, A. and Viari, A. (1999) Imagene: an integrated computer environment for sequence annotation and analysis. *Bioinformatics*, **15** (1), 2–15.

63 Evans, S.J., Choudary, P.V., Vawter, M.P., Li, J., Meador-Woodruff, J.H., Lopez, J.F., Burke, S.M., Thompson, R.C., Myers, R.M., Jones, E.G. Bunney, W.E., Watson, S.J. and Akil, H. (2003) DNA microarray analysis of functionally discrete human brain regions reveals divergent transcriptional profiles. *Neurobiology of Disease*, **14** (2), 240–250.

64 Lu, T., Pan, Y., Kao, S.-Y., Li, C., Kohane, I., Chan, J. and Yankner, B. (2004) Gene regulation and DNA damage in the ageing human brain. *Nature*, **429** (6994), 883–891.

65 Ghazalpour, A., Doss, S., Zhang, B., Wang, S., Plaisier, C., Castellanos, R., Brozell, A., Schadt, E.E., Drake, T.A., Lusis, A.J. and Horvath, S. (2006) Integrating genetic and network analysis to characterize genes related to mouse weight. *PLoS Genetics*, **28**, 1182–1192.

66 Reimers, M. and Carey, V. (2006) Bioconductor: an open source framework for bioinformatics and computational biology. *Methods in Enzymology*, **411**, 119–134.

67 Hosack, D., Dennis, G., Sherman, B., Lane, H. and Lempicki, R. (2003) Identifying biological themes within lists of genes with EASE. *Genome Biology*, **4** (10), R70.1–R70.8.

68 Subramanian, A., Tamayo, P., Mootha, V.K., Mukherjee, S., Ebert, B.L., Gillette, M.A., Paulovich, A., Pomeroy, S.L., Golub, T.R., Lander, E.S. and Mesirov, J.P. (2005) From the cover: Gene set enrichment analysis: a knowledge-based approach for interpreting genome-wide expression profiles. *Proceedings of the National Academy of Sciences of the United States of America*, **102** (43), 15545–15550.

69 Zhang, B., Kirov, S. and Snoddy, J. (2005) WebGestalt: an integrated system for exploring gene sets in various biological contexts. *Nucleic Acids Research*, **33** (Web Server issue, W741–W748).

70 Chen, H. and Sharp, B. (2004) Content-rich biological network constructed by mining PubMed abstracts. *BMC Bioinformatics*, **5** (1), 1–13.

71 Rebhan, M., Chalifa-Caspi, V., Prilusky, J. and Lancet, D. (1997) GeneCards: encyclopedia for genes proteins and diseases. World Wide Web URL:http://wwwgenecardsorg/.

72 Barabasi, A. and Oltvai, Z. (2004) Network biology: understanding the cell's functional organization. *Nature Reviews. Genetics*, **5** (2), 101–113.

73 Jeong, H., Mason, S., Barabasi, A. and Oltvai, Z. (2001) Lethality and centrality in protein networks. *Nature*, **411** (6833), 41–42.

74 Oldham, M., Horvath, S. and Geschwind, D. (2006) Conservation and evolution of gene co-expression networks in human and chimpanzee brain. *Proceedings of the National Academy of Sciences of the United States of America*, **103**, 17973–17978.

75 Zhang, B. and Horvath, S. (2005) A general framework for weighted gene co-expression network analysis. *Statistical Applications in Genetics and Molecular Biology*, **4** (1), 1–43.

76 Horvath, S., Zhang, B., Carlson, M., Lu, K.V., Zhu, S., Felciano, R.M., Laurance, M.F., Zhao, W., Qi, S., Chen, Z., Lee, Y., Scheck, A.C., Liau, L.M., Wu, H., Geschwind, D.H., Febbo, P.G., Kornblum, H.I., Cloughesy, T.F., Nelson, S.F. and Mischel, P.S. (2006) Analysis of oncogenic signaling networks in glioblastoma identifies ASPM as a molecular target. *Proceedings of the National Academy of Sciences of the United States of America*, **103** (46), 17402–17407.

77 Bustin, S. (2000) Absolute quantification of mRNA using real-time reverse transcription polymerase chain reaction assays. *Journal of Molecular Endocrinology*, **25** (2), 169–193.

78 Lock, C., Hermans, G., Pedotti, R., Brendolan, A., Schadt, E., Garren, H., Langer-Gould, A., Strober, S., Cannella, B., Allard, J., Klonowski, P., Austin, A., Lad, N., Kaminski, N., Galli, S.J., Oksenberg, J.R., Raine, C.S., Heller, R. and Steinman, L. (2002) Gene-microarray analysis of multiple sclerosis lesions yields new targets validated in autoimmune encephalomyelitis. *Nature Medicine*, **8** (5), 500–508.

79 Karsten, S.L., Sang, T.K., Gehman, L.T., Chatterjee, S., Liu, J., Lawless, G.M., Sengupta, S., Berry, R.W., Pomakian, J., Oh, H.S. Schulz, C., Hui, K.S., Wiedau-Pazos, M., Vinters, H.V., Binder, L.I., Geschwind, D.H. and Jackson, G.R. (2006) A genomic screen for modifiers of tauopathy identifies puromycin-sensitive aminopeptidase as an inhibitor of tau-induced neurodegeneration. *Neuron*, **51** (5), 549–560.

80 Lee, H., Hsu, A., Sajdak, J., Qin, J. and Pavlidis, P. (2004) Coexpression analysis of human genes across many microarray data sets. *Genome Research*, **14** (6), 1085–1094.

81 Bailey, P. and Cushing, H. (1928) *A Classification of the Tumors of the Glioma Group on a Histogenic Basis with a Correlated Study of Prognosis*, Lippincott.

82 Shai, R., Shi, T., Kremen, T., Horvath, S., Liau, L., Cloughesy, T., Mischel, P. and Nelson, S. (2003) Gene expression profiling identifies molecular subtypes of gliomas. *Oncogene*, **22** (31), 4918–4923.

83 Freije, W., Castro-Vargas, F., Fang, Z., Horvath, S., Cloughesy, T., Liau, L., Mischel, P. and Nelson, S. (2004) Gene expression profiling of gliomas strongly predicts survival. *Cancer Research*, **64** (18), 6503–6510.

84 Sarkar, C., Deb, P. and Sharma, M. (2006) Medulloblastomas: new directions in risk stratification. *Neurology India*, **54** (1), 16–23.

85 Gajjar, A., Hernan, R., Kocak, M., Fuller, C., Lee, Y., McKinnon, P.J., Wallace, D., Lau, C., Chintagumpala, M., Ashley, D.M., Kellie, S.J., Kun, L. and Gilbertson, R.J. (2004) Clinical, histopathologic, and molecular markers of prognosis: toward a new disease risk stratification system for medulloblastoma. *Journal of Clinical Oncology*, **22** (6), 984–993.

86 Pomeroy, S.L., Tamayo, P., Gaasenbeek, M., Sturla, L.M., Angelo, M., Mclaughlin, M.E., Kim, J.Y., Goumnerova, L.C., Black, P.M., Lau, C., Allen, J.C., Zagzag, D., Olson, J.M., Curran, T., Wetmore, C., Biegel, J.A., Poggio, T., Mukherjee, S., Rifkin, R., Califano, A., Stolovitzky, G., Louis, D.N., Mesirov, J.P., Lander, E.S. and Golub, T.R. (2002) Prediction of central nervous system embryonal tumour outcome based on gene expression. *Nature*, **415** (6870), 436–442.

87 Sowar, K., Straessle, J., Donson, A., Handler, M. and Foreman, N. (2006) Predicting which children are at risk for ependymoma relapse. *Journal of Neuro-Oncology*, **78** (1), 41–46.

88 Gyorffy, B., Surowiak, P., Kiesslich, O., Denkert, C., Schäfer, R., Dietel, M. and Lage, H. (2005) Gene expression profiling of 30 cancer cell lines predicts resistance towards 11 anticancer drugs at clinically achieved concentrations. *International Journal of Cancer*, **118** (7), 1699–1712.

89 Staunton, J.E., Slonim, D.K., Coller, H.A., Tamayo, P., Angelo, M.J., Park, J., Scherf, U., Lee, J.K., Reinhold, W.O., Weinstein, J.N., Mesirov, J.P., Lander, E.S. and Golub, T.R. (2001) Chemosensitivity prediction by transcriptional profiling. *Proceedings of the National Academy of Sciences of the United States of America*, **98** (19), 10787–10792.

90 Stegmaier, K., Ross, K., Colavito, S., O'Malley, S., Stockwell, B. and Golub, T. (2004) Gene expression-based high-throughput screening (GE-HTS) and application to leukemia differentiation. *Nature Genetics*, **36** (3), 257–263.

91 Cheok, M., Yang, W., Pui, C., Downing, J., Cheng, C., Naeve, C., Relling, M. and Evans, W. (2003) Treatment-specific changes in gene expression discriminate *in vivo* drug response in human leukemia cells. *Nature Genetics*, **34** (1), 85–90.

92 Sharp, F.R., Xu, H., Lit, L., Walker, W., Apperson, M., Gilbert, D.L., Glauser, T.A., Wong, B., Hershey, A., Liu, D.Z. Pinter, J., Zhan, X., Liu, X. and Ran, R. (2006) The future of genomic profiling of neurological diseases using blood. *Archives of Neurology*, **63** (11), 1529–1536.

93 Sharp, F.R., Lit, L., Xu, H., Apperson, M., Walker, W., Wong, B., Gilbert, D.L., Hershey, A. and Glauser, T.A. (2006) Genomics of brain and blood: progress and pitfalls. *Epilepsia*, **47** (10), 1603–1607.

94 Ohmori, T., Morita, K., Saito, T., Ohta, M., Ueno, S. and Rokutan, K. (2005) Assessment of human stress and depression by DNA microarray analysis. *The Journal of Medical Investigation*, **52** (Suppl.), 266–271.

95 Tang, Y., Lu, A., Aronow, B. and Sharp, F. (2001) Blood genomic responses differ after stroke seizures, hypoglycemia, and hypoxia: blood genomic fingerprints of disease. *Annals of Neurology*, **50** (6), 699–707.

96 Tang, Y., Lu, A., Aronow, B., Wagner, K. and Sharp, F. (2002) Genomic responses of the brain to ischemic stroke intracerebral haemorrhage, kainate seizures, hypoglycemia, and hypoxia. *The European Journal of Neuroscience*, **15** (12), 1937–1952.

97 Moore, D.F., Li, H., Jeffries, N., Wright, V., Cooper, R.A. Jr, Elkahloun, A., Gelderman, M.P., Zudaire, E., Blevins, G., Yu, H., Goldin, E. and Baird, A.E. (2005) Using peripheral blood mono-nuclear cells to determine a gene expression profile of acute ischemic stroke: a pilot investigation. *Circulation*, 111 (2), 212–221.

98 Tang, Y., Xu, H., Du, X., Lit, L., Walker, W., Lu, A., Ran, R., Gregg, J.P., Reilly, M., Pancioli, A., Khoury, J.C., Sauerbeck, L.R., Carrozzella, J.A., Spilker, J., Clark, J., Wagner, K.R., Jauch, E.C., Chang, D.J., Verro, P., Broderick, J.P. and Sharp, F.R. (2006) Gene expression in blood changes rapidly in neutrophils and monocytes after ischemic stroke in humans: a microarray study. *Journal of Cerebral Blood Flow and Metabolism*, **26** (8), 1089–1102.

99 Tang, Y., Gilbert, D., Glauser, T., Hershey, A. and Sharp, F. (2005) Blood gene expression profiling of neurologic diseases: a pilot microarray study. *Archives of Neurology*, **62** (2), 210–215.

100 Kurlan, R. and Kaplan, E. (2004) The pediatric autoimmune neuropsychiatric disorders associated with streptococcal infection (PANDAS) etiology for tics and obsessive-compulsive symptoms: hypothesis or entity? Practical considerations for the clinician. *Pediatrics*, **113** (4), 883–886.

101 Tang, Y., Schapiro, M.B., Franz, D.N., Patterson, B.J., Hickey, F.J., Schorry, E.K., Hopkin, R.J., Wylie, M., Narayan, T., Glauser, T.A., Gilbert, D.L., Hershey, A.D. and Sharp, F.R. (2004) Blood expression profiles for tuberous sclerosis complex 2, neurofibromatosis type 1, and Down's syndrome. *Annals of Neurology*, **56** (6), 808–814.

102 Achiron, A. and Gurevich, M. (2006) Peripheral blood gene expression signature mirrors central nervous system disease: the model of multiple sclerosis. *Autoimmunity Reviews*, **5** (8), 517–522.

103 Kálmán, J., Palotás, A., Juhász, A., Rimanóczy, A., Hugyecz, M., Kovács, Z., Galsi, G., Szabó, Z., Pákáski, M., Fehér, L.Z., Janka, Z. and Puskás, L.G. (2005) Impact of venlafaxine on gene expression profile in lymphocytes of the elderly with major depression evolution of antidepressants and the role of the neuro-immune system. *Neurochemical Research*, **30** (11), 1429–1438.

104 Shukla, S. and Dolan, M. (2005) Use of CEPH and non-CEPH lymphoblast cell lines in pharmacogenetic studies. *Pharmacogenomics*, **6** (3), 303–310.

105 Geschwind, D.H., Gregg, J., Boone, K., Karrim, J., Pawlikowska-Haddal, A., Rao, E., Ellison, J., Ciccodicola, A., D'Urso, M., Woods, R., Rappold, G.A., Swerdloff, R. and Nelson, S.F. (1998) Klinefelter's syndrome as a model of anomalous cerebral laterality: testing gene dosage in the X chromosome pseudoautosomal region using a DNA microarray. *Developmental Genetics*, **23** (3), 215–229.

106 Cheung, V.G., Nowak, N., Jang, W., Kirsch, I.R., Zhao, S., Chen, X.N., Furey, T.S., Kim, U.J., Kuo, W.L., Olivier, M. Conroy, J., Kasprzyk, A., Massa, H., Yonescu, R., Sait, S., Thoreen, C., Snijders, A., Lemyre, E., Bailey, J.A., Bruzel, A., Burrill, W.D., Clegg, S.M., Collins, S., Dhami, P., Friedman, C., Han, C.S., Herrick, S., Lee, J., Ligon, A.H., Lowry, S., Morley, M., Narasimhan, S., Osoegawa, K., Peng, Z., Plajzer-Frick, I., Quade, B.J., Scott, D., Sirotkin, K., Thorpe, A.A., Gray, J.W., Hudson, J., Pinkel, D., Ried, T., Rowen, L., Shen-Ong, G.L., Strausberg, R.L., Birney, E., Callen, D.F., Cheng, J.F., Cox, D.R., Doggett, N.A., Carter, N.P., Eichler, E.E., Haussler, D., Korenberg, J.R., Morton, C.C., Albertson, D., Schuler, G., de Jong, P.J. and Trask, B.J.,BAC Resource Consortium. (2001) Integration of cytogenetic landmarks into the draft sequence of the human genome. *Nature*, **409** (6822), 953–958.

107 Slater, H., Bailey, D., Ren, H., Cao, M., Bell, K., Nasioulas, S., Henke, R., Choo, K. and Kennedy, G. (2005) High-resolution identification of chromosomal abnormalities using oligonucleotide arrays containing 116204 SNPs. *American Journal of Human Genetics*, **77** (5), 709–726.

108 Fan, J.-B., Chee, M. and Gunderson, K. (2006) Highly parallel genomic

assays. *Nature Reviews. Genetics*, **7** (8), 632–644.

109 Lalande, M. (1996) Parental imprinting and human disease. *Annual Review of Genetics*, **30**, 173–195.

110 Gunderson, K.L., Kuhn, K.M., Steemers, F.J., Ng, P., Murray, S.S. and Shen, R. (2006) Whole-genome genotyping of haplotype tag single nucleotide polymorphisms. *Pharmacogenomics*, **7** (4), 641–648.

111 Komura, D., Shen, F., Ishikawa, S., Fitch, K.R., Chen, W., Zhang, J., Liu, G., Ihara, S., Nakamura, H., Hurles, M.E. Lee, C., Scherer, S.W., Jones, K.W., Shapero, M.H., Huang, J. and Aburatani, H. (2006) Genome-wide detection of human copy number variations using high-density DNA oligonucleotide arrays. *Genome Research*, 16 (12), 1575–1584.

112 Weeraratna, A., Nagel, J., de Mello-Coelho, V. and Taub, D. (2004) Gene expression profiling: from microarrays to medicine. *Journal of Clinical Immunology*, **24** (3), 213–224.

113 Redon, R., Ishikawa, S., Fitch, K.R., Feuk, L., Perry, G.H., Andrews, T.D., Fiegler, H., Shapero, M.H., Carson, A.R., Chen, W., Cho, E.K., Dallaire, S., Freeman, J.L., Gonzalez, J.R., Gratacos, M., Huang, J., Kalaitzopoulos, D., Komura, D., MacDonald, J.R., Marshall, C.R., Mei, R., Montgomery, L., Nishimura, K., Okamura, K., Shen, F., Somerville, M.J., Tchinda, J., Valsesia, A., Woodwark, C., Yang, F., Zhang, J., Zerjal, T., Zhang, J., Armengol, L., Conrad, D.F., Estivill, X., Tyler-Smith, C., Carter, N.P., Aburatani, H., Lee, C., Jones, K.W., Scherer, S.W. and Hurles, M.E.,((2006) Global variation in copy number in the human genome. *Nature*, 444 (7118), 444–454.

114 Sebat, J., Lakshmi, B., Troge, J., Alexander, J., Young, J., Lundin, P., Maner, S., Massa, H., Walker, M., Chi, M., Navin, N., Lucito, R., Healy, J., Hicks, J., Ye, K., Reiner, A., Gilliam, T.C., Trask,

B., Patterson, N., Zetterberg, A. and
Wigler, M. (2004) Large-scale copy
number polymorphism in the human
genome. *Science*, **305** (5683), 525–528.

115 Nishimura, Y., Martin, C., Vazquez-
Lopez, A., Spence, S., Alvarez-Retuerto,
A., Sigman, M., Steindler, C., Pellegrini,
S., Schanen, N., Warren, S. and
Geschwind, D. (2004) Genome-wide
expression profiling of lymphoblastoid
cell lines distinguishes different forms
of autism and reveals shared pathways.
Human Molecular Genetics, **16** (14),
1682–1698.

2

A Meta-Analysis of Large-Scale Gene Expression Studies of the Injured PNS: Toward the Genetic Networks That Govern Successful Regeneration

Floor J. Stam, Matthew R.J. Mason, August B. Smit, and Joost Verhaagen

2.1
Introduction

Injury to the spinal cord results in either complete or incomplete disruption of the nerve tracts that lie within the vertebral column. Because of the inability of neurons to regrow and cross a lesion site in the adult central nervous system (CNS), spinal cord injury (SCI) results in permanent disability. The clinical consequences of SCI depend on the level of the lesion and may include paralysis of the legs, trunk instability, paralysis of the arms, bowel, bladder, and sexual dysfunction, and inability to breathe independently. An important goal of SCI research is to find ways to enhance the regeneration of injured neurons. In this respect, it is of great interest that injured neurons of the adult peripheral nervous system (PNS) retain their capacity to extend long neurites and reestablish functional connections. The idea that knowledge of the mechanisms that enable PNS neurons to regenerate may be used to enhance regeneration in the injured CNS has inspired a vast amount of research in the last 25–30 years. In fact, the molecular changes induced by neural injury constitute a tightly controlled gene expression program that is essential for successful regeneration. The advent of new high-throughput screening technologies has facilitated the exploration of such programs, thereby providing insights that may be the basis of future clinical therapy. In this chapter, we review the literature on neuronal gene expression profiles during peripheral nerve regeneration. We present a meta-analysis of the combined data from four studies that provide large-scale expression data in rats, in terms of common findings and gene ontology clusters of the regulated genes. Finally, we discuss the efforts that are required in the future to elucidate the genetic network underlying successful regeneration.

2.2
Lesion Models in the Peripheral Nervous System

Regeneration of damaged axons occurs successfully in both somatic and autonomic peripheral nervous systems. The three injury models used most frequently are the

Neural Degeneration and Repair: Gene Expression Profiling, Proteomics, and Systems Biology
Edited by Hans Werner Müller
Copyright © 2008 WILEY-VCH Verlag GmbH & Co. KGaA, Weinheim
ISBN: 978-3-527-31707-3

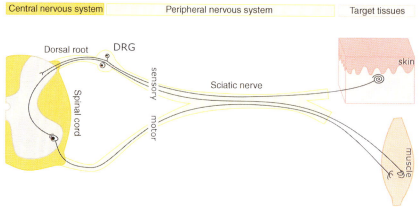

Figure 2.1 Schematic representation of the sciatic nerve lesion model. Sciatic nerve injury axotomizes both motor and sensory neurons located in the ventrolateral spinal cord and dorsal root ganglion, respectively. In addition, DRG neurons can be axotomized centrally by injuring the dorsal root.

sciatic nerve (SN), the facial nerve, and the postganglionic trunk of the superior cervical ganglion.

2.2.1
Sciatic Nerve

The most common model system for regeneration studies is the SN (Figure 2.1). This is a mixed nerve, containing both motor and sensory axons. The motor neurons, whose cell bodies lie in the ventrolateral spinal cord, innervate the hind limb muscles. The sensory neurons contributing to the SN are located in the L4, L5, and L6 dorsal root ganglia (DRG) and innervate the skin and muscle of the hind limb. The DRG neurons extend a short stem axon and then bifurcate, with one neurite extending into the periphery and the other into the dorsal root and subsequently into the spinal cord. Experimental injury is usually carried out at mid-thigh level. Although both sensory and motor neurons are affected by sciatic nerve crush, changes in gene expression are most often assessed in the dorsal root ganglion, as the cell bodies of these neurons are easily accessible.

2.2.2
Facial Nerve

The facial nerve contains the axons of facial nucleus neurons, which are located in the brain stem. These motor neurons innervate the facial musculature. For regeneration studies, the facial nerve is injured just distal from its exit from the skull through the stylomastoid foramen.

2.2.3
Postganglionic Trunk of the Superior Cervical Ganglion

The superior cervical ganglion (SCG) is part of the sympathetic autonomic nervous system. SCG neurons receive input from visceral motor neurons located in the mediolateral spinal cord. The postganglionic fibers innervate the lacrimal and salivary glands and the smooth muscle of the eye. The postganglionic trunk of the superial cervical ganglion is accessible from the ventral side of the neck.

2.2.4
Injury Types

In regeneration studies, these nerves are subjected either to crush, where the surrounding Schwann cell tube remains connected, or transection, resulting in complete discontinuity of the nerve. Transection of the sciatic nerve or ligation of the spinal nerves has also been used to study molecular changes associated with neuropathic pain. As the gene expression data from the DRG in these studies are relevant to regeneration, they will also be discussed in this chapter.

2.3
Cellular Events After Injury

The events that occur after an SN lesion can be divided into several partially overlapping phases. First, the nerve distal from the lesion degenerates within hours to days after injury. Multiple sprouts are formed from each parent axon at the node of Ranvier proximal to the lesion site, starting as early as 9 hours after axotomy [1]. At 27 hours, approximately one third of all injured axons form sprouts [2]. Sprout formation is followed by the elongation of neurites over long distances. Newly formed neurites elongate between the basal lamina sheath and the Schwann cell column, both of which provide contact support by means of cell adhesion molecules. In addition, Schwann cells promote regeneration by secreting growth factors (reviewed by Fawcett and Keynes [3] and Ide [4]). After an initial lag phase, the velocity of regrowth in the distal stump increases to 2.7–4.4 mm/day [5,6]. If the bands of Büngner stay intact, as is the case after a crush injury, neurites elongate within their original basal lamina tubes and the original branching patterns are restored [7]. Axons that regrow into denervated target areas form functional contacts at their original sites [8–11]. Functional recovery is less complete after nerve cut, as a large number of regenerating fibers grow into the connective tissue surrounding the nerve and subsequently stall [5,7]. After complete peripheral nerve transection, in which retraction of the proximal and distal nerve stump results in a gap between the nerve stumps, a nonpermissive fibroblastic scar is formed, which prevents successful regeneration [12]. The extent to which function is restored depends on the time lag between denervation and reinnervation, but is generally not complete.

2.3.1
Regeneration After Dorsal Root Lesion is Limited Due to a Weak Neuronal Response to Axotomy

DRG neurons extend a second neurite branch toward and into the spinal cord. These axons can be injured by a dorsal root crush or transection. In contrast to the peripheral neurite, the regrowing dorsal root axons encounter two different environments. First, they grow through the permissive dorsal root (DR), which contains Schwann cells. Subsequently, these neurites arrive at the growth-inhibitory CNS environment of the dorsal root entry zone (DREZ), where they stop. The outgrowth that occurs after DR injury alone is slower and involves less neurites than injury of the peripheral process of the same neurons [6,13–16]. The difference in outgrowth rate between the peripheral and central processes of the same neuron is thought to be caused by a differential reaction of the neuronal cell body to these injuries and not by differences in growth support by the DR and SN environments. First, the DR and SN environments are thought not to differ greatly. A recent report showed that dissociated DRG neurons grow equally well on SN tissue as they do on DR explants [17]. The cyto-architecture of the DR is similar to that of the peripheral nerve, and several studies show similar behavior of macrophages in the SN and DR after lesion [18]. Both similarities and differences between lesion-induced gene expression changes in these tissues have been reported [17,19–22]. A second, strong argument to attribute the difference in regenerative response to intrinsic neuronal factors is the observation that when a peripheral crush lesion precedes or accompanies the central crush, growth of the central neurites is greatly enhanced. This results in an increased number and speed of growing neurites [15,16,23,24]. Chong *et al.* [16] showed that this conditioning effect is also present when a piece of peripheral nerve is grafted to the central branch. In addition, the conditioning lesion enables these neurites to grow over larger distances into the inhibitory environment of the CNS at the DREZ [25] and into the injured spinal cord [26]. Taken together, these studies show that DRG neurons display differential growth responses to injury of the central and peripheral branches. Therefore, the intrinsic regenerative capacity of DRG neurons is thought to be a key determinant for the success of regeneration.

2.3.2
Injury Signals

In injured neurons, the lesion usually occurs at a large distance from the nucleus. Therefore, for a transcriptional response to be initiated, an injury signal has to travel from the lesion site to the cell body. Several possibilities for the nature of this injury signal have been suggested. An acute disruption of the retrograde transport of target-derived neurotrophins may play a role [27–29], although it has not been established unequivocally that this ''negative'' signal is involved in initiating the regenerative program. Evidence is emerging for a ''positive signal'' formed by retrograde transport of multiple activated proteins from the site of the lesion to the cell body (reviewed by Hanz and Fainzilber [30]). For example, STAT3 is phosphorylated at the lesion site in injured sciatic nerve axons and then retrogradely transported. It appears in the neuronal nuclei within hours of axotomy [31,32] and increases the growth capacity of DRG neurons after a conditional lesion [33]. Retrograde transport of JNK, several of its upstream kinases, and ATF3 was also seen in injured sciatic nerve [34]. Furthermore, the nuclear transport factors importin α and β have been found in injured axons where they form a nuclear localization signal (NLS) binding complex [35]. Thus, several candidate retrograde signaling molecules as well as a mechanism of transporting NLS-containing proteins from the axon to the nucleus have been found.

In addition, cyclic nucleotides have been reported to be important regulators of the regenerative state of injured neurons. Microinjection of a membrane permeable analog of cAMP into the adult DRG enhanced regeneration after a dorsal column lesion *in vivo* and neurite outgrowth after dissection and dissociation *in vitro* [36,37]. Moreover, inhibitors of a downstream effector of cAMP blocked growth enhancement by a conditioning lesion [37]. Thus, cAMP elevation mimics several aspects of the conditioning lesion effect, that is, increased outgrowth speed *in vitro* and enhanced capacity to elongate neurites in a nonpermissive environment. However, in other reports, cAMP injection did not lead to increased growth of the central neurite into a PNS graft [24] or to the upregulation of classical growth-associated proteins [38]. cAMP elevation may not be sufficient by itself to fully stimulate the conditioning lesion effect, but cAMP signaling is probably an important contributor to the intrinsic regenerative response.

2.3.3
Regeneration-Associated Gene Expression

Because the neuronal response to axotomy is clearly a major determinant of successful regeneration, it has long been considered to be of interest to identify the changes in gene expression that comprise this response. Proteins that are upregulated are expected to be important for axon growth, especially those where a functional connection can be made, such as growth-cone proteins or transcription factors. The archetypal growth-associated protein GAP-43 was discovered by analyzing the axonally transported proteins in the crushed optic nerve of the toad by radioactive labeling and subsequent 1D and 2D gel electrophoreses [39]. Many other proteins have been shown to be associated with regeneration, ranging from cytoskeletal components [40–43] to the neuropeptides NP-Y, substance P, galanin, and CGRP [44,45], to cell adhesion molecules [46–48] and transcription factors including c-Jun [49–51] and ATF3 [52,53] (for a review, see [54]). The gene expression changes in axotomized neurons reflect the intrinsic regenerative response discussed above; thus, although peripheral nerve injury induces (by definition) the full complement of regeneration-associated genes (RAGs), dorsal root injury induces only minimal changes in these genes [19,53,55]. A subset of the proteins found to be regulated by peripheral nerve injury were indeed found to enhance or facilitate regeneration or neurite outgrowth *in vitro*, for example, integrin α4 and GAP-43/CAP-23 [47,56], although no single protein has been shown to be essential for regeneration. The molecular machinery required to grow a new axon is likely to be highly complex and to involve a large number of previously unidentified RAGs. The advent of high-throughput gene expression profiling techniques enables a more thorough and open screening for novel RAGs. In addition, this approach may also be instrumental in the elucidation of the regulatory mechanisms controlling the process of regenerative neurite outgrowth.

2.4
Large-Scale Screening Efforts to Find Novel Regeneration-Associated Genes

In several recent studies, gene expression changes in neurons after injury were characterized at a large scale, as summarized in Table 2.1. In these studies, a wide variety of neuronal tissues, lesion types, time points, and array platforms were used. Notwithstanding these differences, several changes observed are common to all or most studies. To assess gene expression changes found by multiple studies, we combined the data sets described in the four papers that present large-scale *Rattus norvegicus* gene expression results [58,59,61,63] (Table 2.2). In addition, the biological processes that may be active during regeneration based on these gene expression changes were analyzed (Table 2.3). Large-scale studies that did not include GenBank accession numbers or that were performed in species other than the rat were not included, as unifying the gene identifier presents difficulties in this case.

2.4.1
Global Gene Expression Changes After Neuronal Injury Found by Gene Expression Profiling Studies

A number of the genes that are highly regulated in all or most studies have been previously identified by low-throughput studies, whereas a great majority of more subtly regulated transcripts are novel RAGs. The marked upregulation of neuro-peptide genes such as galanin, NP-Y, vasoactive intestinal peptide (VIP), and Substance P are among the most dramatic effects found. Galanin not only has antinociceptive effects when infused intrathecally [69] but also affects neurite out-growth *in vivo* and *in vitro* [70]. NP-Y and VIP have been associated with survival and neurite extension in developing neurons [71,72]. In addition, VIP can promote secretion of IL-6 and laminin by macrophages and Schwann cells, respectively [73,74]. In addition, genes related to inflammation, such as MHC molecules and complement factors, are found to be upregulated by most studies summarized in Table 2.2. This phenomenon may be largely due to an influx of immune cells and macrophages into the DRG [63]. This appears to be a common feature of regenerating systems, as immune cell influx is also found in the axotomized facial nucleus [75,76] and macrophages enter the SCG [77]. Several genes involved in neurotransmission, that is, ion channels and transporters, neurotransmitter receptors, and proteins belonging to the vesicle fusion machinery are downregulated, which likely

Table 2.1 Gene expression profiling studies of the peripheral nervous system.

Study	Platform	Lesion model	Time points	Main findings
[57]	Incyte mouse cDNA array	SN transection	7 d	16 genes > twofold, Sprr1A promotes neurite outgrowth
[58]	Affymetrix RGU34A	SCG postganglionic trunk transection	6 h, 48 h	60 and 320 genes regulated at 6 and 48 h, respectively
[59]	Affymetrix RGU34A	Spinal nerve ligation	13 d	148 genes > twofold and $P \leq 0.05$
[60]	Human cDNA	SN crush	7 d	546 genes > twofold
[61]	Affymetrix RGU34A	SN transection	7 d	240 genes regulated
[62]	DD PCR	FN transection, SC hemi-section	7 d	129 genes regulated: 69 known, 60 unknown
[63]	Reverse Northern, Clontech macroarray	SN transection	2, 7, 14, 28 d	173 regulated genes and ESTs
[64]	Affymetrix U74ABC	SN transection	7 d	36 genes > fivefold, Fn14 promotes neurite outgrowth
[65]	Clontech membrane 0.6K	SN crush	3 d	80 regulated genes
[66]	SAGE	SN transection	3 d	971 up-regulated and 444 downregulated tags
[67]	Affymetrix Mu74A	SN transection	12 h, 24 h	48 genes upregulated > twofold

DD PCR: differential display polymerase chain reaction, SAGE: serial analysis of gene expression,
SN: sciatic nerve, SCG: superior cervical ganglion, FN: facial nerve, SC: spinal cord.

Table 2.2 Genes found to be regulated by two or more studies.

↑/↓	Name	Gene symbol	References
↑	Galanin	Gal	[58,59,61,63]
↓	Tachykinin 1	Tac1	[58,59,61,63]
↑	Vasoactive intestinal polypeptide	Vip	[58,59,61,63]
↓	Apolipoprotein D	Apod	[59,61,63]
↑	Arginase 1	Arg1	[58,59,61]
↓	Activating transcription factor 3	Atf3	[58,59,61]
↓	Benzodiazepine receptor, peripheral	Bzrp	[59,61,63]
↑	Calcium channel, voltage-dependent, alpha2/delta subunit 1	Cacna2d1	[59,61,63]
↑	Cysteine and glycine-rich protein 3	Csrp3	[59,61,63]
↑	Growth arrest and DNA-damage-inducible 45 alpha	Gadd45a	[59,61,63]
↑	GDNF family receptor alpha 1	Gfra1	[59,61,63]
↑	Insulin-like growth factor binding protein 3	Igfbp3	[58,59,63]
↑	Neuropeptide Y	Npy	[59,61,63]
↓	Pancreatitis-associated protein	Pap	[58,59,61]
↓	Protein tyrosine phosphatase, nonreceptor type 5	Ptpn5	[59,61,63]
↑	RT1 class II, locus Da	RT1-Da	[59,61,63]
↑	Sodium channel, voltage-gated, type 10, alpha polypeptide	Scn10a	[59,61,63]
↑	Synaptic vesicle glycoprotein 2b	Sv2b	[59,61,63]
↑	Tissue inhibitor of metallopeptidase 1	Timp1	[58,59,61]
↑	VGF nerve growth factor inducible	Vgf	[59,61,63]
↑	Visinin-like 1	Vsnl1	[58,59,63]
↑	Adenylate cyclase activating polypeptide 1	Adcyap1	[59,61]
↓	Allograft inflammatory factor 1	Aif1	[59,61]
↑	Ankyrin repeat domain 1 (cardiac muscle)	Ankrd1	[58,61]
↓	Actin-related protein 2/3 complex, subunit 1B	Arpc1b	[59,61]
↓	ATPase, Ca^{2+} transporting, plasma membrane 2	Atp2b2	[58,61]
↑	ATPase, Ca^{2+} transporting, plasma membrane 3	Atp2b3	[58,59]
↓	Complement component 1q, beta polypeptide	C1qb	[59,61]
↓	Complement component 4a	C4a	[59,61]
↓	Calcitonin/calcitonin-related polypeptide, alpha	Calca	[61,63]
↓	Calcium/calmodulin-dependent protein kinase II, delta	Camk2d	[61,63]
↓	CD74 antigen (invariant polypeptide of MHC II)	Cd74	[59,61]
↑	CCAAT/enhancer binding protein (C/EBP), delta	Cebpd	[58,61]
↑	Cholinergic receptor, nicotinic, alpha polypeptide 3	Chrna3	[58,59]
↑	Cellular retinoic acid binding protein 2	Crabp2	[59,61]
↑	Cathepsin S	Ctss	[59,61]
↑	Chemokine (C-X-C motif) ligand 14	Cxcl14	[59,61]
↑	Dihydrofolate reductase	Dhfr	[59,61]
↑	Dihydropyrimidinase-like 4	Dpysl4	[59,61]
↓	Endothelin converting enzyme-like 1	Ecel1	[58,61]
↓	Early growth response 1	Egr1	[58,59]
↑	Fatty acid binding protein 3	Fabp3	[59,61]
↑	Fc receptor, IgG, low affinity III	Fcgr3	[59,61]
↑	Growth arrest specific 7	Gas7	[59,61]
↑	Guanylate nucleotide binding protein 2	Gbp2	[58,59]
↑	GTP cyclohydrolase 1	Gch	[59,61]

Table 2.2 (*Continued*)

↑/↓	Name	Gene symbol	References
↑	Glutamate receptor, ionotropic, kainate 1	Grik1	[59,61]
↑	Glutamate receptor, metabotropic 4	Grm4	[61,63]
↓	Glycogenin 1	Gyg1	[59,61]
↓	Major histocompatibility complex, class II, DM beta	Hla-dmb	[59,61]
↑	Heat shock 27 kDa protein 1	Hspb1	[61,63]
↑	5-hydroxytryptamine (serotonin) receptor 3a	Htr3a	[58,61]
↓	Similar to Cornifin A (Small proline-rich protein 1A)	LOC499660	[59,61]
↑	Lysozyme	Lyz	[59,61]
↑	Macrophage erythroblast attacher	Maea	[61,63]
↑	Macrophage galactose *N*-acetyl-galactosamine spec. lectin 1	Mgl1	[59,61]
↓	Neurofilament 3, medium	Nef3	[58,63]
↓	Neurofilament, heavy polypeptide	Nefh	[58,63]
↑	Neurofilament, light polypeptide	Nefl	[58,63]
↓	Neuritin	Nrn1	[58,59]
↑	PDZ and LIM domain 1 (elfin)	Pdlim1	[61,63]
↑	Phospholipase C, delta 4	Plcd4	[59,63]
↓	Parathyroid hormone-like peptide	Pthlh	[58,59]
↓	Protein tyrosine phosphatase 4a1	Ptp4a1	[61,63]
↑	Protein tyrosine phosphatase, receptor type, O	Ptpro	[59,61]
↓	Poliovirus receptor	PVR	[59,61]
↑	RAB3A, member RAS oncogene family	Rab3a	[59,63]
↑	Similar to Tescalcin (predicted)	RGD1566317	[59,61]
↑	Regulator of G-protein signaling 4	Rgs4	[59,61]
↓	RT1 class II, locus Bb	RT1-Bb	[59,63]
↑	Secretogranin 2	Scg2	[58,61]
↑	Sodium channel, voltage-gated, type I, alpha	Scn1a	[58,59]
↑	Secretin receptor	Sctr	[58,63]
↑	Serine (or cysteine) proteinase inhibitor, member 1	Serpina1	[61,63]
↑	Solute carrier family 1 member 3	Slc1a3	[58,61]
↓	Stathmin-like 4	Stmn4	[59,61]
↓	Transglutaminase 1	Tgm1	[59,61]
↑	Tetraspanin 8	Tspan8	[59,61]
↓	Tubulin, alpha 6	Tuba6	[58,61]
↑	UDP glycosyltransferase 1 family, polypeptide A6	Ugt1a6	[59,61]
↑	Vesicle-associated membrane protein 1	Vamp1	[59,63]

↑: upregulated, ↓: downregulated.

reflects a transition from a mature, information-transmitting state to a state of growth. During regenerative neurite outgrowth, the neuron has less need for these proteins. Three studies also report upregulation of cell cycle related transcripts [58–60], possibly reflecting proliferation of macrophages in the lesioned tissue [77]. Among the most interesting genes not previously found by low-throughput studies is Arginase 1, which plays a role in the biosynthesis of polyamines, which, in turn, promote regeneration [78]. In addition, Csrp3, also termed MLP, is a highly regulated gene encoding a protein that shuttles from the cytoskeleton to the nucleus

Table 2.3 Gene ontology clusters (biological process level 6 [68])
present in combined data of four large-scale gene expression
studies of rat peripheral nerve regeneration.

Gene ontology cluster	Regulated genes within cluster (gene symbols)	Count
Cellular protein metabolism	Adam17↑ Anxa1↑ Apobec1↑ Btg1↑ C1qb↑ C1r↑ C1s↑ Ccnd1↑ Cd74↑ Cdc2a↑ Clk3↓ Col2a1↓ Dnajb9↑ Dpp6↓ Dusp6↓ Ece1↓ Ecel1↑ Eef2↑ Eif4ebp1↑ Fcgr3↑ Fgf2↑ Gas7↑ Gria2↓ Gzmb↑ Gzmm↓ Hla-dmb↑ Hspa1a↑ Hspb1↑ Inha↓ Kit↓ Limk1↓ Mcpt8↓ Nfkb1↑ Nrg1↓ Ntrk1↓ Pja2↓ Prkg2↓ Ptp4a1↑ Ptpro↑ Rapgef4↓ Ripk3↑ Rpl36a↑ Rpl5↑ Rpl7↑ RT1-Aw2↓ S100a9↑ Serping1↑ Tfrc↓ Tgm1↑ Timp1↑ Tuba6↑ Tubb5↑ Ube2g1↓ Ugt1a6↑	54
Apoptosis	Adam17↑ Bcap31↓ Bcl2l1↑ Bok↑ Btg1↑ Cck↑ Cd74↑ Cdc2a↑ Dnajb9↑ Fcgr3↑ Fgf2↑ Gal↑ Hspb1↑ Igfbp3↓ Inha↓ Litaf↑ Mgmt↓ Ngfr↓ Ntf3↓ RGD1311350↓ Ripk3↑ Serinc3↓ Tegt↑	23
Biopolymer modification	Anxa1↑ Apobec1↑ Btg1↑ Ccnd1↑ Cdc2a↑ Clk3↓ Dusp6↓ Ece1↓ Fgf2↑ Kit↓ Limk1↓ Ntrk1↓ Pja2↓ Prkg2↓ Ptp4a1↑ Ptpro↑ Rapgef4↓ Ripk3↑ RT1-Aw2↓ Tgm1↑ Ube2g1↓ Ugt1a6↑	22
G-PCR signaling pathway	Adra2c↓ Arl3↓ Calca↓ Cckbr↑ Cxcr4↓ Dgkz↓ Ecel1↑ Entpd2↑ Gabbr2↓ Gal↑ Gnao↓ Gpr176↓ Lgr4↓ Npy↑ Npy5r↑ Nsg1↑ Oprm1↓ P2ry1↑ Pthlh↑ Tac1↓ Tegt↑	21
Transcription	Ankrd1↑ Apobec1↑ Atf3↑ Btg1↑ Crem↑ Egr1↑ Fgf2↑ Hmgb2↑ Jun↑ Kcnh2↓ Kcnh6↓ Litaf↑ Mcm6↑ Myt1l↓ Nfkb1↑ Ntf3↓ Pdlim1↑ Prrxl1↓ Pura_predicted↓ Rere↓ Sox11↑	20
Neurogenesis	C1s↑ Cck↑ Cxcr4↓ Dpysl4↓ Fgf2↑ Gap-43↑ Limk1↓ Mcm6↑ Ngfr↓ Nog↓ Nrg1↓ Ntf3↓ Prrxl1↓ Pura_predicted↓ Thbs4↑ Vgf↑	16
Synaptic transmission	Cabp1↓ Fcgr3↑ Fgf2↑ Gria2↓ Grik1↓ Lin7b↓ Npy↑ Npy5r↑ Nrg1↓ Ntf3↓ Sv2b↓ Syn2↓ Syt4↑ Tac1↓	14
Phosphate metabolism	Ccnd1↑ Cdc2a↑ Clk3↓ Dusp6↓ Fgf2↑ Inha↓ Kit↓ Limk1↓ Ntrk1↓ Prkg2↓ Ptp4a1↑ Ptpro↑ Rapgef4↓ Ripk3↑	14
Cellular lipid metabolism	Acox1↑ Cd36↑ Cd74↑ Cpt1a↓ Ech1↓ Fgf2↓ Idi1↓ Ldlr↑ Nudt4↓ Oprs1↑ Pctp↓ Rbp1↓ Serinc3↓ Timp1↑	14
Intracellular transport	Bcap31↓ Cd74↑ Fgf2↑ Fgf9↓ Lin7b↓ Nudt4↓ Nupl1↓ Rhoc_predicted↑ RT1-Bb↓ Trappc3↑ Tuba6↑ Tubb5↑ Vamp1↓	13
Cation transport	Cacna2d1↑ Kcna4↓ Kcnab1↓ Kcnh2↓ Kcnh6↓ Kcnj4↓ Kcns1↓ Kcns3↓ Scn10a↓ Scn11a↑ Scn2b↑ Slc24a2↓ Trpv1↓	13

Table 2.3 (Continued)

Gene ontology cluster	Regulated genes within cluster (gene symbols)	Count
Inflammatory response	A2m↑ C1qb↑ C1s↑ Calca↓ Fcgr2b↑ Fcgr3↑ Gal↑ Pap↑ Reg3a↑ Scg2↓ Serping1↑ Tac1↓	12
Cytoskeleton organization and biogenesis	Aif1↑ Dbn1↑ Gas7↑ Nef3↓ Nefh↓ Nefl↓ Racgap1_predicted↓ Rhoc_predicted↑ S100a9↑ Tuba6↑ Tubb5↑	11
Regulation of progression through cell cycle	Apc↑ Bin1↑ Ccnb1↑ Ccnd1↑ Ccnd2↑ Cdc2a↑ Fgf2↑ Fgf9↑ Gadd45a↑ Inha↓ Jun↑	11
Carboxylic acid metabolism	Acox1↑ Arg1↑ Ass↓ Atf3↑ Bcat1↑ Cd36↑ Cd74↑ Cpt1a↓ Ech1↓ Fgf2↑ Mthfd1↓	11
Generation of neurons	Cck↑ Cxcr4↓ Dpysl4↓ Limk1↓ Ngfr↓ Nog↓ Ntf3↓ Prrxl1↓ Racgap1_predicted↓ Thbs4↑ Vgf↑	11
Macromolecule biosynthesis	Atf3↑ Eef2↑ Eif4ebp1↑ Fcgr3↑ Gyg1↓ Inha↓ Nfkb1↑ Rpl36a↑ Rpl5↑ S100a9↑	11

↑: upregulated, ↓: downregulated.

in overstretched muscle cells. Csrp3 is thought to induce gene expression changes necessary to meet an increased mechanical demand upon the myocyte cytoskeleton [79]. Its upregulation in regenerating neurons may reflect a common need for increased cytoskeletal protein production in both cases.

2.4.2
Biological Processes Affected by Peripheral Nerve Injury

The large number of regulated genes found by each study and the range of gene functions found within the data sets indicate that a wide range of cellular processes is activated during successful regeneration. We have analyzed the gene ontology (GO) clusters present in the combined data sets of these studies to gain insight into the biological processes that are activated after injury. These combined data sets represent 625 messengers, of which 138 do not represent a Unigene cluster at present. The remaining messengers map to 325 unique gene clusters. Genes may belong to more than one GO cluster. GO clusters with more than 10 members are listed, and clusters with more than 80% overlap were merged. Several of these GO clusters relate to processes already known to be important during regeneration, although in many cases the genes identified are largely novel RAGs. For example, the largest cluster to emerge is "cellular protein metabolism." In this cluster, many genes are involved in immunological responses (MHC-associated proteins and complement factors, all upregulated). In addition, a number of upregulated genes involved in translation are present within this cluster. This, along with the appearance of the cluster "macromolecule biosynthesis," probably reflects the requirement to produce large quantities of growth-related proteins. The second largest cluster consists of apoptosis-related genes. Of these 22 genes, 9 are known as positive regulators of apoptosis, while 7 are known as negative regulators. Of the former group, five are downregulated and four are upregulated, whereas in the latter group all genes are upregulated. This is a strong indication that the prevention of apoptosis is a regeneration-associated process in DRG neurons. This is most likely necessary to counter the common and well-established tendency for axotomy to induce neuronal apoptosis. The cluster "cytoskeleton organization and biogenesis" is likewise not an unexpected finding, although the members listed are all novel RAGs. The class of "G protein coupled receptor protein signaling pathway" includes the previously discussed neuropeptides and their receptors. Three transcription-related gene ontology clusters were combined in the cluster "transcription." Several known regeneration-associated transcription factors are present in this class, such as ATF3 and c-Jun. Potentially, novel regulators of the transcriptional response to injury may be present in this class. For example, Ankyrin domain repeat protein, Elfin, and Early growth response 1 are each found by multiple studies and have not previously been studied in neurite outgrowth assays.

The appearance of the gene ontologies "neurogenesis" and "generation of neurons" are particularly intriguing, as this lends support to the idea that injured neurons dedifferentiate to enter a state of growth, and that developmentally regulated proteins may play a role in this process. The combined data sets show 14 genes involved in phosphate metabolism, which encode, for the largest part, kinases and phosphatases. The regulated genes within this cluster may be involved in signaling processes during neurite outgrowth or target recognition and may therefore represent interesting novel players in the regenerative process. Several genes present in the lipid metabolism class are involved in synthesis or binding of steroids and could therefore be involved in injury- or regeneration-associated signaling. Three enzymes involved in mitochondrial fatty acid oxidation are regulated (Cpt1a, Ech1, and Acox1), indicating a differential energy demand upon injury.

2.4.3
Identification of Novel Regeneration-Associated Genes by Microarray Analysis

Microarray studies contributed substantially in revealing genes that are potentially important for growth enhancement. To date, two studies have combined the acquisition of large-scale gene expression data with functional characterization of promising novel targets. These studies have identified Sprr1a and Fn14 as enhancers of neurite outgrowth in primary culture and PC12 cells, respectively [57,64]. Many other genes indicated by gene expression analysis await functional studies to reveal their contribution to the regeneration process.

The relatively low number of novel RAGs that, to date, have been shown to enhance regeneration or neurite outgrowth could reflect the fact that nerve regeneration is a complex process organized by a large number of proteins interacting with each other. Increasing expression of a single gene, for instance, will not necessarily lead to enhanced neurite outgrowth. This is illustrated by the effect of GAP-43 overexpression. Regeneration improves after SN crush and rhizotomy [80], although long distance axon regeneration does not occur in the CNS of these mice [81]. Interestingly, overexpression of both GAP-43 and a second growth-associated protein, CAP-23, in double transgenics leads to a significantly stronger regenerative response, which partially mimics the effect of the conditioning lesion on the regeneration of the central DRG neurites [56], indicating that these proteins act synergistically and that both are needed to obtain a regenerative response. A second factor complicating the identification of novel regeneration-enhancing proteins from large-scale gene expression profiling efforts is the fact that follow-up experiments that establish a role in neurite outgrowth are very time consuming. New methodology, which will allow for high-throughput functional screening, is required to link newly discovered genes to the neurite outgrowth process.

2.5
Developing New Insights into the Molecular Biology of Regenerative Neurite Outgrowth: From Single Gene to Genetic Networks

In the preceding paragraphs, an overview of the most important molecular changes induced by nerve injury has been presented. Of these changes, no single gene has been found that is essential for regeneration. In addition, the multitude of genes found to be regulated by neuronal injury paradigms illustrate that the regenerative process is not controlled by a single gene or a small set of genes. It is likely that a transcriptional regulatory network is activated by neuronal injury that governs a complex cascade of gene expression changes necessary for the sequential stages of neurite outgrowth and reestablishment of functional contacts. Investigation of this hypothesis and elucidation of the properties of the network requires genome-wide analysis of the transcriptome and/or proteome at multiple time points after nerve injury, in combination with analysis of promoter regions of regulated genes and identification of target genes of TFs that are activated by nerve injury. The latter two analyses have not been performed to date.

2.5.1
Strategies to Enhance the Revenue of Profiling Regenerating Neurons

The gene expression analyses described in this chapter appoint a number of genes as targets for functional studies, but they do not provide insights into the genetic network underlying regeneration. Single snapshots of the highly complex biological process of regeneration do not allow association of genes with a particular stage of the outgrowth process. To this end, expression analysis of either proteins or transcripts should be genome-wide and conducted in a high-resolution time course. In addition, the biological interpretation of gene expression data is facilitated to a great extent if multiple, related processes are analyzed [82]. In this respect, the DRG neuron offers the unique opportunity to compare gene expression changes during a robust outgrowth response (sciatic nerve crush) and a weak outgrowth response (dorsal root crush). This comparison holds the advantage that the tissue samples that will be analyzed are very similar to each other, the only biological difference being the localization of the injury inflicted to the neurons. Also, stress- and injury-related

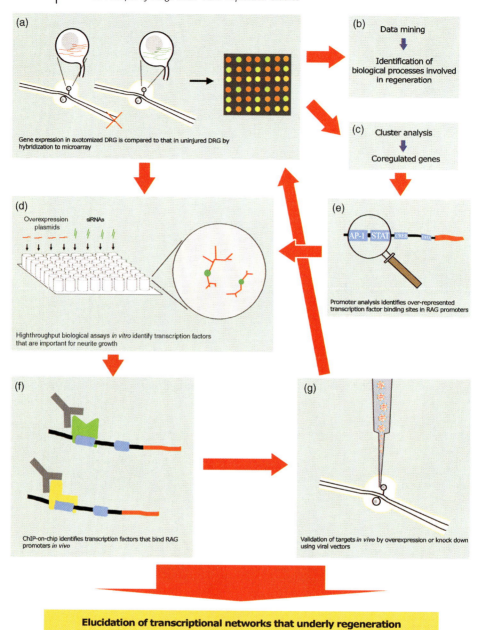

Elucidation of transcriptional networks that underly regeneration

Figure 2.2 (legend see p. 49)

gene expression changes could be similar in both paradigms. If genes that are regulated in a similar fashion by both stress and injuries are excluded from further analysis, true regeneration-associated genes may be enriched. Therefore, a high-resolution time course analysis of gene expression changes after DR and SN crush will increase our understanding of the molecular aspects of successful regeneration.

2.5.2
Open Screening for Regeneration-Associated Changes in the Transcriptome and (Phospho)Proteome

It is not likely that microarray analysis will identify the first signals leading to initiation of the regenerative response. This injury-induced "master switch" will probably involve posttranslational modification of proteins present at the lesion site and subsequent transport to the nucleus. In this respect, high-throughput (phospho)proteomics analysis of injured neurons can generate valuable data. Recent advances have been made using proteomics approaches [83–85]. Further work will be greatly accelerated by optimization of protein-labeling techniques such as iTRAQ and subsequent high-throughput tandem mass spectrometry for small samples [86]. The combination of these techniques is likely to identify many additional target genes (Figure 2.2a).

Figure 2.2 Unraveling transcriptional control of the regeneration program. Among the most interesting targets are transcription factors that may regulate the regeneration-associated gene expression program. These may be identified and studied in ways outlined in the flow diagram: (a) Open screening for changes in mRNA levels, protein levels or the phosphorylation states of proteins will identify regeneration-associated genes. In this example, RNA is extracted from axotomized and uninjured DRG neurons. The RNA is reverse transcribed and labeled with Cy3 (green) or Cy5 (red). Competitive hybridization to a microarray reveals gene expression differences between the two samples. (b and c) Analysis of the regulated genes by gene ontology class reveals what cellular processes are affected by axotomy, while cluster analysis reveals groups of genes with similar expression profiles over time. These genes may therefore be regulated by similar mechanisms. (d) High-throughput screening. To avoid biased selection of targets for validation, high-throughput screening is necessary. Overexpression plasmids or siRNAs can be transfected into neuron-like cell lines in a 96-well plate format. This is followed by automated image capture, analysis, and neurite growth quantification. (e and f) Promoter analysis by *in silico* and ChIP-on-chip approaches. The promoters of the many genes that are regulated during regeneration are studied to find out which transcription factors control their expression. Promoter analysis reveals transcription factor binding motifs that are over-represented in the regulated genes. Using ChIP-on-chip, DNA fragments that are actually bound by specific TFs are immunoprecipitated; these fragments are then hybridized to a promoter array to identify them. (g) After the most promising targets have been identified, they need to be validated *in vivo*. Viral vector mediated delivery of overexpression cassettes or short hairpin RNAs to knock down expression can be combined with sciatic nerve injury or dorsal root injury models to study the roles of these targets *in vivo*. When transcription factor expression has been perturbed, gene expression profiling can be applied again to study the effects on expression of down stream genes.

2.5.3
High-Throughput Screening for the Function of Target Genes

The development of high-throughput gene and protein expression technologies in the past decade has created vast opportunities for exploratory research. The unbiased nature of these experiments enables discoveries leading to novel insights and new hypotheses. However, testing these hypotheses is a challenging task for cell biologists as the data derived from gene expression analyses in a wide range of cell types, organisms, and treatments accumulate. Conventional cell biological techniques are aimed at studying the function of one or a few proteins in detail, which might take years. For practical reasons, therefore, gene expression profiling is often followed by a reduction of the "genes of interest" to a feasible number. However, this trimming down compromises the unprejudiced nature of large-scale screening techniques as the selection is usually guided by data available in the literature or in databases based on literature such as gene ontology [68] and KEGG [87] (Figure 2.2b). To fully exploit the power of exploratory research, an a priori gene selection should be avoided. To achieve this, a high-throughput semi-automated approach to biological assays should be taken.

Recent developments have enabled automated analysis of biological images. Analysis of variables such as axonal outgrowth in live cells can now be performed in 96-well format. In combination with the generation of species-specific genome-wide RNAi libraries, these advances enable assessment of the effect of hundreds of gene products on a parameter of interest. Application of these techniques is, after transcriptome and proteome analysis, the second step toward elucidation of the transcriptional regulatory network underlying regeneration (Figure 2.2d).

2.5.4
Finding Target Genes of Regeneration-Associated Transcription Factors

The combined efforts of assessing altered transcription, translation, transport, or phosphorylation of transcription factors and subsequent high-throughput functional screening of their effect on neurite outgrowth will result in a set of possible regulators of the regenerative response. As a next step, their target genes could be identified by ChIP-on-chip techniques (Figure 2.2f). ChIP-on-chip combines chromatin-immunoprecipitation with DNA-chip analysis. For these experiments, a (tagged) transcription factor and the stretches of DNA it is bound to are coprecipitated. The DNA is subsequently amplified, labeled, and hybridized to an array with genomic DNA sequences [88,89]. In *Saccharomyces cerevisiae*, this technique was applied to a high number of transcription factors in the genome, generating a wealth of information on possible interactions between TFs and target genes [90]. However, protein–DNA interactions are dynamic in nature and depend on the biological processes that are active in a particular situation. In addition, the accessibility of promoter regions for TFs is highly dependent on the chromatin structure, which is altered by acetylation and methylation of histones and methylation of DNA [91,92]. In the most recent studies, transcription factor binding analyses are performed in mammalian cells under conditions relevant to the biological question of interest [93,94]. A second, complementary approach is to perturb the expression of given TFs in regenerating neurons and study the changes in the gene expression profile that occur as a result (Figure 2.2g). It is expected that this would give significant insight into which genes are regulated by each TF and what sort of cellular processes are influenced. Application of these techniques to regeneration-associated transcription factors in the context of growing neurons will further extend our understanding of how successful regeneration is achieved in the PNS.

2.5.5
In Silico Approaches to Transcriptional Regulatory Network Elucidation

In the last paragraphs, we approached the task of elucidating the transcriptional regulatory network by first identifying regeneration-associated transcription factors and subsequently their target genes. Possibilities for the reverse approach are increasing with the progression of the genome-sequencing efforts and expanding knowledge regarding transcription factor binding sites. The underlying assumption is that coregulated genes, as identified by microarray analysis (Figure 2.2c), are likely to be controlled by the same combination of transcription factors. Therefore, the upstream sequences of coregulated genes should be enriched for particular transcription factor binding sites (Figure 2.2e). Several studies have shown that this *in silico* approach has predictive value in *S. cerevisiae* [95–97]. However, as transcription factor binding sites are often short and degenerate, the use of sequence information alone does not lead to a high sensitivity and specificity. In addition, *cis*-regulatory sequences in metazoan genomes can be several kilobases remote from the transcription start site, and this approach is therefore not sufficient to extract meaningful information from eukaryotic species other than yeast. Assuming that *cis*-regulatory motifs are more likely to be conserved between related species than other noncoding DNA sequences, the progression of the genome-sequencing projects has generated new opportunities for the *in silico* approach to regulatory network elucidation. Comparative genomics was used to identify regulatory motifs in both yeast [98,99] and vertebrate eukaryotes [100,101]. Identifying orthologous regulatory stretches of DNA in different genomes is, however, not a trivial task. Moreover, the discovery of *cis*-regulatory motifs does not automatically lead to identification of transcription factors that bind to them. In summary, predicting regulatory modules from the combination of mRNA expression data and genome sequences remains a challenge. The rapid development of novel algorithms that integrate mRNA quantitation data, sequence information, and ChIP-on-chip data holds promising perspectives for this field of research (for reviews, see [102,103]).

2.5.6
From Transcriptional Regulatory Network to Regeneration

Strategies to promote regeneration after CNS lesions include attempts to modify the growth-inhibitory environment of the CNS, to neutralize axon repellent properties of the neuronal scar [104,105], and to enhance the intrinsic regenerative capacity of the injured neuron by the use of viral vectors or mutant mice [56,106]. So far, these findings have not yet resulted in effective therapies for CNS injury. The effectiveness of such strategies will increase if target genes are selected on the basis of their ability to play a regulatory role in the regenerative process and their involvement in the early stages of the process. Elucidation of the transcriptional regulatory network underlying successful regeneration by means of genome- or proteome-wide time course gene expression profiling, followed by high-throughput functional assays and ChIP studies of candidate regeneration-associated transcription factors, is an important next step in spinal cord injury research.

Acknowledgments

The work in the laboratory of Joost Verhaagen was supported by grants from SenterNovem, the Prinses Beatrix Fund, the International Paraplegia Foundation (Geneva, Swiss), and the International Spinal Research Trust (London, UK). Work in the laboratory of August Smit was supported by grants from SenterNovem and the Center for Medical Systems Biology (CMSB).

References

1 McQuarrie, I.G. (1985) Effect of conditioning lesion on axonal sprout formation at nodes of Ranvier. *The Journal of Comparative Neurology*, **231**, 239–249.

2 Friede, R.L. and Bischhausen, R. (1980) The fine structure of stumps of transected nerve fibers in subserial sections. *Journal of the Neurological Sciences*, **44**, 181–203.

3 Fawcett, J.W. and Keynes, R.J. (1990) Peripheral nerve regeneration. *Annual Review of Neuroscience*, **13**, 43–60.

4 Ide, C. (1996) Peripheral nerve regeneration. *Neuroscience Research*, **25**, 101–121.

5 Pan, Y.A., Misgeld, T., Lichtman, J.W. and Sanes, J.R. (2003) Effects of neurotoxic and neuroprotective agents on peripheral nerve regeneration assayed by time-lapse imaging *in vivo*. *Journal of Neuroscience*, **23**, 11479–11488.

6 Wujek, J.R. and Lasek, R.J. (1983) Correlation of axonal regeneration and slow component B in two branches of a single axon. *Journal of Neuroscience*, **3**, 243–251.

7 Nguyen, Q.T., Sanes, J.R. and Lichtman, J.W. (2002) Pre-existing pathways promote precise projection patterns. *Nature Neuroscience*, **5**, 861–867.

8 Nurse, C.A., Macintyre, L. and Diamond, J. (1984) Reinnervation of the rat touch dome restores the Merkel cell population reduced after denervation. *Neuroscience*, **13**, 563–571.

9 Zelena, J. (1984) Multiple axon terminals in reinnervated Pacinian corpuscles of adult rat. *Journal of Neurocytology*, **13**, 665–684.

10 Barker, D., Scott, J.J. and Stacey, M.J. (1985) Sensory reinnervation of cat peroneus brevis muscle spindles after nerve crush. *Brain Research*, **333**, 131–138.

11 Rich, M.M. and Lichtman, J.W. (1989) *in vivo* visualization of pre- and postsynaptic changes during synapse

elimination in reinnervated mouse muscle. *Journal of Neuroscience*, **9**, 1781–1805.

12 Sunderland, S. (1978) *Nerve and Nerve Injuries*, Churchill Livingstone, London.

13 Komiya, Y. (1981) Axonal regeneration in bifurcating axons of rat dorsal root ganglion cells. *Experimental Neurology*, **73**, 824–826.

14 Oblinger, M.M. and Lasek, R.J. (1984) A conditioning lesion of the peripheral axons of dorsal root ganglion cells accelerates regeneration of only their peripheral axons. *Journal of Neuroscience*, **4**, 1736–1744.

15 Richardson, P.M. and Verge, V.M. (1987) Axonal regeneration in dorsal spinal roots is accelerated by peripheral axonal transection. *Brain Research*, **411**, 406–408.

16 Chong, M.S., Woolf, C.J., Turmaine, M., Emson, P.C. and Anderson, P.N. (1996) Intrinsic versus extrinsic factors in determining the regeneration of the central processes of rat dorsal root ganglion neurons: the influence of a peripheral nerve graft. *The Journal of Comparative Neurology*, **370**, 97–104.

17 Fun, W., Costigan, M., Fawcett, J. and Woolf, C.J. (2005) The expression profile of dorsal root Schwann cells is different from that in sciatic nerve. *Society for Neuroscience*, Program no. 439.11, Washington, DC.

18 Avellino, A.M., Hart, D., Dailey, A.T., MacKinnon, M., Ellegala, D. and Kliot, M. (1995) Differential macrophage responses in the peripheral and central nervous system during Wallerian degeneration of axons. *Experimental Neurology*, **136**, 183–198.

19 Chong, M.S., Reynolds, M.L., Irwin, N., Coggeshall, R.E., Emson, P.C., Benowitz, L.I. and Woolf, C.J. (1994) GAP-43 expression in primary sensory neurons following central axotomy. *Journal of Neuroscience*, **14**, 4375–4384.

20 Zhang, Y., Roslan, R., Lang, D., Schachner, M., Lieberman, A.R. and Anderson, P.N. (2000) Expression of CHL1 and L1 by neurons and glia following sciatic nerve and dorsal root injury. *Molecular and Cellular Neurosciences*, **16**, 71–86.

21 Zhang, Y., Tohyama, K., Winterbottom, J.K., Haque, N.S., Schachner, M., Lieberman, A.R. and Anderson, P.N. (2001) Correlation between putative inhibitory molecules at the dorsal root entry zone and failure of dorsal root axonal regeneration. *Molecular and Cellular Neurosciences*, **17**, 444–459.

22 Hunt, D., Hossain-Ibrahim, K., Mason, M.R., Coffin, R.S., Lieberman, A.R., Winterbottom, J. and Anderson, P.N. (2004) ATF3 upregulation in glia during Wallerian degeneration: differential expression in peripheral nerves and CNS white matter. *BMC Neuroscience*, **5**, 9.

23 Richardson, P.M. and Issa, V.M. (1984) Peripheral injury enhances central regeneration of primary sensory neurones. *Nature*, **309**, 791–793.

24 Han, P.J., Shukla, S., Subramanian, P.S. and Hoffman, P.N. (2004) Cyclic AMP elevates tubulin expression without increasing intrinsic axon growth capacity. *Experimental Neurology*, **189**, 293–302.

25 Chong, M.S., Woolf, C.J., Haque, N.S. and Anderson, P.N. (1999) Axonal regeneration from injured dorsal roots into the spinal cord of adult rats. *The Journal of Comparative Neurology*, **410**, 42–54.

26 Neumann, S. and Woolf, C.J. (1999) Regeneration of dorsal column fibers into and beyond the lesion site following adult spinal cord injury. *Neuron*, **23**, 83–91.

27 Wong, J. and Oblinger, M.M. (1991) NGF rescues substance P expression but not neurofilament or tubulin gene expression in axotomized sensory neurons. *Journal of Neuroscience*, **11**, 543–552.

28 Ji, R.R., Zhang, Q., Pettersson, R.F. and Hokfelt, T. (1996) aFGF bFGF and NGF

differentially regulate neuropeptide expression in dorsal root ganglia after axotomy and induce autotomy. *Regulatory Peptides*, **66**, 179–189.

29 Shadiack, A.M., Sun, Y. and Zigmond, R.E. (2001) Nerve growth factor antiserum induces axotomy-like changes in neuropeptide expression in intact sympathetic and sensory neurons. *Journal of Neuroscience*, **21**, 363–371.

30 Hanz, S. and Fainzilber, M. (2006) Retrograde signaling in injured nerve – the axon reaction revisited. *Journal of Neurochemistry*, **99**, 13–19.

31 Schwaiger, F.W., Hager, G., Schmitt, A.B., Horvat, A., Streif, R., Spitzer, C., Gamal, S., Breuer, S., Brook, G.A., Nacimiento, W. and Kreutzberg, G.W. (2000) Peripheral but not central axotomy induces changes in Janus kinases (JAK) and signal transducers and activators of transcription (STAT). *The European Journal of Neuroscience*, **12**, 1165–1176.

32 Lee, N., Neitzel, K.L., Devlin, B.K. and MacLennan, A.J. (2004) STAT3 phosphorylation in injured axons before sensory and motor neuron nuclei: potential role for STAT3 as a retrograde signaling transcription factor. *The Journal of Comparative Neurology*, **474**, 535–545.

33 Qiu, J., Cafferty, W.B., McMahon, S.B. and Thompson, S.W. (2005) Conditioning injury-induced spinal axon regeneration requires signal transducer and activator of transcription 3 activation. *Journal of Neuroscience*, **25**, 1645–1653.

34 Lindwall, C. and Kanje, M. (2005) Retrograde axonal transport of JNK signaling molecules influence injury induced nuclear changes in p-c-Jun and ATF3 in adult rat sensory neurons. *Molecular and Cellular Neurosciences*, **29**, 269–282.

35 Hanz, S., Perlson, E., Willis, D., Zheng, J.Q., Massarwa, R., Huerta, J.J., Koltzenburg, M., Kohler, M., van-

Minnen, J., Twiss, J.L. and Fainzilber, M. (2003) Axoplasmic importins enable retrograde injury signaling in lesioned nerve. *Neuron*, **40**, 1095–1104.

36 Neumann, S., Bradke, F., Tessier-Lavigne, M. and Basbaum, A.I. (2002) Regeneration of sensory axons within the injured spinal cord induced by intraganglionic cAMP elevation. *Neuron*, **34**, 885–893.

37 Qiu, J., Cai, D., Dai, H., McAtee, M., Hoffman, P.N., Bregman, B.S. and Filbin, M.T. (2002) Spinal axon regeneration induced by elevation of cyclic AMP. *Neuron*, **34**, 895–903.

38 Andersen, P.L., Webber, C.A., Kimura, K.A. and Schreyer, D.J. (2000) Cyclic AMP prevents an increase in GAP-43 but promotes neurite growth in cultured adult rat dorsal root ganglion neurons. *Experimental Neurology*, **166**, 153–165.

39 Skene, J.H. and Willard, M. (1981) Changes in axonally transported proteins during axon regeneration in toad retinal ganglion cells. *The Journal of Cell Biology*, **89**, 86–95.

40 Oblinger, M.M. and Lasek, R.J. (1988) Axotomy-induced alterations in the synthesis and transport of neuro-filaments and microtubules in dorsal root ganglion cells. *Journal of Neuroscience*, **8**, 1747–1758.

41 Woodhams, P.L., Calvert, R. and Dunnett, S.B. (1989) Monoclonal antibody G10 against microtubule-associated protein 1× distinguishes between growing and regenerating axons. *Neuroscience*, **28**, 49–59.

42 Moskowitz, P.F. and Oblinger, M.M. (1995) Sensory neurons selectively upregulate synthesis and transport of the beta III-tubulin protein during axonal regeneration. *Journal of Neuroscience*, **15**, 1545–1555.

43 Ma, D., Connors, T., Nothias, F. and Fischer, I. (2000) Regulation of the expression and phosphorylation of microtubule-associated protein 1B during regeneration of adult dorsal root ganglion neurons. *Neuroscience*, **99**, 157–170.

44 Villar, M.J., Wiesenfeld-Hallin, Z., Xu, X.J., Theodorsson, E., Emson, P.C. and Hokfelt, T. (1991) Further studies on galanin-, substance P-, and CGRP-like immunoreactivities in primary sensory neurons and spinal cord: effects of dorsal rhizotomies and sciatic nerve lesions. *Experimental Neurology*, **112**, 29–39.

45 Wakisaka, S., Kajander, K.C. and Bennett, G.J. (1991) Increased neuropeptide Y (NPY)-like immuno-reactivity in rat sensory neurons following peripheral axotomy. *Neuroscience Letters*, **124**, 200–203.

46 Werner, A., Willem, M., Jones, L.L., Kreutzberg, G.W., Mayer, U. and Raivich, G. (2000) Impaired axonal regeneration in alpha7 integrin-deficient mice. *Journal of Neuroscience*, **20**, 1822–1830.

47 Vogelezang, M.G., Liu, Z., Relvas, J.B., Raivich, G., Scherer, S.S. and ffrench-Constant, C. (2001) Alpha4 integrin is expressed during peripheral nerve regeneration and enhances neurite outgrowth. *Journal of Neuroscience*, **21**, 6732–6744.

48 Wallquist, W., Zelano, J., Plantman, S., Kaufman, S.J., Cullheim, S. and Hammarberg, H. (2004) Dorsal root ganglion neurons up-regulate the expression of laminin-associated integrins after peripheral but not central axotomy. *The Journal of Comparative Neurology*, **480**, 162–169.

49 Jenkins, R. and Hunt, S.P. (1991) Long-term increase in the levels of c-jun mRNA and jun protein-like immuno-reactivity in motor and sensory neurons following axon damage. *Neuroscience Letters*, **129**, 107–110.

50 Kenney, A.M. and Kocsis, J.D. (1997) Temporal variability of jun family transcription factor levels in peripherally or centrally transected adult rat dorsal

root ganglia. *Brain Research. Molecular Brain Research*, **52**, 53–61.

51 Raivich, G., Bohatschek, M., Da Costa, C., Iwata, O., Galiano, M., Hristova, M., Nateri, A.S., Makwana, M., Riera-Sans, L., Wolfer, D.P., Lipp, H.P., Aguzzi, A., Wagner, E.F. and Behrens, A. (2004) The AP-1 transcription factor c-Jun is required for efficient axonal regeneration. *Neuron*, **43**, 57–67.

52 Tsujino, H., Kondo, E., Fukuoka, T., Dai, Y., Tokunaga, A., Miki, K., Yonenobu, K., Ochi, T. and Noguchi, K. (2000) Activating transcription factor 3 (ATF3) induction by axotomy in sensory and motoneurons: a novel neuronal marker of nerve injury. *Molecular and Cellular Neurosciences*, **15**, 170–182.

53 Seijffers, R., Allchorne, A.J. and Woolf, C.J. (2006) The transcription factor ATF-3 promotes neurite outgrowth. *Molecular and Cellular Neurosciences*, **32**, 143–154.

54 Vogelaar, C.F., Hoekman, M.F., Gispen, W.H. and Burbach, J.P. (2003) Homeobox gene expression in adult dorsal root ganglia during sciatic nerve regeneration: is regeneration a recapitulation of development? *European Journal of Pharmacology*, **480**, 233–250.

55 Jenkins, R., McMahon, S.B., Bond, A.B. and Hunt, S.P. (1993) Expression of c-Jun as a response to dorsal root and peripheral nerve section in damaged and adjacent intact primary sensory neurons in the rat. *The European Journal of Neuroscience*, **5**, 751–759.

56 Bomze, H.M., Bulsara, K.R., Iskandar, B.J., Caroni, P. and Skene, J.H. (2001) Spinal axon regeneration evoked by replacing two growth cone proteins in adult neurons. *Nature Neuroscience*, **4**, 38–43.

57 Bonilla, I.E., Tanabe, K. and Strittmatter, S.M. (2002) Small proline-rich repeat protein 1A is expressed by axotomized neurons and promotes axonal outgrowth. *Journal of Neuroscience*, **22**, 1303–1315.

58 Boeshore, K.L., Schreiber, R.C., Vaccariello, S.A., Sachs, H.H., Salazar,

R., Lee, J., Ratan, R.R., Leahy, P. and Zigmond, R.E. (2004) Novel changes in gene expression following axotomy of a sympathetic ganglion: a microarray analysis. *Journal of Neurobiology*, **59**, 216–235.

59 Wang, H., Sun, H., Della Penna, K., Benz, R.J., Xu, J., Gerhold, D.L., Holder, D.J. and Koblan, K.S. (2002) Chronic neuropathic pain is accompanied by global changes in gene expression and shares pathobiology with neurodegenerative diseases. *Neuroscience*, **114**, 529–546.

60 Cameron, A.A., Vansant, G., Wu, W., Carlo, D.J. and Ill, C.R. (2003) Identification of reciprocally regulated gene modules in regenerating dorsal root ganglion neurons and activated peripheral or central nervous system glia. *Journal of Cellular Biochemistry*, **88**, 970–985.

61 Costigan, M., Befort, K., Karchewski, L., Griffin, R.S., D'Urso, D., Allchorne, A., Sitarski, J., Mannion, J.W., Pratt, R.E. and Woolf, C.J. (2002) Replicate high-density rat genome oligonucleotide microarrays reveal hundreds of regulated genes in the dorsal root ganglion after peripheral nerve injury. *BMC Neuroscience*, **3**, 16.

62 Schmitt, A.B., Breuer, S., Liman, J., Buss, A., Schlangen, C., Pech, K., Hol, E.M., Brook, G.A., Noth, J. and Schwaiger, F.W. (2003) Identification of regeneration-associated genes after central and peripheral nerve injury in the adult rat. *BMC Neuroscience*, **4**, 8.

63 Xiao, H.S., Huang, Q.H., Zhang, F.X., Bao, L., Lu, Y.J., Guo, C., Yang, L., Huang, W.J., Fu, G., Xu, S.H., Cheng, X.P., Yan, Q., Zhu, Z.D., Zhang, X., Chen, Z. and Han, Z.G. (2002) Identification of gene expression profile of dorsal root ganglion in the rat peripheral axotomy model of neuropathic pain. *Proceedings of the National Academy of Sciences of the United States of America*, **99**, 8360–8365.

64 Tanabe, K., Bonilla, I., Winkles, J.A. and Strittmatter, S.M. (2003) Fibroblast growth factor-inducible-14 is induced in axotomized neurons and promotes neurite outgrowth. *Journal of Neuroscience*, **23**, 9675–9686.

65 Fan, M., Mi, R., Yew, D.T. and Chan, W.Y. (2001) Analysis of gene expression following sciatic nerve crush and spinal cord hemisection in the mouse by microarray expression profiling. *Cellular and Molecular Neurobiology*, **21**, 497–508.

66 Mechaly, I., Bourane, S., Piquemal, D., Al-Jumaily, M., Venteo, S., Puech, S., Scamps, F., Valmier, J. and Carroll, P. (2006) Gene profiling during development and after a peripheral nerve traumatism reveals genes specifically induced by injury in dorsal root ganglia. *Molecular and Cellular Neurosciences*, **32**, 217–229.

67 Nilsson, A., Moller, K., Dahlin, L., Lundborg, G. and Kanje, M. (2005) Early changes in gene expression in the dorsal root ganglia after transection of the sciatic nerve: effects of amphiregulin and PAI-1 on regeneration. *Brain Research. Molecular Brain Research*, **136**, 65–74.

68 Ashburner, M., Ball, C.A., Blake, J.A., Botstein, D., Butler, H., Cherry, J.M., Davis, A.P., Dolinski, K., Dwight, S.S., Eppig, J.T., Harris, M.A., Hill, D.P., Issel-Tarver, L., Kasarskis, A., Lewis, S., Matese, J.C., Richardson, J.E., Ringwald, M., Rubin, G.M. and Sherlock, G. (2000) Gene ontology: tool for the unification of biology. The Gene Ontology Consortium. *Nature Genetics*, **25**, 25–29.

69 Hao, J.X., Shi, T.J., Xu, I.S., Kaupilla, T., Xu, X.J., Hokfelt, T., Bartfai, T. and Wiesenfeld-Hallin, Z. (1999) Intrathecal galanin alleviates allodynia-like behaviour in rats after partial peripheral nerve injury. *The European Journal of Neuroscience*, **11**, 427–432.

70 Holmes, F.E., Mahoney, S., King, V.R., Bacon, A., Kerr, N.C., Pachnis, V., Curtis, R., Priestley, J.V. and Wynick, D. (2000)

Targeted disruption of the galanin gene reduces the number of sensory neurons and their regenerative capacity. *Proceedings of the National Academy of Sciences of the United States of America*, **97**, 11563–11568.

71 White, D.M. and Mansfield, K. (1996) Vasoactive intestinal polypeptide and neuropeptide Y act indirectly to increase neurite outgrowth of dissociated dorsal root ganglion cells. *Neuroscience*, **73**, 881–887.

72 DiCicco-Bloom, E., Deutsch, P.J., Maltzman, J., Zhang, J., Pintar, J.E., Zheng, J., Friedman, W.F., Zhou, X. and Zaremba, T. (2000) Autocrine expression and ontogenetic functions of the PACAP ligand/receptor system during sympathetic development. *Developmental Biology*, **219**, 197–213.

73 Zhang, Q.L., Lin, P.X., Shi, D., Xian, H. and Webster, H.D. (1996) Vasoactive intestinal peptide: mediator of laminin synthesis in cultured Schwann cells. *Journal of Neuroscience Research*, **43**, 496–502.

74 Martinez, C., Delgado, M., Pozo, D., Leceta, J., Calvo, J.R., Ganea, D. and Gomariz, R.P. (1998) VIP and PACAP enhance IL-6 release and mRNA levels in resting peritoneal macrophages: *in vitro* and *in vivo* studies. *Journal of Neuroimmunology*, **85**, 155–167.

75 Olsson, T., Diener, P., Ljungdahl, A., Hojeberg, B., van der Meide, P.H. and Kristensson, K. (1992) Facial nerve transection causes expansion of myelin autoreactive T cells in regional lymph nodes and T cell homing to the facial nucleus. *Autoimmunity*, **13**, 117–126.

76 Raivich, G., Jones, L.L., Kloss, C.U., Werner, A., Neumann, H. and Kreutzberg, G.W. (1998) Immune surveillance in the injured nervous system: T-lymphocytes invade the axotomized mouse facial motor nucleus and aggregate around sites of neuronal degeneration. *Journal of Neuroscience*, **18**, 5804–5816.

77 Schreiber, R.C., Vaccariello, S.A., Boeshore, K., Shadiack, A.M. and Zigmond, R.E. (2002) A comparison of the changes in the non-neuronal cell populations of the superior cervical ganglia following decentralization and axotomy. *Journal of Neurobiology*, **53**, 68–79.

78 Cai, D., Deng, K., Mellado, W., Lee, J., Ratan, R.R. and Filbin, M.T. (2002) Arginase I and polyamines act down-stream from cyclic AMP in overcoming inhibition of axonal growth MAG and myelin *in vitro*. *Neuron*, **35**, 711–719.

79 Knoll, R., Hoshijima, M., Hoffman, H.M., Person, V., Lorenzen-Schmidt, I., Bang, M.L., Hayashi, T., Shiga, N., Yasukawa, H., Schaper, W., McKenna, W., Yokoyama, M., Schork, N.J., Omens, J.H., McCulloch, A.D., Kimura, A., Gregorio, C.C., Poller, W., Schaper, J., Schultheiss, H.P. and Chien, K.R. (2002) The cardiac mechanical stretch sensor machinery involves a Z disc complex that is defective in a subset of human dilated cardiomyopathy. *Cell*, **111**, 943–955.

80 Aigner, L., Arber, S., Kapfhammer, J.P., Laux, T., Schneider, C., Botteri, F., Brenner, H.R. and Caroni, P. (1995) Overexpression of the neural growth-associated protein GAP-43 induces nerve sprouting in the adult nervous system of transgenic mice. *Cell*, **83**, 269–278.

81 Buffo, A., Holtmaat, A.J., Savio, T., Verbeek, J.S., Oberdick, J., Oestreicher, A.B., Gispen, W.H., Verhaagen, J., Rossi, F. and Strata, P. (1997) Targeted overexpression of the neurite growth-associated protein B-50/GAP-43 in cerebellar Purkinje cells induces sprouting after axotomy but not axon regeneration into growth-permissive transplants. *Journal of Neuroscience*, **17**, 8778–8791.

82 Nagarajan, R., Le, N., Mahoney, H., Araki, T. and Milbrandt, J. (2002) Deciphering peripheral nerve

myelination by using Schwann cell expression profiling. *Proceedings of the National Academy of Sciences of the United States of America*, **99**, 8998–9003.

83 Perlson, E., Hanz, S., Medzihradszky, K.F., Burlingame, A.L. and Fainzilber, M. (2004) From snails to sciatic nerve: retrograde injury signaling from axon to soma in lesioned neurons. *Journal of Neurobiology*, **58**, 287–294.

84 Perlson, E., Hanz, S., Ben-Yaakov, K., Segal-Ruder, Y., Seger, R. and Fainzilber, M. (2005) Vimentin-dependent spatial translocation of an activated MAP kinase in injured nerve. *Neuron*, **45**, 715–726.

85 Willis, D., Li, K.W., Zheng, J.Q., Chang, J.H., Smit, A., Kelly, T., Merianda, T.T., Sylvester, J., van Minnen, J. and Twiss, J.L. (2005) Differential transport and local translation of cytoskeletal injury-response, and neurodegeneration protein mRNAs in axons. *Journal of Neuroscience*, **25**, 778–791.

86 Zhang, Y., Wolf-Yadlin, A., Ross, P.L., Pappin, D.J., Rush, J., Lauffenburger, D.A. and White, F.M. (2005) Time-resolved mass spectrometry of tyrosine phosphorylation sites in the epidermal growth factor receptor signaling network reveals dynamic modules. *Molecular and Cellular Proteomics*, **4**, 1240–1250.

87 Ogata, H., Goto, S., Sato, K., Fujibuchi, W., Bono, H. and Kanehisa, M. (1999) KEGG: Kyoto Encyclopedia of Genes and Genomes. *Nucleic Acids Research*, **27**, 29–34.

88 Ren, B., Robert, F., Wyrick, J.J., Aparicio, O., Jennings, E.G., Simon, I., Zeitlinger, J., Schreiber, J., Hannett, N., Kanin, E., Volkert, T.L., Wilson, C.J., Bell, S.P. and Young, R.A. (2000) Genome-wide location and function of DNA binding proteins. *Science*, **290**, 2306–2309.

89 Iyer, V.R., Horak, C.E., Scafe, C.S., Botstein, D., Snyder, M. and Brown, P.O. (2001) Genomic binding sites of the yeast cell-cycle transcription factors SBF and MBF. *Nature*, **409**, 533–538.

90 Lee, T.I., Rinaldi, N.J., Robert, F., Odom, D.T., Bar-Joseph, Z., Gerber, G.K., Hannett, N.M., Harbison, C.T., Thompson, C.M., Simon, I., Zeitlinger, J., Jennings, E.G., Murray, H.L., Gordon, D.B., Ren, B., Wyrick, J.J., Tagne, J.B., Volkert, T.L., Fraenkel, E., Gifford, D.K. and Young, R.A. (2002) Transcriptional regulatory networks in Saccharomyces cerevisiae. *Science*, **298**, 799–804.

91 Colvis, C.M., Pollock, J.D., Goodman, R.H., Impey, S., Dunn, J., Mandel, G., Champagne, F.A., Mayford, M., Korzus, E., Kumar, A., Renthal, W., Theobald, D.E. and Nestler, E.J. (2005) Epigenetic mechanisms and gene networks in the nervous system. *Journal of Neuroscience*, **25**, 10379–10389.

92 Hsieh, J. and Gage, F.H. (2005) Chromatin remodeling in neural development and plasticity. *Current Opinion in Cell Biology*, **17**, 664–671.

93 Boyer, L.A., Lee, T.I., Cole, M.F., Johnstone, S.E., Levine, S.S., Zucker, J.P., Guenther, M.G., Kumar, R.M., Murray, H.L., Jenner, R.G., Gifford, D.K., Melton, D.A., Jaenisch, R. and Young, R.A. (2005) Core transcriptional regulatory circuitry in human embryonic stem cells. *Cell*, **122**, 947–956.

94 Carroll, J.S., Liu, X.S., Brodsky, A.S., Li, W., Meyer, C.A., Szary, A.J., Eeckhoute, J., Shao, W., Hestermann, E.V., Geistlinger, T.R., Fox, E.A., Silver, P.A. and Brown, M. (2005) Chromosome-wide mapping of estrogen receptor binding reveals long-range regulation requiring the forkhead protein Fox A1. *Cell*, **122**, 33–43.

95 Roth, F.P., Hughes, J.D., Estep, P.W. and Church, G.M. (1998) Finding DNA regulatory motifs within unaligned noncoding sequences clustered by whole-genome mRNA quantitation. *Nature Biotechnology*, **16**, 939–945.

96 van Helden, J., Andre, B. and Collado-Vides, J. (1998) Extracting regulatory sites from the upstream region of yeast

genes by computational analysis of oligonucleotide frequencies. *Journal of Molecular Biology*, **281**, 827–842.

97 Sinha, S. and Tompa, M. (2002) Discovery of novel transcription factor binding sites by statistical over-representation. *Nucleic Acids Research*, **30**, 5549–5560.

98 Cliften, P., Sudarsanam, P., Desikan, A., Fulton, L., Fulton, B., Majors, J., Waterston, R., Cohen, B.A. and Johnston, M. (2003) Finding functional features in Saccharomyces genomes by phylogenetic footprinting. *Science*, **301**, 71–76.

99 Kellis, M., Patterson, N., Endrizzi, M., Birren, B. and Lander, E.S. (2003) Sequencing and comparison of yeast species to identify genes and regulatory elements. *Nature*, **423**, 241–254.

100 Boffelli, D., McAuliffe, J., Ovcharenko, D., Lewis, K.D., Ovcharenko, I., Pachter, L. and Rubin, E.M. (2003) Phylogenetic shadowing of primate sequences to find functional regions of the human genome. *Science*, **299**, 1391–1394.

101 Thomas, J.W., Touchman, J.W., Blakesley, R.W., Bouffard, G.G., Beckstrom-Sternberg, S.M., Margulies, E.H., Blanchette, M., Siepel, A.C., Thomas, P.J., McDowell, J.C., Maskeri, B., Hansen, N.F., Schwartz, M.S., Weber, R.J., Kent, W.J., Karolchik, D., Bruen, T.C., Bevan, R., Cutler, D.J., Schwartz, S., Elnitski, L., Idol, J.R., Prasad, A.B., Lee-Lin, S.Q., Maduro, V.V., Summers, T.J., Portnoy, M.E., Dietrich, N.L., Akhter, N., Ayele, K., Benjamin, B., Cariaga, K., Brinkley, C.P., Brooks, S.Y., Granite, S., Guan, X., Gupta, J., Haghighi, P., Ho, S.L., Huang, M.C., Karlins, E., Laric, P.L., Legaspi, R., Lim, M.J., Maduro, Q.L., Masiello, C.A., Mastrian, S.D., McCloskey, J.C., Pearson, R., Stantripop, S., Tiongson, E.E., Tran, J.T., Tsurgeon, C., Vogt, J.L., Walker, M.A., Wetherby, K.D., Wiggins, L.S., Young, A.C., Zhang, L.H., Osoegawa, K., Zhu, B., Zhao, B., Shu, C.L., De Jong, P.J., Lawrence, C.E., Smit, A.F., Chakravarti, A., Haussler, D., Green, P., Miller, W. and Green, E.D. (2003) Comparative analyses of multi-species sequences from targeted genomic regions. *Nature*, **424**, 788–793.

102 Li, H. and Wang, W. (2003) Dissecting the transcription networks of a cell using computational genomics. *Current Opinion in Genetics and Development*, **13**, 611–616.

103 Siggia, E.D. (2005) Computational methods for transcriptional regulation. *Current Opinion in Genetics and Development*, **15**, 214–221.

104 Schwab, M.E. (2002) Repairing the injured spinal cord. *Science*, **295**, 1029–1031.

105 Pasterkamp, R.J. and Verhaagen, J. (2006) Semaphorins in axon regeneration: developmental guidance molecules gone wrong? *Philosophical Transactions of the Royal Society of London. Series B: Biological Sciences*, **361**, 1499–1511.

106 Wong, L.F., Yip, P.K., Battaglia, A., Grist, J., Corcoran, J., Maden, M., Azzouz, M., Kingsman, S.M., Kingsman, A.J., Mazarakis, N.D. and McMahon, S.B. (2006) Retinoic acid receptor beta2 promotes functional regeneration of sensory axons in the spinal cord. *Nature Neuroscience*, **9**, 243–250.

3

Analyzing Complex Gene Expression Profiles in Sensorimotor Cortex Following Spinal Cord Injury and Regeneration Promoting Treatment

Fabian Kruse, Nicole Brazda, Patrick Küry, Frank Bosse, and Hans W. Müller

3.1
Introduction

Damage of pyramidal tract motor axons in rat spinal cord leads to permanent loss of locomotor functions and atrophy or death of a substantial proportion of cortical motoneurons. Moreover, injured axons fail to regenerate due to inhibitory cues in the lesion environment, for example, fibrous lesion scar [1]. This latter growth barrier consists of a collagen type IV network (basement membrane) that binds and accumulates inhibitory molecules and thereby prevents axonal regeneration across the lesion site. Transient suppression of scar formation triggered by a pharmacological intervention promotes long distance axonal growth beyond the lesion site, resulting in significant functional recovery [2]. To study regeneration in the central nervous system, we applied Affymetrix microarray technology to a rat animal model in which we examined the genetic responses of cortical tissues after spinal cord injury (SCI) with and without such a pharmacological intervention.

Previous work in our laboratory showed that the transient scar suppression due to local application of an antiscarring treatment (AST) using iron chelators and cyclic AMP not just enables long distance axon regeneration and functional recovery after transection of the corticospinal tract (CST). It has also been shown that lesion to the CST leads to the loss of up to 30–40% of pyramidal cells in layer V of the sensorimotor cortex 4 weeks after injury [3]. But in animals that received the AST treatment, the entire pyramidal cell population could be rescued from cell death [2].

To characterize mRNA expression profiles of sham-operated, lesion-only, and AST-treated adult rats, we prepared a comprehensive series of gene chip hybridizations at distinct time points after lesion to identify stage-specific molecular responses. The time points cover the following stages: acute reactions, axon sprouting, axonal contact with the scar tissue, regeneration failure (lesion only), and axonal regrowth beyond the lesion site (AST treated). Given the complex task of assessing genetic profiles at multiple conditions and stages from such a heterogeneous tissue,

Neural Degeneration and Repair: Gene Expression Profiling, Proteomics, and Systems Biology
Edited by Hans Werner Müller
Copyright © 2008 WILEY-VCH Verlag GmbH & Co. KGaA, Weinheim
ISBN: 978-3-527-31707-3

like the cerebral cortex, the experimental setup as well as the subsequent data processing and statistical analysis procedures had to be adjusted to cope with the expected variations. Especially the method applied for data analysis, including a procedure to combine multiple preprocessing algorithms and adequate statistical testing, will be discussed in detail.

3.2
Scar-Suppressing Treatment of SCI

After CNS injury a collagen-rich wound-healing scar forms at the lesion site in the brain [4] and spinal cord [5,6]. This fibrous scar is composed of extracellular matrix and cellular components such as fibroblasts, inflammatory cells, and blood cells (for review see [1,7,8]). Collagen type IV is one of the major components of the fibrous scar since it forms a dense meshwork to which numerous molecules can bind [1], such as NG2 [9–12] and other chondroitin sulfate proteoglycans (CSPG) [7,13], semaphorins [14,15], and ephrins [16]. The accumulation of, for example, the growth inhibitory NG2 molecule correlates with the formation of the dense collagen IV network in the lesion core [2]. After spinal cord injury collagen is expressed by different cell types, such as meningeal fibroblasts [17], astrocytes [18], and endothelial cells [19]. It was previously shown that axons, which are able to sprout spontaneously after injury, stop at the border of the fibrous scar in spinal cord [2,10] and brain injury [20,21]. The intrinsic capacity of axons to regrow after spinal cord injury is obviously not potent enough to allow axonal regeneration through and beyond the fibrous scar. Furthermore, *in vitro* studies showed that axon growth was inhibited at astrocyte/meningeal cell interfaces [22]. Axon growth was previously observed in white matter of adult rat spinal cord following the atraumatic injection of dissociated adult rat dorsal root ganglion neurons [23] or a single sharp spinal transection [24]. These findings in lesion models that caused very little or no scar formation are in support of our hypothesis that fibrous scarring is a major regeneration barrier in CNS injury.

Our therapeutic approach to brain and spinal cord injury is based on the transient suppression of collagen biosynthesis and, therefore, the inhibition of fibrous scarring. The key component of this treatment is an iron chelator that is applied immediately after injury to inhibit the prolyl 4-hydroxylase, a key enzyme of collagen biosynthesis. Bipyridin (BPY) proved to be very efficient in the brain lesion model in suppressing fibrous scar formation and allowing axonal regeneration and functional reconnection of the postcommissural fornix to its target, the mammillary body [4,21]. Recently, this treatment was successfully reproduced in another brain lesion model [25]. Following spinal cord transection, the more potent iron chelator BPY–dicarboxylate (BPY–DCA) was applied in combination with cAMP to suppress proliferation of meningeal fibroblasts [26]. Injection of BPY–DCA and cAMP immediately after lesion to the spinal cord injury site proved to be a highly effective treatment to transiently inhibit fibrous scar formation and NG2 accumulation in spinal cord injury [2,27]. The treatment retrogradely rescued projecting primary motoneurons in layer V of sensorimotor cortex 1 month after lesion [2]. This effect is most likely due to increased local protection against oxidative stress by the iron chelator [28] through inhibition of the Fenton's reaction, thus protecting cells at the lesion site, which normally die after spinal cord injury [29–31].

In conclusion, the scar-suppressing treatment opened a time window of 12–14 days for regenerating axons that were not confronted by the inhibitory fibrous scar during this period. Elongation of anterogradely traced corticospinal tract axons could be observed for long distances (up to 1.5–2 cm after 10–12 weeks [2]) showing terminal arborizations in distal gray matter. Interestingly, we detected axon regeneration both in gray and white matter and submeningeally in injured animals receiving the scar-suppressing treatment. Axon growth in myelin-rich white matter indicates that at least a proportion of CST axons may be insensitive to myelin-derived inhibitors, such as NOGO, MAG, or MOG [32,33], possibly due to lack of the respective receptors. Finally, functional tests proved that the scar-suppressing treatment resulted in significant functional recovery of the lesioned animals. Rats receiving a transection lesion at thoracic level 8 and scar-suppressing treatment showed significant functional recovery according to the BBB open field score [34], the horizontal ladder [35], and the CatWalk device [36] during a period of 15 weeks.

3.3
Experimental Design

3.3.1
Treatment Paradigms and Animal Groups

To study changes in neocortical mRNA expression after axotomy of the CST in the thoracic spinal cord and to identify alterations in gene expression due to AST treatment, three experimental animal groups were examined and compared:

1. *Sham-operated* animals underwent laminectomy and opening of the dura but received no transection of the CST.
2. *Lesion-only* animals further received a CST transection resulting in a nonregenerating condition.
3. *AST-treated* animals received a CST transection followed by a combined treatment with BPY–DCA and cAMP resulting in complex regenerating reactions.

The animals were sacrificed 1, 7, 21, or 60 days post operation (dpo). These time points were chosen to obtain genetic profiles of distinct states of spinal cord injury and repair. One day post lesion represents an acute phase, whereas 7 days post lesion represents a phase of spontaneous axonal sprouting. At 21 dpo growth cones had reached the border of the lesion site and, in the case of the AST-treated animals, axons entered the lesion area. At 60 dpo commencement of functional recovery could be observed in AST-treated animals [2].

We used heterogeneous cortical tissue and, therefore, we had to compensate for the expected higher variations by increasing the number of test animals per experimental group and the type of analysis applied. For this reason, four to five biological replicates (minimum three) per condition were routinely analyzed. Samples were not pooled, but each subject was hybridized to a separate microchip. Considerations concerning replicate numbers and pooling strategies can be found in Section 3.4.3. In addition, further technical aspects of our experiment required attention to achieve valuable data, for example, reproducibility of spinal cord axotomy, speed and accuracy of tissue preparation, extraction of quality RNA, optimal conditions for reverse transcription, labeling, and hybridization.

3.3.2
Corticospinal Tract Transection

Transection of the CST was carried out as previously described in [2]. In brief, laminectomy of vertebrae Th8 and Th9 was performed under isoflurane-mediated anesthesia. The dura was opened with spring scissors and the dorsal columns and dorsal CST were cut with a Scouten wire knife (Bilaney, Germany). In animals with antiscarring treatment, the iron chelator 2,2′-bipyridine-5,5′-dicarboxylic acid (BPY–DCA, 40 mM in Tris-buffer) was injected both into the lesion site (four injections of 0.2 µl) and at 1 mm proximal to the lesion site (two injections). After injection, 2 mg of 8-Br-cAMP were applied to the lesion area before the dura was sutured. Control animals received injections of Tris-buffer without cAMP application. The lesion of treated animals was covered with a piece of ELVAX (ethylene-vinyl-) copolymer sheet loaded with BPY–DCA for slow release, whereas ELVAX copolymer in control animals contained Tris-buffer alone. Finally, the animals were sutured and treated with antibiotics (Baytril) for 1 week. If necessary, the bladders were emptied manually.

3.3.3
Cortical Tissue Preparation and Total RNA Isolation

For this study, we dissected the complete layer V of the sensorimotor cortex to prepare total RNA. Alternatively, individual pyramidal cells from layer V of the cerebral cortex could be collected via laser microdissection. Although the advantage of laser microdissection is the cellular purity of the resulting samples and the gene regulations detected by subsequent array analysis can be ascribed to neurons directly affected by the transection. The drawback of this approach is, however, the necessity of RNA amplification due to the limited amount of collected material, which inevitably leads to additional technical variations. On the contrary, using a tissue block to harvest a defined cortical layer may give insight into not only the reactions of pyramidal neurons but also the response of the surrounding glial cells. For this reason as well as to refrain from RNA amplification, we preferred the tissue block preparation method.

The adequate cortical area for tissue preparation of pyramidal cells in layer V of the sensory-motor cortex was determined via retrograde labeling with FluoroGold. For tissue collection the brains were removed in a cold room ($\sim$4 °C) and directly frozen in isopropanol at -45 to -55 °C. Using a cryotome, 40 serial coronal brain slices of 50 μm thickness were cut. The area of layer V containing the primary motor neurons and the subjacent part of layer VI were dissected at -20 °C and collected in Qiazol. Cortical slices from lesioned adult rats (lesion-only and AST-treated), as well as from sham-operated rats were prepared. Tissue was rapidly removed and processed using the RNeasy Lipid Tissue Mini Kit (Qiagen). In addition, DNAse-I treatment and the RNeasy-clean up protocol (Qiagen) were applied in combination to avoid contamination with genomic DNA.

3.3.4
Probe Labeling and Array Hybridization

Briefly, approximately 2 μg of total RNA were converted into labeled cRNA consecutively using Superscript Double-Stranded cDNA Synthesis Kit (Invitrogen) and BioArray High Yield RNA Transcript Labeling Kit (Enzo) for each condition. Following hybridization and several washing steps according to the manufacturer's protocol, the hybridized Rat 230A microarrays (Affymetrix) were exposed to a scanner and the signals were digitalized. Signal intensities were determined and raw data quality was independently evaluated using ArrayAssist 4.2.0 Software (Stratagene).

3.4
Data Analysis

3.4.1
Affymetrix GeneChip Technology

Over the past 10 years, Affymetrix microarrays have become a standard in mRNA expression profiling. Using solid-phase chemical synthesis and photolithographic techniques employed in the semiconductor industry, 25-mer oligonucleotides are directly synthesized at specific locations on coated glass slides as probes for cRNA fragments [37,38]. Given the high density of probes due to their small feature size (from 50 to 2 μm), chips with the size of a human thumbnail holding the whole transcribed genome of species such as rat, mouse, or human are available today [39]. To assess nonspecific binding, each *perfect match* (*PM*) oligonucleotide sequence is accompanied by a *mismatch* (*MM*) probe in which an incorrect nucleotide is introduced at position 13 of the 25-mer oligonucleotide. A PM probe and its reference MM probe make up a *probe pair*. To obtain reliable gene expression measures and background estimations, multiple probe pairs are used for each mRNA expression measurement. Typically, on current Affymetrix arrays 11 different probe pairs make up such a so-called probe set, related to a common gene or a fraction of a gene. Using the information of the multiple measurements of hybridization in each *probe set* allows a more robust measure of expression. However, calculating the expression is much more complex as compared to spotted arrays where each gene is represented by just one probe.

3.4.2
Variations

The measurand in microarray experiments is the amount of a specific transcript in a present sample from prepared tissue or cells of interest. The selective binding of cRNA fragments to their complementary chip probes is a function of this mRNA amount. Unfortunately, this function holds a number of unknown variables that lead to background noise. Among these variables are variations in the RNA extraction and reverse transcription efficiency, chip fabrication tolerances, background intensity fluctuations, nonuniform target labeling, pipetting errors, scanning deviations, and so forth. The sources of these variations can be separated in three layers: biological variations, technical variations, and measurement errors [40]. The biological variations are of interest for the investigator. This type of variation is intrinsic to all biological organisms and can be influenced by factors such as tissue heterogeneity, genetic polymorphism, environmental factors, and pooling of samples as well as by any type of treatment [41–44]. Technical variations accumulate during handling of the biological samples such as extraction, RNA preparation, labeling, and probe hybridization. Measurement errors originate from the process of reading the fluorescence signals on the array. A complete elaboration of the different sources of variation can be found in Hartemink *et al.* [45]. Given the fact that the ratio of interesting variations to obscuring variations has a significant impact on the usability of microarray data, minimizing the technical variations by controlling the quality of the RNA samples and using well-proven and efficient labeling and hybridization methods is crucial [46–48].

3.4.3
Impact of the Experimental Setup

The experimental setup has a great impact on the statistical power of the resulting data. This includes the choice of tissue and tissue preparation, number and kind of replicates, as well as the fact whether or not samples are pooled. Although multiple replicates for each condition may tremendously increase the cost of a broad experimental setup, choosing too few replicates to bring down costs may render a still expensive study into an investigation lacking a reliable result. Various articles have assessed the effect of replicate numbers on the false-positive rate [49,50] or to estimate the statistical power of experiments a priori [51]. Hariharan [49] showed that the number of false positives included catching all 14 spike-in genes in the Affymetrix Latin Square data set drops from 2000 (two replicates) to 50 (four replicates).

Pooling biological samples seems to be appropriate for reducing the total number of microchips. The concept of pooling is to minimize subject-to-subject variations in order to identify substantial differences between the experimental groups [40,52,53].

Drawback of this approach is the inability to identify and remove outliers and to approximate the variation within the population. Although there are ways to minimize this effect by adequate pooling strategies where each group is split into overlapping subgroups, the advantages of pooling are limited to larger study designs and high amounts of samples [54–56].

3.4.4
Low-Level Analyses

To separate biological variations of interest from obscuring variations, the collected raw data have to be preprocessed. This so-called low-level analysis normally includes background adjustment, normalization, PM correction, and summarization. While background adjustment removes nonspecific background from scanned images for each single array, normalization reduces nonspecific, nonbiological variations between multiple chips. PM correction is supposed to reduce the effects of nonspecific binding or cross-hybridization by MM probe subtraction. The usefulness of this procedure is still controversially discussed in the literature, as several studies have shown that ignoring MM probes can lead to a lower variance [57–64]. Finally, the summarization step generates a single expression value out of the multiple intensities of each probe set. Depending on the algorithm used, this can be done with a single chip or by including the data of multiple chips from one project. The steps of low-level analysis cannot be separated by a clear-cut approach, as there are algorithmic approaches to solve two or more of these measures at once. There also are approaches that skip one or more steps such as the background adjustment or, especially, the controversial issue of PM correction [58].

In recent years it became more and more obvious that the way the oligonucleotide array data are preprocessed dramatically influences the results that can be extracted from the experiments [62,65–67]. Several studies tried to evaluate the performance of different preprocessing methods, mainly using "spike-in" and "dilution" experiments [57,58,61,62,64–66,68–72]. Given the many different ways to perform the respective parts of low-level analysis and their countless combinations, making the right choice for preprocessing has become a scientific field of its own. Obviously, though coefficients such as accuracy, precision, and bias from a set of preprocessing combinations can be assessed, the overall "performance" is difficult to measure. The performance of low-level analyses mainly depends on the type of data to be processed, factors such as the number of chips, the type of tissue that is to be analyzed, and the scientific goal that is pursued.

3.4.4.1 Microarray Suite (MAS)
Until 2001, GeneChip MAS 4.0 software used the average of the difference (AvDiff) of corresponding PM and MM intensities to calculate expression values. AvDiff is defined as

$$\text{AvDiff} = |A|^{-1} \sum_{\{j \in A\}} (\text{PM}_j - \text{MM}_j), \tag{3.1}$$

where A is a set of suitable probe pairs. In about one third of the probe pairs of an average array, MM $\geq$ PM [61]. Thus, adjusting for nonspecific binding and background noise by the PM–MM transformation leads to two obvious problems: about 5% of the resulting intensities of the probe sets are negative and data including negative values cannot be log transformed to account for the multiplicative measurement error. With the introduction of MAS 5.0 in 2001, the *signal* was calculated as follows:

$$\text{Signal} = \text{Tukey biweight}\{\log(\text{PM}_j - \text{MM}_j^*)\}, \tag{3.2}$$

where MM* is a modified MM value to prevent adjusted expression values to become less or equal to 0. Each probe pair has a "vote" in determining the signal; the probe pairs are weighted based on their distance from the probe set mean. Using the weighted intensity values, the adjusted mean for the probe set is determined (for detailed information on MAS 5.0, see Affymetrix [73]). For background adjustment each chip is divided into 16 zones correcting the probe values by using (1) the second percentile of the probe values in that zone as background and (2) the distance of the probe to the center of its zone as a weight. To normalize the data of multiple chips, MAS 5.0 uses linear regression, scaling the overall intensities of all chips to the same user-defined target intensity.

3.4.4.2 Model-Based Expression Indexes (MBEI)

In 2001, Li and Wong [74] showed that there are huge differences in the intensities of probes in the same probe set, though they all bind different segments of the same gene. However, the so-called probe set patterns of genes are generally the same compared between different chips (Figure 3.1). The MBEI method, implemented in the dChip software package, uses this information to account for individual probe-specific effects as well as for the detection of outliers and image artifacts [69]. The *invariant set*, a large number of ad hoc selected genes as references for nonlinear normalization instead of a fixed catalog of "housekeeping genes", is used for

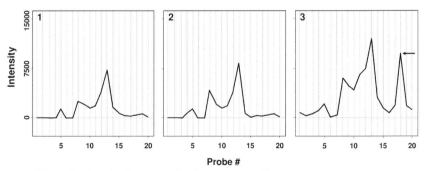

Figure 3.1 Outlier detection by means of probe set patterns. The 20 PM intensity values of one probe set on three different arrays plotted against their probe numbers show almost the same profile. Irregular probes (black arrow) or chips can be identified. Figure modified from Li and Wong [74].

normalization [74]. Both PMMM and PM modes are implemented in dChip, meaning that either the PM–MM differences are evaluated (PMMM) or ignored (PM).

Several other low-level analyses have been developed from different groups. Most of them are based on the findings of Li and Wong [74], namely, strong probe effects in PMMM-adjusted intensity values, advantages of multiarray summaries for signal estimation as well as outlier detection, and need for nonlinear normalization. Here we focus on five algorithms: MAS 5 and MBEI (mentioned above), as well as robust multiarray average (RMA), GC–RMA, and PLIER.

3.4.4.3 Robust Multiarray Average

In 2003, Irizarry *et al.* introduced RMA as a new method for low-level analysis [61,75]. It is based on the discoveries made by Li and Wong [74], but uses different algorithms for each preprocessing step. Only PM values are used for the calculation, the MM values are ignored. The assumption is made that the observed PM intensity distribution is a combination of an exponentially distributed signal and a normally distributed background (Figure 3.2). The resulting background corrected probe intensities are then normalized using *quantile normalization*. Bolstad *et al.* [57] demonstrated that data-driven quantile normalization is a fast and simple way of normalization. Moreover, quantile normalization showed good performance when compared to two other, already established methods (*cyclic loess* and *contrast based*). All three normalization methods are referred to as "complete data methods", meaning that the data of all chips in an experiment are combined to form the normalization relation. Quantile normalization adjusts the data of all arrays to the same distribution (Figure 3.3). The method is based on the idea that a quantile–quantile plot of two data vectors shows a straight diagonal line if the distributions of the two vectors are the same. This suggests that projecting the data points of all n arrays in a n-dimensional quantile–quantile plot onto the n-dimensional diagonal identity line leads to an equally distributed data set. Table 3.1 shows a simplified example: the expression values of each chip make up a column of a spreadsheet, each row representing a specific gene. Now each column is sorted in increasing order, and the values of every cell are replaced with the row average. Finally, the columns are unsorted, each row representing a gene again. This method works well with most types of data sets and is stable against outliers. However, an extreme probe intensity value of a gene on a certain chip can influence the calculated expression values of

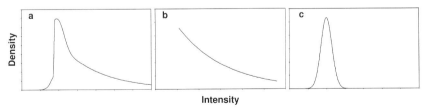

Figure 3.2 Components of the measured intensity distribution.
Detected density of probe intensities (a) includes two
components, an exponentially distributed signal (b) and
a normally distributed background (c).

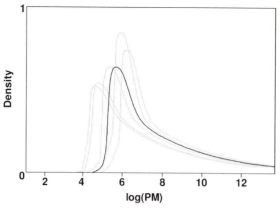

Figure 3.3 Densities of PM probe intensities for spike-in data sets. Distributions before (gray) and after (black) quantile normalization are plotted. Figure modified from Bolstad *et al.* [57].

different genes in the data set of all the other chips. Therefore, quantile normalization should be performed before summarization to prevent such rare cases. Moreover, certain kinds of experimental setups can lead to a high error rate due to the assumption that there are no distribution changes in all chips.

After performing quantile normalization, RMA fits the background-adjusted, normalized and $\log_2$-transformed PM intensities, denoted by Y, to a linear additive model:

Table 3.1 Example for quantile normalization.

	Chip 1	Chip 2	Chip 3	mean	Chip 1	Chip 2	Chip 3
Gene 1	4	5	6	4	4	2	6
Gene 2	8	11	9	6	4	5	9
Gene 3	7	10	10	9	7	10	10
Gene 4	4	2	14	11	8	11	14

	Chip 1	Chip 2	Chip 3	mean	Chip 1	Chip 2	Chip 3
Gene 1	4	6	4	4	4	4	4
Gene 2	11	11	6	6	6	6	6
Gene 3	9	9	9	9	9	9	9
Gene 4	6	4	11	11	11	11	11

Columns representing chip data are sorted in ascending order, the values in each row replaced by the rows' mean and finally the columns unsorted. After quantile normalization each chip shows the same distribution, due to the same values in every column. For example, gene 2 seems to be lower expressed in the sample on chip 3, though the original values do not show that directly. Extreme outliers can influence corrected values of other genes on other chips.

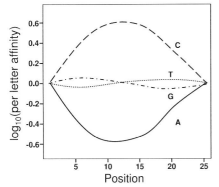

Figure 3.4 Effect of bases A, T, G, and C in position k on the affinity and brightness of probes. Position 1 corresponds to the first base on the glass slide. Figure modified from Naef and Magnasco [79] and Wu et al. [78].

$$Y_{ijn} = \mu_{in} + \alpha_{jn} + \varepsilon_{ijn}, \quad i = 1, \ldots, I, j = 1, \ldots, J, n = 1, \ldots, n, \qquad (3.3)$$

where α_j stands for a probe affinity effect and ε_{ij} is an independent identical error term with mean 0. An estimated μ_i represents the log scale expression level for probe set n on array i. The assumption that the average of each probe set is a representative measurement of the associated gene's expression leads to $\sum_j \alpha_j = 0$.

The model parameters are estimated using the robust *median polish* [76] procedure. A detailed comparison of MAS 5.0, MBEI, and RMA methods is given in Irizarry *et al.* [77].

3.4.4.4 GC–RMA

In 2004, Wu *et al.* [78] added a new way of background adjustment to the RMA method, using probe sequence information to estimate the affinity of the probe for nonspecific binding (NSB). This approach, called GC–RMA, was designed to resolve the drawback of RMA. While the precision of RMA is high, it lacks accuracy in estimating fold changes. The new GC–RMA method does not simply use the GC content but the position of each base type (A, T, G, or C) in the 25-mer oligonucleotide sequence to determine the affinity of each probe. Two effects come into play here. First, G–C pairs form three hydrogen bonds as opposed to two in the case of A–T pairs, leading to a stronger hybridization of the former. Second, the purines U and C in the mRNA are labeled, leading to weaker hybridization [79] (Figure 3.4). The original model introduced by Naef and Magnasco [79] described the probe affinity α as the sum of position-dependent base effects:

$$\alpha = \sum_{k=1}^{25} \sum_{j \in \{A,T,G,C\}} \mu_{j,k} 1_{b_k=j} \quad \text{with} \quad \mu_{j,k} = \sum_{l=0}^{3} \beta_{j,l} k^l, \qquad (3.4)$$

where $k = 1, \ldots, 25$ represents the position along the probe, j indicates the base letter, b_k indicates the base at position k, $1_{b_k=j}$ is 1 when the kth base is of type j and 0 otherwise, and $\mu_{j,k}$ indicates the contribution to affinity of base j in position k. The effect $\mu_{j,k}$ for fixed j is assumed to be a polynomial of degree 3. This model is adapted to describe the NSB in GC–RMA. It is assumed that PM is the sum of optical noise O_{PM}, NSB noise N_{PM}, and the signal S, while MM is the sum of optical noise O_{MM} and NSB noise N_{MM} only. *Maximum likelihood estimate* (MLE) or *empirical Bayes estimate* (EB) is used to estimate S. GC–RMA implementing an empirical Bayes approach outperforms RMA for low expressed genes [78].

3.4.4.5 Probe Logarithmic Intensity ERror (PLIER)

Affymetrix introduced PLIER in the year 2005 [80]. Because of the complex interactions leading to measured intensities, the analyzed parameters are termed as *feature responses* instead of *probe affinities* as in Irizarry *et al.* [77]. The PLIER algorithm does not utilize probe sequence information. It rather generates an empirical probe set specific *feature response pattern* that is supposed to incorporate not only the different thermodynamic properties and binding efficiencies but also other factors such as labeling, nonequilibrium washes, and density of synthesis. This feature response pattern can be compared to the *probe set pattern* introduced in MBEI. Feature response patterns across multiple arrays are utilized to identify poorly performing features with erratic hybridization characteristics. The PLIER algorithm additionally accounts for heteroskedacity of the data. It is assumed that in probe sets with a mean close to the background, probes with the highest feature response are those most informative. In the process of signal generation, each feature receives a weight, the most informative features providing the strongest contribution to the signal. The weight is depending on the consistency of the feature over multiple arrays and the median feature intensity, favoring higher feature responses at the low end of target abundance. The error estimation also includes abundance information. Although at low abundance the largest component of the measured intensity is most likely background, at high abundance it is a specific target response. This is also true for the error contained in the intensity. To avoid underestimation of error at the lower end of abundance, PLIER implements an error model, which smoothly transitions between a low abundance "arithmetic" and a high abundance "multiplicative" form. This design leads to a high sensitivity for low expressors and a low false-positive rate [72]. A detailed description of the underlying *M*-estimator calculation can be found at: http://www.affymetrix.com/support/technical/technotes/plier_technote.pdf.

3.4.5
Combination of Preprocessing Methods

We described five of the most commonly used preprocessing methods above. Depending on multiple factors, all algorithms will be able to find more or less overlapping and accurate groups of regulated genes. Using only one preprocessing algorithm will lead to biased data depending on the accuracy and precision of the algorithm and the type of background adjustment, normalization, and summarization steps. To narrow down the group of false negatives without including too many false positives, a combination of multiple analysis methods appears beneficial in the majority of cases [62].

For each experiment, a reasonable balance between *type I* and *type II* errors (see Box) has to be found, based on the data and the scientific aim. If only a few new candidate genes are to be identified, a higher false-negative rate can be accepted. In a systemic approach, on the contrary, a slightly higher false-positive rate will not disturb the overall regulation pattern, but, for example, an algorithm-specific non-sensitivity for low-level expression changes will do so. We developed a method implementing five well-described algorithms with different weights on the vote for regulation that can be used to utilize the advantages of all algorithms while holding the disadvantages in check. As multiple statistical tests based on the resulting data of each preprocessing method are performed, the *P*-value thresholds need to be adapted to compensate for the resulting *type I* error increase.

3.4.6

Box: Error types

Two different types of errors can be differentiated, *statistical* and *systematic errors*. Although the statistical error is caused by random variations, the systematic error is the result of nonrandom variations of an unknown source.

The statistical error can be divided into two types:

- Type I is the error of accepting a difference when in truth there is none (false positive).
- Type II is the error of accepting the null hypothesis when in truth there is a difference (false negative).

Statistical Analysis

Once the data have been background corrected, transformed into log scale, normalized, and summarized, expression values for every gene are obtained. The main purpose for microarray experiments is to assess information about differences of gene expression. Thus, a decision has to be made which genes will be accounted for as regulated/differently expressed based on their expression values. The easiest way is to calculate the ratio of the group's mean expression values, the so-called fold change, and set a threshold above which the genes will be considered as regulated. This method was widely used at the beginning of the microarray era. The fold-change cutoff, however, has major drawbacks, because it does not accommodate for either the actual level of expression values or their variance. Although at small intensities slight changes of the signal due to background noise can already lead to a massive fold change, highly expressed, truly regulated genes, on the contrary, may not reach the fold-change cutoff, as they may run into a saturation effect. Furthermore, the resulting fold-change value is highly dependent on the preceding low-level analysis. By changing the type of background adjustment, the fold change could change dramatically [58,72].

Additionally, comparison of actual RNA amounts to resulting fold changes measured in spike-in experiments showed that the ratios assessed by microarray data greatly underestimate the actual RNA fold changes [64]. Taking into account that these changes could be caused by only a subgroup of cells in heterogeneous tissue samples, biologically relevant gene regulations may show fold changes lower than 1.5.

The *t*-test can be used to prove significance in differential gene expression between two experimental groups. The *t*-statistic t_g is calculated for each gene g with e_1, e_2 representing the mean expression values, s_1, s_2 the standard deviations, and n_1, n_2 the number of arrays for group 1 and group 2:

$$t_g = \frac{e_1 - e_2}{\sqrt{\dfrac{s_1^2}{n_1} + \dfrac{s_2^2}{n_2}}}. \tag{3.5}$$

The t_g value can be transformed into a more convenient *P*-value using the *Student's t-distribution*. The assumption is made that the expression values in each group are normally distributed and the variances of these two distributions are the same. Thousands of genes are tested at once, leading to a severe inflation of the *type I error rate* increasing the chance for false positives. To neutralize this effect, several *P*-value correction methods have been introduced. On the contrary, these *P*-value correction methods tend to be rather conservative, leading to a higher number of false negatives.

If more than two conditions have to be analyzed, a comparison of all possible individual pairs of conditions could be performed using the *t*-test. But increasing the number of tests will subsequently rise the number of false positives. Another parametric test, the *analysis of variance* (ANOVA), is not bound to a comparison of only two groups and might thus be beneficial in such a study. The ANOVA follows the null hypothesis according to which the population means μ for all conditions are the same:

$$H_0 : \mu_1 = \mu_2 = \cdots = \mu_k, \tag{3.6}$$

where H_0 is the null hypothesis and k is the number of conditions. Basically, ANOVA compares two estimates of variance (σ^2), the *mean square error* (MSE) and the *mean square between* (MBE). The MSE is based on the variances within the sample's mean and is an estimate of σ^2 no matter if the null hypothesis is true or not. The MSB is based on the differences among the samples' means and is only an estimate of σ^2 if the null hypothesis is true, otherwise it will be larger. Therefore, if $MSB \gg MSE$, it is likely that at least one mean of the population is different to the rest. The ratio of MSB and MSE can be used to calculate the corresponding *P*-value for this difference using the *F* distribution. Just like the *t*-test, the ANOVA assumes independence, normal distribution, and homogeneity of variance. Although the distribution of microarray data of interest may not be known, ANOVA is quite robust to violations of these assumptions, tending to be rather conservative. To completely avoid these problems, nonparametric methods like *Mann–Whitney U* for two conditions or *Kruskal–Wallis* for more then two conditions are suitable tests for statistical analysis.

3.4.7
From Raw Data to Biological Meaning

Our comprehensive study on differential genomic responses in sensorimotor cortex after CST transection with or without pharmacological intervention implies several factors that complicated the identification of differentially expressed genes. As noted above we studied heterogeneous cortical tissue, a fact that implies the advantageous potential to analyze both neuronal and glial reactions to CST lesion. However, this approach leads to a decrease in signal detection, because gene expression changes in one particular cell type are diluted by the other cells. Also, counteracting responses in different cell types may mask each other. In the case of the CST lesion, only a proportion of cells in the analyzed cortical tissue, the primary motor neurons of layer V, is directly affected by the lesion. Furthermore, only a subpopulation of these neurons will regenerate, depending on the condition examined. Nevertheless, to assure accurate and reproducible results, an increased number of biological replicates per condition were used, and in the subsequent data analysis a broad spectrum of preprocessing methods was implemented. Gene regulations involved in regeneration processes, apoptosis, and survival were identified and distinct AST-treatment-mediated modifications were observed.

Initial data analyses have been performed using the Stratagene softwares *ArrayAssist* and *PathwayArchitect*. Using ArrayAssist the investigator can choose between the five well-established algorithms for low-level analysis, MAS 5, MBEI, PLIER, RMA, and GC–RMA. To ensure a fast and flexible workflow, we developed Python-based scripts to automatically and reproducibly process the information of different sets of arrays. The raw data were imported separating the chips into groups according to their experimental conditions. For all five algorithms the corresponding set of background correction, normalization, variance stabilization, and log transformation were performed and statistical analyses were carried out. The resulting data sets were exported to Excel file format. Further analysis was done in Excel using a package of self-provided *visual basic for applications* (VBA)-based tools, which we termed *ChipChat*.

3.4.7.1 Chip Chat
By incorporating the whole data derived from the five different preprocessing methods used into our ChipChat tool, we were able to directly compare the five resulting lists of regulated genes. Moreover, the setting of separately changeable thresholds for crucial criteria, such as *P*-values and fold changes, enables widespread analyses and comparisons. Overlaps of lists were calculated and information regarding ranks or percentages of genes that have a proper *P*-value but do not meet the fold-change threshold can be assessed. In the vote for regulated gene expression, the different algorithms could be rated by selectable weightings. A concluding result sheet was then generated representing the calculated expression information of all algorithms for each regulated gene, including the respective fold

changes and *P*-values. For each gene in each comparison, a *regulation index* is calculated based on the number of preprocessing methods that account for the gene to be regulated, the weights given for the respective analysis type, and the direction of regulation. This regulation index offers an excellent capability for fast semiautomated identification of genes that, for example, satisfied specific threshold criteria in at least three of the preprocessing procedures. Additionally, genes comprising similar regulation patterns can be identified. These calculations can be performed with multiple worksheets at once, which enable the user of ChipChat to quickly compare different data sets and further simplifies an informed decision as to which data are reliable.

3.4.7.2 Implemented Thresholds

Using the ANOVA statistical test, we generated additional lists of genes that were significantly regulated at least in one of the analyzed conditions. To specify the time point and experimental condition at which a particular gene is regulated, *t*-tests were applied. Using the information gained from *t*-test cross-comparisons, genes were classified as (1) regulated in response to the injury, (2) boosted by AST, (3) counterregulated due to AST treatment when compared to lesion-only, or (4) exclusively regulated in the AST-treated group (Figure 3.5). The results shown here were acquired using a one-way ANOVA for the 7, 21, and 60 dpo time points (with a *P*-value threshold of 0.02 after GC–RMA and PLIER low-level analysis). The 1 dpo time point contained only two conditions; therefore, *t*-tests were run at *P*-value thresholds of 0.02 and fold-change thresholds of 1.2. At 1 dpo a gene was considered to be regulated if the calculations met the thresholds in at least two of the five low-level analysis methods described, and if one of the fulfilling methods was GC–RMA or PLIER.

3.4.8
Biological Pathways and Ontology Information

Fitting a list of regulated genes to already known pathway maps of biological processes provides an approach toward the understanding of the biological function of the observed gene regulations. Projects like the *Kyoto Encyclopedia of Genes and Genomes* (KEGG database of biological systems; http://www.genome.jp/kegg/) may help to unravel putative molecular interactions and signaling networks. Tools like PathwayArchitect use known connections between genes, and their products elucidate putative functional pathways out of a given group of genes.

In information science, ontology describes a set of individuals and the relationships between these individuals within a domain. In the case of gene ontology (GO) the individuals are different genes that belong to certain classes, such as "cytoskeleton" or "neurotransmitter secretion." Linked by the two relationships *is-a* and *part-of*, these GO classes build a tree-like structure holding information about biological processes, cellular components, and molecular functions in a species-independent manner. While annotation binds biological information to specific genes, ontology provides a framework of structured, controlled vocabulary to do this.

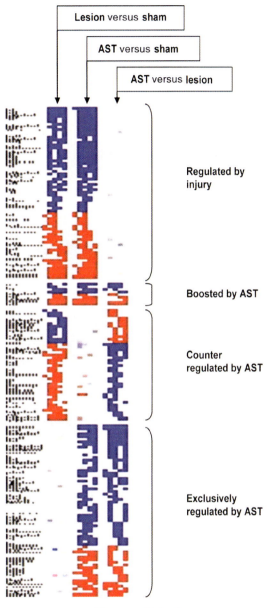

Blue = up   Red = down

Figure 3.5 Heat map of genes sorted for certain regulation profiles. Color indicates direction of regulation; color depth corresponds to *P*-value quality. For each gene in each cross-comparison, the result of every analysis method (in the order: MAS 5, MBEI, PLIER, RMA, GC–RMA) is plotted. For example, genes regulated after injury that are not changed due to AST are clustered at the top of the list. These genes fulfill the rules: significant regulation in the same direction of lesioned-only and treated compared to sham animals and no regulation of treated compared to lesioned-only animals.

Using gene ontology annotation information is a simple way for a high-level analysis of gene functions based on microarray data. Web-based tools such as *David* (http://david.abcc.ncifcrf.gov) or *L2L* (http://depts.washington.edu/l2l/) enable the scientist to identify functional annotations that are significantly enriched in a given list of probe set IDs as described in the following example: imaging a functional group *F* that is represented by 100 genes on a chip with 10 000 different probe sets hitting at least one of the terms in the GO database. By chance, about 1% of the genes in a list of regulated genes belongs to *F*. If the outcome of a virtual array experiment results in a much higher proportion of regulated genes of that functional group *F*, there would be a strong evidence for a possible biological function of that specific group in the analyzed paradigm. One handicap of this procedure is that only one gene list is analyzed at a time. Changes in regulation patterns over time that might not be significant at one specific time point but would deliver significant results when different time points are compared cannot be directly assessed. For a more detailed description of high-level analysis measures see Chapter 1.1x(1)

3.5
Results and Discussion

3.5.1
Expression Patterns

To characterize mRNA expression profiles of sham-operated, lesion-only, and AST-treated adult rats, we identified significantly regulated genes at distinct time points after lesion to classify stage-specific molecular responses over a period of 60 days. Out of 15 000 probe set IDs examined, approximately 2700 probe sets were detected that showed a significant regulation. In spite of the remarkable distance between the lesion site (at thoracic level 8) and the analyzed sensorimotor cortex of several centimeters, 384 significantly regulated probe sets were identified as early as 1 day after CST transection (Figure 3.6). At 1 week, the number of regulated genes remained constant ($\sim$400 regulated IDs; Figure 3.6). At later time points (21 and 60 dpo) the number of regulated genes markedly increased and showed a maximum at 3 weeks after injury (1.117 regulated probe set IDs; Figure 3.6).

When comparing the groups of regulated genes between the different time points examined, we found only small overlaps of regulated genes suggesting distinct time-point-specific injury-induced regulations (Figure 3.6). Never were more than 10% of such genes observed to be regulated at two consecutive time points. Interestingly, not a single gene was regulated over the whole period of 60 days in comparison to sham controls. The observation of distinct injury-induced temporal regulation patterns is in-line with results of previous studies from our laboratory, including an analysis of subicular tissue after fornix transection [81–83].

A comparison of the lesion-only group with the AST-treated group reveals an increase in the proportion of differentially regulated genes over time. At 7 dpo,

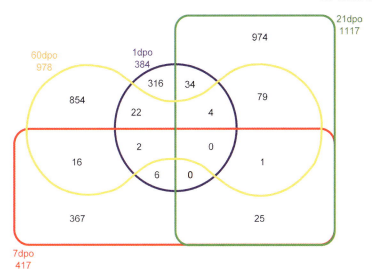

Figure 3.6 Venn diagram showing the overlap of regulated genes
at the four different time points 1 dpo (blue), 7 dpo (red), 21 dpo
(green), and 60 dpo (yellow).

approximately 50% of the detected gene regulations showed differences in their
mRNA expression between sham animals and lesioned animals (lesion-only and
AST-treated) but no changes between lesioned-only and AST-treated animals. At
later time points the proportion of genes showing injury- but not AST-dependent
regulation consistently decreases to approximately 25% at 21 dpo and 20% at 60 dpo
(Figure 3.7). Our observation of increasing divergence in gene regulation indicates
a strong impact of the AST treatment on the transcriptional response of lesion-
affected pyramidal neurons in sensorimotor cortex. The latter cells showed successful axonal regeneration in spinal cord and participation in functional recovery
promoted by AST treatment [2].

When compared to lesion-induced gene regulation, AST-triggered alterations of
gene expression may lead to an even higher expression level of the respective gene
(AST-boosted) or to a counterregulation back to or beyond the basal sham expression
level (AST-counter).

Interestingly, the group of AST-boosted genes comprised a proportion of approximately 10% of the regulated genes at all time points examined (Figure 3.7). In
contrast, the number of AST-counterregulated genes clearly increased over time.
Thus, more than 60% of the gene pool regulated at 60 dpo are AST-counterregulated
genes (Figure 3.7), revealing a significant and long-lasting influence of the expression profile by AST.

This aspect suggests that many of the "normal" lesion-induced cortical reactions
to CST-lesion were reversed by AST. Interestingly, we observed a decrease in the
proportion of AST-specific regulated genes over time. At 7 dpo, approximately 40%
of the regulated genes are AST-specific regulated, whereas at 60 dpo the AST-specific
proportion declined to ~25% (Figure 3.7). These observations revealed an AST-

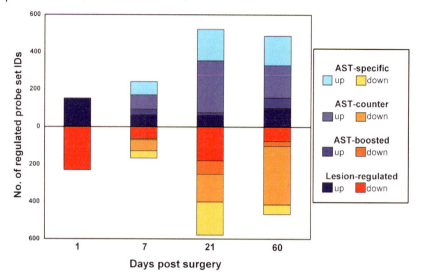

Figure 3.7 Numbers of significantly regulated probe set IDs over time. Four distinct regulation patterns are distinguished: (1) genes regulated in lesion-only and AST-treated compared to sham animals, with no change between lesioned-only and AST-treated animals (lesion-regulated); (2) regulations of genes in lesioned-only compared to sham animals that are significantly stronger, regulated in the same direction as AST animals (AST-boosted); (3) counterregulated by AST back to or beyond sham expression level (AST-counter); (4) genes regulated in AST-treated compared to sham and lesioned-only, but not between lesioned-only and sham animals (AST-specific). In the AST-counter group upregulation stands for a downregulation in lesioned-only compared to sham and an upregulation in AST-treated compared to lesioned-only animals.

promoted adjustment of the late cortical gene expression profile toward the sham profile, which is in-line with the observed capacity of AST-treated animals for axonal regeneration. These findings have also been confirmed by *principal component analysis* (PCA) plots (data not shown).

To understand the processes that were activated after CST-transection and during AST-mediated axonal regeneration, we identified the GO clusters within the time-point-specific groups of regulated genes. Unfortunately, as mentioned above, temporal ontology annotation analyses can hardly be assessed if the compositions of the gene pools show little or no overlap. Therefore, we used a modified approach to evaluate changes in functional gene classes by assessing the number of regulated genes at each time point that fit to a given set of ontology classes. To avoid stochastic effects, ontologies that were not well represented on the array were not considered. We screened for regulated genes that were associated with the generic terms "survival/cell death" and "differentiation/regeneration" (Figure 3.8).

To our surprise, the number of genes associated with survival/cell death showed an oscillatory profile with a steady increase from 7 to 60 dpo (Figure 3.8). In-depth analysis of known functional roles of regulated genes revealed a high proportion of stress–response-related genes in the GO classes of survival/cell death at 1 dpo, while at later time points an increasing number of apoptotic and antiapoptotic genes

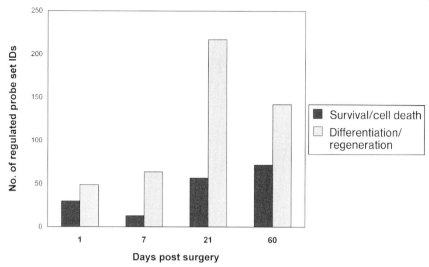

Figure 3.8 Numbers of regulated probe set IDs matching ontology classes associated with survival/cell death or differentiation/ regeneration.

were regulated. In contrast, the number of genes associated with differentiation/ regeneration peaked at 21 days postlesion.

Further evaluation with particular consideration of the direction of regulation revealed that survival/cell death associated genes were mainly downregulated at 21 days after injury in both lesion-only and AST-treated gene pools (Figure 3.9). However, we observed a general switch from a status of downregulation at 21 dpo to a predominant status of upregulation of the genes at 60 dpo. This suggests that the stage-specific distinct regulation patterns described above are dissimilar not only with respect to the regulated genes but also in the general direction of regulation of functional groups of genes.

The differentiation/regeneration associated GO group showed an expression profile that differs from the GO classes of survival/cell death associated genes. The lesioned-only animals illustrated a less pronounced regulation profile, and the numbers of upregulated and downregulated genes presented a peak at 21 dpo. In contrast, in AST-treated animals the examination of the affected sensorimotor cortex revealed that the numbers of upregulated genes that were associated with the GO classes differentiation/regeneration continuously increased over time (Figure 3.9). This cumulative induction of differentiation/regeneration associated genes coincides with the observed axonal regeneration of CST fibers in the injured spinal cord following AST treatment.

As shown in Figure 3.10, the progression of survival/cell death associated gene regulations after AST treatment were mainly caused by an increase in AST-counterregulated and AST-specific-regulated genes, reflecting a distinct AST-mediated cell survival-promoting switch in the injury-induced gene regulation program of these GO classes. Interestingly, the predominant effect of AST to the

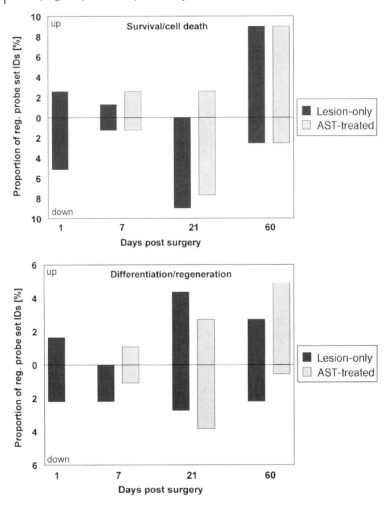

Figure 3.9 Direction of regulation of genes matching ontology classes associated with survival/cell death and differentiation/ regeneration. Percentages of the total number of probe set IDs in ontology classes sets are plotted.

regulation of the differentiation/regeneration associated genes is different (Figure 3.10). This latter functional gene group mainly showed a continuous increase in the AST-boosted genes, whereas the proportion of AST-counterregulated genes continuously declines and the proportion of AST-specific genes remains constant (Figure 3.10). Our observations indicate that the normal transection-induced genetic programs of affected cortical cells involving survival/cell death-related genes are mainly counteracted, whereas gene programs facilitating cell differentiation/regeneration are consolidated in AST-treated animals to promote axonal regeneration.

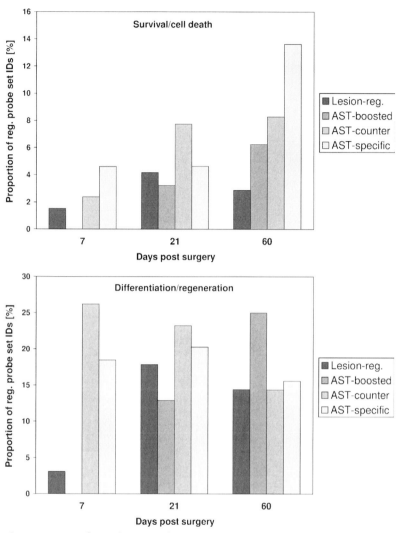

Figure 3.10 AST-influenced gene regulations. Diagrammed are the percentages of regulated genes matching the ontology sets of classes of survival/cell death and differentiation/regeneration compared to the time-point- and regulation-pattern-specific total regulated probe set numbers.

3.5.2
Summary

We have applied gene microarray profiling as a molecular systemic approach to investigate transcriptional responses of primary motor neurons in the sensorimotor cortex of adult rat following axotomy of the corticospinal tract in thoracic spinal cord.

In addition, we have applied a pharmacological treatment recently developed in our laboratory to promote axon regeneration and to improve functional recovery. Comparison of gene expression profiles between sham, lesioned-only and treated animals clearly revealed treatment-specific genetic programs. With respect to the transcriptional profiles of genes with functions related to (1) survival/cell death and (2) differentiation/regeneration distinct stage-specific alterations in the genetic program could be detected. Furthermore, while the lesion-induced changes in survival/cell death-related gene expression are counteracted by the regeneration-promoting treatment, the gene programs facilitating cell differentiation and regeneration are largely consolidated by the treatment.

Acknowledgments

The authors would like to thank C. Vogelaar for critical reading of the manuscript, and the Deutsche Forschungsgemeinschaft (SFB 590, C2) and the Deutsche Stiftung Querschnittlähmung for financial support to H.W. Müller.

References

1 Klapka, N. and Muller, H.W. (2006) Collagen matrix in spinal cord injury. *Journal of Neurotrauma*, **23**, 422–436.

2 Klapka, N., Hermanns, S., Straten, G., Masanneck, C., Duis, S., Hamers, F.P., Muller, D., Zuschratter, W. and Muller, H.W. (2005) Suppression of fibrous scarring in spinal cord injury of rat promotes long-distance regeneration of corticospinal tract axons, rescue of primary motoneurons in somatosensory cortex and significant functional recovery. *The European Journal of Neuroscience*, **22**, 3047–3058.

3 Hains, B.C., Black, J.A. and Waxman, S.G. (2003) Primary cortical motor neurons undergo apoptosis after axotomizing spinal cord injury. *The Journal of Comparative Neurology*, **462**, 328–341.

4 Stichel, C.C., Niermann, H., D'Urso, D., Lausberg, F., Hermanns, S. and Müller, H.W. (1999) Basal membrane-depleted scar in lesioned CNS: characteristics and relationships with regenerating axons. *Neuroscience*, **93**, 321–333.

5 Hermanns, S., Reiprich, P. and Müller, H.W. (2001) A reliable method to reduce collagen scar formation in the lesioned rat spinal cord. *Journal of Neuroscience Methods*, **110**, 141–146.

6 Hermanns, S. and Müller, H.W. (2001) Preservation and detection of lesion-induced collagenous scar in the CNS depend on the method of tissue processing. *Brain Research. Brain Research Protocols*, **7**, 162–167.

7 Morgenstern, D.A., Asher, R.A. and Fawcett, J.W. (2002) Chondroitin sulphate proteoglycans in the CNS injury response. *Progress in Brain Research*, **137**, 313–332.

8 Silver, J. and Miller, J.H. (2004) Regeneration beyond the glial scar. *Nature Reviews. Neuroscience*, **5**, 146–156.

9 Davies, J.E., Tang, X., Denning, J.W., Archibald, S.J. and Davies, S.J. (2004) Decorin suppresses neurocan, brevican, phosphacan and NG2 expression and promotes axon growth across adult rat spinal cord injuries. *The European Journal of Neuroscience*, **19**, 1226–1242.

10 Jones, L.L., Yamaguchi, Y., Stallcup, W.B. and Tuszynski, M.H. (2002) NG2 is a major chondroitin sulfate proteoglycan produced after spinal cord injury and is expressed by macrophages and oligo-dendrocyte progenitors. *Journal of Neuroscience*, **22**, 2792–2803.

11 Hasegawa, K., Chang, Y.W., Li, H., Berlin, Y., Ikeda, O., Kane-Goldsmith, N. and Grumet, M. (2005) Embryonic radial glia bridge spinal cord lesions and promote functional recovery following spinal cord injury. *Experimental Neurology*, **193**, 394–410.

12 Mey, J., Morassutti, J., Brook, G., Liu, R.H., Zhang, Y.P., Koopmans, G. and McCaffery, P. (2005) Retinoic acid synthesis by a population of NG2-positive cells in the injured spinal cord. *The European Journal of Neuroscience*, **21**, 1555–1568.

13 Jones, L.L., Margolis, R.U. and Tuszynski, M.H. (2003) The chondroitin sulfate proteoglycans neurocan, brevican, phos-phacan, and versican are differentially regulated following spinal cord injury. *Experimental Neurology*, **182**, 399–411.

14 De Winter, F., Oudega, M., Lankhorst, A.J., Hamers, F.P., Blits, B., Ruitenberg, M.J., Pasterkamp, R.J., Gispen, W.H. and Verhaagen, J. (2002) Injury-induced class 3 semaphorin expression in the rat spinal cord. *Experimental Neurology*, **175**, 61–75.

15 Niclou, S.P., Franssen, E.H., Ehlert, E.M., Taniguchi, M. and Verhaagen, J. (2003) Meningeal cell-derived semaphorin 3A inhibits neurite outgrowth. *Molecular and Cellular Neurosciences*, **24**, 902–912.

16 Bundesen, L.Q., Scheel, T.A., Bregman, B.S. and Kromer, L.F. (2003) Ephrin-B2 and EphB2 regulation of astrocyte-meningeal fibroblast interactions in response to spinal cord lesions in adult rats. *Journal of Neuroscience*, **23**, 7789–7800.

17 Berry, M., Maxwell, W.L., Logan, A., Mathewson, A., McConnell, P., Ashhurst, D.E. and Thomas, G.H. (1983) Deposition of scar tissue in the central nervous system. *Acta Neurochirurgica. Supplement (Wien)*, **32**, 31–53.

18 Liesi, P. and Kauppila, T. (2002) Induction of type IV collagen and other basement-membrane-associated proteins after spinal cord injury of the adult rat may participate in formation of the glial scar. *Experimental Neurology*, **173**, 31–45.

19 Schwab, J.M., Beschorner, R., Nguyen, T.D., Meyermann, R. and Schluesener, H.J. (2001) Differential cellular accu-mulation of connective tissue growth factor defines a subset of reactive astro-cytes, invading fibroblasts, and endot-helial cells following central nervous system injury in rats and humans. *Journal of Neurotrauma*, **18**, 377–388.

20 Stichel, C.C. and Müller, H.W. (1998) The CNS lesion scar: new vistas on an old regeneration barrier. *Cell and Tissue Research*, **294**, 1–9.

21 Stichel, C.C., Hermanns, S., Luhmann, H.J., Lausberg, F., Niermann, H., D'Urso, D., Servos, G., Hartwig, H.G. and Müller, H.W. (1999) Inhibition of collagen IV deposition promotes regeneration of injured CNS axons. *The European Journal of Neuroscience*, **11**, 632–646.

22 Shearer, M.C. and Fawcett, J.W. (2001) The astrocyte/meningeal cell interface – a barrier to successful nerve regeneration? *Cell and Tissue Research*, **305**, 267–273.

23 Davies, S.J., Fitch, M.T., Memberg, S.P., Hall, A.K., Raisman, G. and Silver, J. (1997) Regeneration of adult axons in white matter tracts of the central nervous system. *Nature*, **390**, 680–683.

24 Iseda, T., Nishio, T., Kawaguchi, S., Kawasaki, T. and Wakisaka, S. (2003) Spontaneous regeneration of the corticospinal tract after transection in young rats: collagen type IV deposition and astrocytic scar in the lesion site are not the cause but the effect of failure of regeneration. *The Journal of Comparative Neurology*, **464**, 343–355.

25 Kawano, H., Li, H.P., Sango, K., Kawamura, K. and Raisman, G. (2005)

Inhibition of collagen synthesis overrides the age-related failure of regeneration of nigrostriatal dopaminergic axons. *Journal of Neuroscience Research*, **80**, 191–202.

26 Duncan, M.R., Frazier, K.S., Abramson, S., Williams, S., Klapper, H., Huang, X. and Grotendorst, G.R. (1999) Connective tissue growth factor mediates transforming growth factor beta-induced collagen synthesis: down-regulation by cAMP. *FASEB Journal*, **13**, 1774–1786.

27 Hermanns, S., Klapka, N. and Müller, H.W. (2001) The collagenous lesion scar – an obstacle for axonal regeneration in brain and spinal cord injury. *Restorative Neurology and Neuroscience*, **19**, 139–148.

28 Youdim, M.B., Fridkin, M. and Zheng, H. (2004) Novel bifunctional drugs targeting monoamine oxidase inhibition and iron chelation as an approach to neuroprotection in Parkinson's disease and other neurodegenerative diseases. *Journal of Neural Transmission*, **111**, 1455–1471.

29 Beattie, M.S., Farooqui, A.A. and Bresnahan, J.C. (2000) Review of current evidence for apoptosis after spinal cord injury. *Journal of Neurotrauma*, **17**, 915–925.

30 Beattie, M.S., Hermann, G.E., Rogers, R.C. and Bresnahan, J.C. (2002) Cell death in models of spinal cord injury. *Progress in Brain Research*, **137**, 37–47.

31 Park, E., Velumian, A.A. and Fehlings, M.G. (2004) The role of excitotoxicity in secondary mechanisms of spinal cord injury: a review with an emphasis on the implications for white matter degeneration. *Journal of Neurotrauma*, **21**, 754–774.

32 Hunt, D., Coffin, R.S. and Anderson, P.N. (2002) The Nogo receptor, its ligands and axonal regeneration in the spinal cord; a review. *Journal of Neurocytology*, **31**, 93–120.

33 McKerracher, L. and Winton, M.J. (2002) Nogo on the go. *Neuron*, **36**, 345–348.

34 Basso, D.M., Beattie, M.S. and Bresnahan, J.C. (1995) A sensitive and reliable locomotor rating scale for open field testing in rats. *Journal of Neurotrauma*, **12**, 1–21.

35 Metz, G.A., Merkler, D., Dietz, V., Schwab, M.E. and Fouad, K. (2000) Efficient testing of motor function in spinal cord injured rats. *Brain Research*, **883**, 165–177.

36 Hamers, F.P.T., Lankhorst, A.J., Van Laar, T.J., Veldhuis, W.B. and Gispen, W.H. (2001) Automated quantitative gait analysis during overground locomotion in the rat: its application to spinal cord contusion and transection injuries. *Journal of Neurotrauma*, **18**, 187–201.

37 Lockhart, D.J., Dong, H., Byrne, M.C., Follettie, M.T., Gallo, M.V., Chee, M.S., Mittmann, M., Wang, C., Kobayashi, M., Horton, H. and Brown, E.L. (1996) Expression monitoring by hybridization to high-density oligonucleotide arrays. *Nature Biotechnology*, **14**, 1675–1680.

38 Lipshutz, R.J., Fodor, S.P., Gingeras, T.R. and Lockhart, D.J. (1999) High density synthetic oligonucleotide arrays. *Nature Genetics*, **21**, 20–24.

39 Affymetrix. www.affymetrix.com.

40 Churchill, G.A. (2002) Fundamentals of experimental design for cDNA microarrays. *Nature Genetics*, **32** (Suppl.), 490–495.

41 Spruill, S.E., Lu, J., Hardy, S. and Weir, B. (2002) Assessing sources of variability in microarray gene expression data. *Biotechniques*, **33**, 916–920.

42 Whitney, A.R., Diehn, M., Popper, S.J., Alizadeh, A.A., Boldrick, J.C., Relman, D.A. and Brown, P.O. (2003) Individuality and variation in gene expression patterns in human blood. *Proceedings of the National Academy of Sciences of the United States of America*, **100**, 1896–1901.

43 Molloy, M.P., Brzezinski, E.E., Hang, J., McDowell, M.T. and VanBogelen, R.A. (2003) Overcoming technical variation and biological variation in quantitative proteomics. *Proteomics*, **3**, 1912–1919.

44 Oleksiak, M.F., Churchill, G.A. and Crawford, D.L. (2002) Variation in gene expression within and among natural populations. *Nature Genetics*, **32**, 261–266.

45 Hartemink, A.J., Gifford, D.K., Jaakkola, T.S. and Young, R.A. (2001) Maximum likelihood estimation of optimal scaling factors for expression array normalization. *Proceedings of SPIE*, 4266, 132–140.

46 Bakay, M., Chen, Y.W., Borup, R., Zhao, P., Nagaraju, K. and Hoffman, E.P. (2002) Sources of variability and effect of experimental approach on expression profiling data interpretation. *BMC Bioinformatics*, **3**, 4.

47 Brown, J.S., Kuhn, D., Wisser, R., Power, E. and Schnell, R. (2004) Quantification of sources of variation and accuracy of sequence discrimination in a replicated microarray experiment. *Biotechniques*, **36**, 324–332.

48 Dumur, C.I., Nasim, S., Best, A.M., Archer, K.J., Ladd, A.C., Mas, V.R., Wilkinson, D.S., Garrett, C.T. and Ferreira-Gonzalez, A. (2004) Evaluation of quality-control criteria for microarray gene expression analysis. *Clinical Chemistry*, **50**, 1994–2002.

49 Hariharan, R. (2003) The analysis of microarray data. *Pharmacogenomics*, **4**, 477–497.

50 Pan, W., Lin, J. and Le, C.T. (2002) How many replicates of arrays are required to detect gene expression changes in microarray experiments? A mixture model approach. *Genome Biology*, **3**, research0022. Epub, Apr 22, 2002.

51 Seo, J., Gordish-Dressman, H. and Hoffman, E.P. (2006) An interactive power analysis tool for microarray hypothesis testing and generation. *Bioinformatics*, **22**, 808–814.

52 Churchill, G.A. and Oliver, B. (2001) Sex flies and microarrays. *Nature Genetics*, **29**, 355–356.

53 Simon, R.M. and Dobbin, K. (2003) Experimental design of DNA microarray experiments. *Biotechniques*, **34** (3) (Suppl.), 16–21.

54 Kendziorski, C., Irizarry, R.A., Chen, K.S., Haag, J.D. and Gould, M.N. (2005) On the utility of pooling biological samples in microarray experiments. *Proceedings of the National Academy of Sciences of the United States of America*, **102**, 4252–4257.

55 Kendziorski, C.M., Zhang, Y., Lan, H. and Attie, A.D. (2003) The efficiency of pooling mRNA in microarray experiments. *Biostatistics*, **4**, 465–477.

56 Shih, J.H., Michalowska, A.M., Dobbin, K., Ye, Y., Qiu, T.H. and Green, J.E. (2004) Effects of pooling mRNA in microarray class comparisons. *Bioinformatics*, **20**, 3318–3325.

57 Bolstad, B.M., Irizarry, R.A., Astrand, M. and Speed, T.P. (2003) A comparison of normalization methods for high density oligonucleotide array data based on variance and bias. *Bioinformatics*, **19**, 185–193.

58 Irizarry, R.A., Wu, Z. and Jaffee, H.A. (2006) Comparison of Affymetrix GeneChip expression measures. *Bioinformatics*, **22**, 789–794.

59 Naef, F., Hacker, C.R., Patil, N. and Magnasco, M. (2002) Empirical characterization of the expression ratio noise structure in high-density oligonucleotide arrays. *Genome Biology*, **3**, research0018. Epub, Mar 22, 2002.

60 Bolstad, B.M., Collin, F., Simpson, K.M., Irizarry, R.A. and Speed, T.P. (2004) Experimental design and low-level analysis of microarray data. *International Review of Neurobiology*, **60**, 25–58.

61 Irizarry, R.A., Hobbs, B., Collin, F., Beazer-Barclay, Y.D., Antonellis, K.J., Scherf, U. and Speed, T.P. (2003) Exploration, normalization, and summaries of high density oligonucleotide array probe level data. *Biostatistics*, **4**, 249–264.

62 Millenaar, F.F., Okyere, J., May, S.T., van, Z.M., Voesenek, L.A. and Peeters, A.J. (2006) How to decide? Different methods of calculating gene expression from short oligonucleotide array data will give different results. *BMC Bioinformatics*, **7**, 137.

63 Wu, Z. and Irizarry, R.A. (2005) Stochastic models inspired by hybridization theory for short oligonucleotide arrays. *Journal of Computational Biology*, **12**, 882–893.

64 Cope, L.M., Irizarry, R.A., Jaffee, H.A., Wu, Z. and Speed, T.P. (2004) A benchmark for Affymetrix GeneChip expression measures. *Bioinformatics*, **20**, 323–331.

65 Barash, Y., Dehan, E., Krupsky, M., Franklin, W., Geraci, M., Friedman, N. and Kaminski, N. (2004) Comparative analysis of algorithms for signal quantitation from oligonucleotide microarrays. *Bioinformatics*, **20**, 839–846.

66 Seo, J., Bakay, M., Chen, Y.W., Hilmer, S., Shneiderman, B. and Hoffman, E.P. (2004) Interactively optimizing signal-to-noise ratios in expression profiling: project-specific algorithm selection and detection *p*-value weighting in Affymetrix microarrays. *Bioinformatics*, **20**, 2534–2544.

67 Choe, S.E., Boutros, M., Michelson, A.M., Church, G.M. and Halfon, M.S. (2005) Preferred analysis methods for Affymetrix GeneChips revealed by a wholly defined control dataset. *Genome Biology*, **6**, R16.

68 Hill, A.A., Brown, E.L., Whitley, M.Z., Tucker-Kellogg, G., Hunter, C.P. and Slonim, D.K. (2001) Evaluation of normalization procedures for oligonucleotide array data based on spiked cRNA controls. *Genome Biology*, **2**, research0055. Epub. Nov 21, 2001.

69 Schadt, E.E., Li, C., Ellis, B. and Wong, W.H. (2001) Feature extraction and normalization algorithms for high-density oligonucleotide gene expression array data. *Journal of Cellular Biochemistry Supplement*, (Suppl.) 37, 120–125.

70 Shedden, K., Chen, W., Kuick, R., Ghosh, D., Macdonald, J., Cho, K.R., Giordano, T.J., Gruber, S.B., Fearon, E.R., Taylor, J.M. and Hanash, S. (2005) Comparison of seven methods for producing Affymetrix expression scores based on false discovery rates in disease profiling data. *BMC Bioinformatics*, **6**, 26.

71 Qin, L.X., Beyer, R.P., Hudson, F.N., Linford, N.J., Morris, D.E. and Kerr, K.F. (2006) Evaluation of methods for oligo-nucleotide array data via quantitative real-time PCR. *BMC Bioinformatics*, **7**, 23.

72 Seo, J. and Hoffman, E.P. (2006) Probe set algorithms: is there a rational best bet? *BMC Bioinformatics*, **7**, 395.

73 Affymetrix. Statistical Algorithms Reference Guide. (2001)

74 Li, C. and Wong, W.H. (2001) Model-based analysis of oligonucleotide arrays: expression index computation and outlier detection. *Proceedings of the National Academy of Sciences of the United States of America*, **98**, 31–36.

75 Irizarry, R.A., Gautier, L. and Cope, L. (2003) An R package for analysis of Affymetrix oligonucleotide arrays. *The Analysis of Gene Expression Data: Methods and Software*, Springer, Berlin, pp. 102–119.

76 Holder, D., Raubertas, R.F., Pikounis, V.B., Svetnik, V. and Soper, K. (2001) Statistical analysis of high density oligonucleotide arrays: a SAFER approach. *Proceedings of the ASA Annual Meeting*, 2001.

77 Irizarry, R.A., Bolstad, B.M., Collin, F., Cope, L.M., Hobbs, B. and Speed, T.P. (2003) Summaries of Affymetrix GeneChip probe level data. *Nucleic Acids Research*, **31**, e15.

78 Wu, Z., Irizarry, R., Gentleman, R., Murillo, F. and Spencer, F. (2003) A Model Based Background Adjustment for Oligonucleotide Expression Arrays. Technical Report John Hopkins University, Department of Biostatistics Working Papers, Baltimore.

79 Naef, F. and Magnasco, M.O. (2003) Solving the riddle of the bright mismatches: labeling and effective binding in oligonucleotide arrays. *Physical Review – E, Statistical, Nonlinear, and Soft Matter Physics*, **68**, research011906. Epub, Jul 16, 2003.

80 Affymetrix.Guide to Probe Logarithmic Intensity Error (PLIER) Estimation. (2005)

81 Abankwa, D., Kury, P. and Muller, H.W. (2002) Dynamic changes in gene

expression profiles following axotomy of projection fibres in the mammalian CNS. *Molecular and Cellular Neurosciences*, **21**, 421–435.

82 Abankwa, D. and Kury, P. (2004) Traumatic injury to CNS fiber tracts – what are the genes telling us? *Current Drug Targets*, **5**, 647–654.

83 Kury, P., Abankwa, D., Kruse, F., Greiner-Petter, R. and Muller, H.W. (2004) Gene expression profiling reveals multiple novel intrinsic and extrinsic factors associated with axonal regeneration failure. *The European Journal of Neuroscience*, **19**, 32–42.

4

Unraveling Plasticity of Dorsal Root Ganglion and Spinal Cord Neurons Using cDNA Arrays

Xu Zhang, Hua-Sheng Xiao, and Lan Bao

Peripheral nerve injury can cause neuropathic pain. The nerve injury induced phenotypic changes in gene expression in dorsal root ganglion (DRG) and the dorsal horn of the spinal cord contribute to the generation and development of neuropathic pain. In early days, the changes in gene expression of individual molecules, such as neuropeptides and neurotransmitter receptors, were analyzed in rats after a complete transection of the sciatic nerve, which resulted in robust and reproducible effects. Notably, these studies were mainly carried out with immunohistochemistry, *in situ* hybridization, and other methods [1,2]. However, the limiting factor with these methods is the lack of global view of the modified gene expression. Most of the analyzed genes were selected from the genes that are normally expressed in DRGs or spinal cord at various levels. Recent gene array studies have been carried out to identify the regulated genes at the spinal cord level after peripheral nerve injury. The findings of the marked changes in gene expression in both DRG and the dorsal horn of spinal cord indicate that the gene array appears to be a powerful approach to gain a global view of the changes in the gene expression in the pain pathways [3,4].

Complementary DNA (cDNA) array technology is one of the array techniques that have been used to analyze the gene expression profiles. It is based on the specific binding of transcripts from tissue samples to a library of probes, which can be generated by using PCR-amplified inserts of clones isolated from cDNA libraries, immobilized in an orderly array on a solid support such as nylon membranes or glass slides. Thus, the array consists of thousands of probes with known identity by virtue of its position within the array. This is a very sensitive array method especially for the genes expressed at low levels in the tissues, such as receptors for neurotransmitters and ion channels in DRG and spinal cord. In general, PCR and other techniques are often required to confirm the results of cDNA array. To address potential roles of the regulated molecules in either physiology or pathology of neural circuits, cellular localization of the molecules should be carried out by *in situ* hybridization and immunostaining. The results would provide a basis for further physiological or pharmacological studies. In the following sections, we will introduce the progress in cDNA array analysis of gene expression in DRG and dorsal

Neural Degeneration and Repair: Gene Expression Profiling, Proteomics, and Systems Biology
Edited by Hans Werner Müller
Copyright © 2008 WILEY-VCH Verlag GmbH & Co. KGaA, Weinheim
ISBN: 978-3-527-31707-3

spinal cord after peripheral nerve injury, with an expansion of the functional significance of some of the regulated molecules.

4.1
Identification of Regulated Molecules in DRG After Peripheral Nerve Injury

In 2002, Xiao *et al*. [5] published their work with a cDNA array made of 7523 genes and expressed sequence tags (ESTs) mainly from the cDNA libraries of lumbar DRGs of normal rats and the rats 14 days after sciatic nerve transection. Using a twofold change in normal signal intensity as the cutoff line, Xiao *et al*. identified a total of 122 genes and 51 ESTs that are strongly regulated in DRGs in a 2–28-day time course after peripheral nerve injury. In this cDNA array study, 50% of the markedly regulated genes are related to neurotransmission, including neuropeptides, receptors, channels, synaptic proteins, and signal transduction molecules. The regulated expression levels in 80% of these genes were maintained over 28 days, indicating their involvement in the maintenance of the pain. Interestingly, using oligonucleotide microarray, Nilsson *et al*. examined the changes in gene expression in DRGs within 24 hours and found that more transcription factors are regulated [6]. The published data suggest that more receptors, ion channels, and other membrane proteins are identified by the cDNA array than that shown with the oligonucleotide microarray [7–9]. This is consistent with the notion that the cDNA array could be more sensitive for detecting the membrane proteins that are generally expressed at relatively low levels. However, notice that many genes in the list remain to be further studied at the cellular level by *in situ* hybridization and immunohistochemistry.

4.1.1
Neuropeptides and Neuropeptide Receptors

Following peripheral nerve injury, the expression of neuropeptides is strongly altered. Early studies using immunohistochemistry and *in situ* hybridization demonstrated that the expression of several neuropeptides had changed after peripheral nerve injury [1]. The cDNA array confirms that in the rat DRGs, the expression of substance P and calcitonin gene-related peptide is reduced in small DRG neurons, whereas galanin in small neurons and neuropeptide Y (NPY) in large neurons are markedly upregulated (Tables 4.1 and 4.2). However, the regulation of these neuropeptides is so strong that cDNA array might not be much better than other methods to find these regulated neuropeptides. It has to pointed out that galanin is the only neuropeptide that has been found to be markedly upregulated in both monkey and rat [10–12]. In addition to its neurotrophic actions such as promoting neurite outgrowth [12–14], both pro- and antinociceptive effects of galanin have been reported in the rodent, probably via activating different types of galanin receptors [15,16].

The cDNA array also confirms that several neuropeptide receptors are significantly regulated after peripheral nerve injury (Figure 4.1; Tables 4.1 and 4.2). NPY Y1

Table 4.1 Selected upregulated genes in rat DRG after peripheral nerve injury.

Neuropeptides	
Galanin	↑↑↑
Neuropeptide Y	↑↑↑
Vasoactive intestinal polypeptide	↑↑↑
Receptors	
GABA$_A$ receptor α5	↑
Nicotinic acetylcholine receptor α7	↑
Adrenergic receptor α2A	↑
P2Y1 receptor	↑
Peripheral benzodiazepine receptor	↑
Neuropeptide Y Y2 receptor	↑
Neuropeptide Y Y5 receptor	↑
Cholecystokinin $_B$ receptor	↑
Glial cell line-derived neurotrophic factor receptor α	↑
Channels	
Na$^+$ channel β2 subunit	↑
Na$^+$ channel III (Na$_v$1.3)	↑
Ca^{2+} channel α2/δ1 subunit	↑↑
Signal transduction molecules	
Neuronal nitric oxide synthase	↑↑
Tyrosin phosphatase	↑↑
Tyrosine kinase	↑
Synaptic transmission	
Synaptotagmin IV	↑
Others	
Class II MHC α chain RT1.D	↑
Class II MHC β chain RT1.D	↑
Brain prostaglandin D synthase	↑

↑↑↑ >10-fold increase, ↑↑ 10–5-fold increase, ↑ five- to twofold increase.

receptor and μ-opioid receptor are downregulated, while NPY Y2 and Y5 receptors and cholecystokinin (CCK) B receptor are upregulated. The CCK B receptor and NPY Y2 receptor are reported to mediate an increase in excitability of axotomized neurons [17,18]. The decrease in inhibitory μ-opioid receptor and NPY Y1 receptor could contribute to the disinhibition of DRG neurons. Since CCK is known as an endogenous inhibitor of opioid-induced analgesia [19], upregulation of CCK, CCK B receptor, and downregulation of μ-opioid receptor in DRG neurons could contribute to the reduction in the efficacy of morphine in neuropathic pain treatment.

4.1.2
Molecules Related to Synaptic Transmission

Modification of the molecular machinery for synaptic transmission in afferent terminals could contribute to the mechanism of neuropathic pain. cDNA array

Table 4.2 Selected downregulated genes in rat DRG after peripheral nerve injury.

Neuropeptides	
Calcitonin gene-related peptide	↓
Substance P	↓
Receptors	
Adrenergic α2B receptor	↓
Metabotropic glutamate receptor 4	↓
μ-Opioid receptor	↓
Neuropeptide Y Y1 receptor	↓
Channels	
Na^+ channel (SNS) ($Na_v1.8$)	↓
K^+ channel 11 (inward rectifier)	↓
K^+ channel RCK4 subunit	↓
Signal transduction molecules	
Neuronal visinin-like Ca^{2+} binding protein	↓
Phospholipase C δ4	↓
ras-related protein 3a	↓
Synaptic transmission	
Vesicle-associated membrane protein-1	↓
Synaptosomal-associated protein 25 kDa	↓
Synaptic vesicle protein 2B	↓

↓ 0.5- to 0.2-fold decrease.

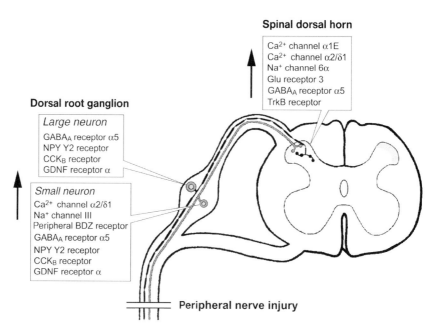

Figure 4.1 The representative receptors and ion channels that are markedly upregulated in the dorsal root ganglion and the dorsal horn of spinal cord of rat after peripheral nerve axotomy.

studies show that the expression of 12 vesicle-associated molecules is strongly changed in rat DRG after peripheral nerve injury [5]. Expression of synaptosomal-associated protein 25 kDa (SNAP-25), synaptic vesicle protein 2B, and vesicle-associated membrane protein 1 (VAMP-1) is downregulated in DRGs after peripheral nerve injury, indicating that the process of docking and fusion of synaptic vesicles could be significantly modified. *In situ* hybridization shows that SNAP-25 and VAMP-1 are normally expressed in large DRG neurons [20], suggesting that the reduction in these proteins might contribute to the modification of the synaptic transmission of Aβ fibers. What are the molecules involved in synaptic transmission of C fibers? The cDNA and immunohistochemistry show that synaptoporin is a major synaptic vesicle protein in nociceptive afferents in both physiological and neuropathic pain states. Synaptoporin and synaptophysin are integral membrane components of synaptic vesicles. Synaptoporin is expressed in subsets of small neurons that contain either neuropeptides or isolectin B4 and is distributed in their afferent terminals in laminae I–II of the spinal cord [20]. Peripheral nerve injury increases synaptoporin expression in small DRG neurons and synaptoporin level in their afferent terminals. However, how synaptoporin is involved in the modulation of synaptic transmission remains unclear.

4.1.3
Neurotransmitter Receptors and Ion Channels

It is known that the stimulus-induced release of the excitatory neurotransmitters from afferent terminals is regulated by intrinsic inhibitory neurons in the dorsal horn of the spinal cord, such as γ-aminobutyric acid (GABA) expressing neurons. GABA$_A$ receptor, known as the central benzodiazepine (BDZ) receptor, is a GABA/drug receptor–Cl$^-$ channel macromolecular complex including binding sites for GABA and BDZs. The BDZs increase the affinity of GABA$_A$ receptor for GABA and the frequency of opening of the Cl$^-$ channel. After peripheral nerve injury, GABA$_A$ receptor α5 subunit is upregulated (Figure 4.1; Table 4.1), which might lead to a formation of the receptor containing α5. In addition, peripheral-type BDZ receptor, a BDZ receptor that is not expressed in normal DRG neurons, is expressed in small DRG neurons after peripheral nerve injury. Since GABA is decreased in the dorsal horn [21], and so far there is no evidence of the presence of an endogenous agonist for peripheral BDZ receptor at the spinal level, administration of exogenous ligands is needed to activate these upregulated receptors. Moreover, expression of nicotinic acetylcholine receptor (nACh) α7, P2Y1 receptor, and adrenergic receptor α2A is also found to be upregulated.

It could be expected that changes in the expression of ion channels would contribute to altered neural excitability. The cDNA array shows a transient upregulation of voltage-dependent Ca^{2+} channel α2/δ1 subunit in DRG neurons (Figure 4.1; Table 4.1). Voltage-dependent Ca^{2+} channels contain three subunits: the α1 channel-forming subunit, the intracellular β subunit, and the α2 subunit consisting of two disulfide-lined polypeptides (α2/δ). The α2/δ1 is thought to increase the current amplitude and activation rate of Ca^{2+} channels. Thus, transient increase of Ca^{2+}

channel α2/δ1 in small DRG neurons suggests an effect on the increased excitability during the early postlesion period. Voltage-gated Na$^+$ channels consist of a pore-forming α subunit and one or more auxiliary β subunits. The Na$^+$ channel β1 and β2 are involved in targeting Na$^+$ channel α subunits to the cell surface [22]. Expression of both Na$^+$ channel III α subunit (Na$_v$1.3) and β2 subunit is increased following peripheral nerve injury. In contrast, K$^+$ channels are generally downregulated (Table 4.2). Therefore, these changes in expression of ion channels may contribute to the increased excitability of sensory neurons.

4.1.4
Molecules for Survival or Regulating Gene Expression

Upregulation of the molecules for survival is consistent with the fact that damaged peripheral nerve can be regenerated. Nilsson *et al.* found that a number of transcription factors or regulatory elements are upregulated in DRGs within 24 hours following peripheral nerve injury [6], including c-Fos, activating transcription factor-3, and Kruppel-like factor 6. Some early upregulated genes are related to transforming growth factor-beta (TGF-β) signaling, such as TGF-β I receptor, follistatin, TG-interacting factor, SMAD-1, and PAI-1. Xiao *et al.* identified that the transcription factor Jun-D and eukaryotic initiation factor-4E, a translation initiation factor having an important role in cell growth and differentiation [23], are upregulated 2 days after peripheral nerve injury [5]. Heat shock protein 27, endoplasmic reticular stress protein, and several growth-associated proteins such as growth-associated protein 43 (GAP-43), nerve growth factor (NGF) inducible protein, growth arrest and DNA damage inducible protein 45, glypican, basic fibroblast growth factor (bFGF), FGF-7 and superior cervical ganglion 10 and brain-derived neurotrophic factor (BDNF) are upregulated. In parallel with the upregulation of glial cell line derived neurotrophic factor (GDNF), the expression of GDNF receptor (GDNFR-α) is increased in small neurons [24] (Figure 4.1; Table 4.1). It has been suggested that GDNF activates a transcriptional program repressing neurite growth in DRG [25]. Upregulation of various tyrosine kinases and tyrosine phosphotases may be involved in virtually every function of neurons, including survival, extension of axons, and synapse formation. The dynamic changes of gene expression ranging from transcriptional factors to structural proteins may reflect the adaptation of neurons to nerve injury.

Axons in the brain and spinal cord have little innate capacity for regeneration. The difference in regeneration outcomes after the central and peripheral injuries may thus be related to the difference in gene expression between these two types of lesion. Differentially expressed growth-associated molecules and receptors may be the key players that are responsible for different regenerative outcomes. Interestingly, nine growth-related genes (bFGF, FGF-7, GDNF, GDNFR-α, GAP-43, NGF-inducible protein, superior cervical ganglion 10, adenomatous polyposis coli protein, and growth arrest and DNA damage inducible protein 45) are upregulated in DRG after peripheral nerve injury but showed either no change or downregulation in the spinal cord after spinal cord injury [26].

4.2
Modification of Gene Expression in the Dorsal Horn of Spinal Cord

Sensory afferents project into the dorsal horn of spinal cord and form the extensive network with the dorsal horn neurons to modulate the sensory inputs. Recent microarray studies show that the spinal cord enriched genes are distinct from that in DRGs [27]. However, the dorsal horn enriched genes have been analyzed [28,29]. Following peripheral nerve injury, the altered neurotransmission of primary afferents may lead to changes in the activity of neural circuits in the spinal dorsal horn. The cDNA array studies show that the expression of the genes encoding 14 channels, 25 receptors, and 42 signal transduction related molecules is strongly regulated in the dorsal horn after sciatice nerve transection [30]. The oligonucleotide microarray has been used to study the differential gene expression in the spinal cord after lumbar 5 spinal nerve transection and lumbar 5 nerve root ligation [31]. Although a large number of genes have been found to be differentially regulated in the spinal cord, only a few receptors and ion channels are shown to be regulated by the oligonucleotide microarray. Our discussion is focused on the changes in the receptors, ion channels, and signal transduction molecules.

4.2.1
Ion Channels

Expression of several Ca^{2+} channel subunits is changed in the dorsal spinal cord after sciatic nerve transection (Figure 4.1; Tables 4.3 and 4.4). The Ca^{2+} channel $\alpha 1E$ subunit is the most strongly upregulated molecule, while Ca^{2+} channel $\alpha 1C$ is downregulated [30]. Since $\alpha 1E$ subunit is the leading candidate of pore-forming subunits for R-type Ca^{2+} channels and $\alpha 1C$ for L-type Ca^{2+} channels, upregulation of R-type Ca^{2+} channel and downregulation of L-type Ca^{2+} channel may imply a change in major properties of Ca^{2+} channels in the dorsal spinal cord. In addition to changes in Ca^{2+} channels, Na^+ channel 6 α subunit (Na_x) is strongly upregulated in the dorsal horn, suggesting its important role in abnormal spinal activity. Similar to their changes in DRGs, K^+ channels are generally downregulated in the dorsal horn.

4.2.2
Neurotransmitter/Neuromodulator Receptors

It has been suggested that the central glutamatergic system is involved in the pathogenesis of neuropathic pain. The AMPA receptors are assembled from four subunits, GluR1, 2, 3, and 4. The AMPA receptor subunits, GluR1, 2, 3, and 4, are expressed in spinal neurons with most labeling in the superficial dorsal horn. Incorporation of GluR2 into heteromeric AMPA receptor reduces the permeability of the receptor channel to Ca^{2+} and modifies current rectification and macroscopic channel conductance. GluR2 is almost universally present at AMPA receptor containing synapses throughout spinal laminae, while GluR1 is present at postsynaptic AMAP receptors in laminae I–II [32], suggesting that majority of AMPA

Table 4.3 Selected upregulated genes in the dorsal spinal cord of the rat after peripheral nerve injury.

Channels	
Ca^{2+} channel α1E	↑↑↑
Ca^{2+} channel α2/δ1	↑↑
Na^+ channel 6α (Na_x)	↑↑↑
Receptors	
$GABA_A$ receptor α5	↑
Ionotropic glutamate receptor, AMPA3	↑↑
Nicotinic acetylcholine receptor β2	↑
P2Y1 receptor	↑↑
Neurotrophic tyrosine kinase receptor, type 2 (TrkB)	↑
Signal transduction molecules	
Stress-activated protein kinase gamma isoform (JNK1)	↑
Stress-activated protein kinase alpha II (JNK2)	↑
Mitogen-activated protein kinase 10 (JNK3)	↑
Mitogen-activated protein kinase 1 (ERK2)	↑
Mitogen-activated protein kinase 6 (ERK3)	↑
Mitogen-activated protein kinase 14 (p38)	↑
Protein kinase C α	↑↑↑
Protein kinase C β1	↑

↑↑↑ >10-fold increase, ↑↑ 10- to 5-fold increase, ↑ five- to twofold increase.

Table 4.4 Selected downregulated genes in the dorsal spinal cord of the rat after peripheral nerve injury.

Channels	
K^+ channel drk1	↓↓
K^+ channel KIR6.2	↓↓
K^+ channel, Isk-related, member 1	↓↓
Ca^{2+} channel α1C	↓↓
Receptors	
P2Y6 receptor	↓
Signal transduction molecules	
Protein phosphatase 2, catalytic subunit, α isoform	↓
Calcium/calmodulin-dependent protein kinase II α	↓↓

↓ 0.5- to 0.2-fold decrease, ↓↓ <0.2-fold decrease.

receptors in spinal dorsal horn have low permeability for Ca^{2+}. Physiological evidences show that AMPA receptors in spinal cord neurons are involved in the increase in neuronal sensitivity after nerve injury [33]. Gene array reveals that peripheral nerve injury increases the expression of AMPA receptor GluR3 and GluR4 in the dorsal spinal cord (Figure 4.1; Table 4.3). These AMPA receptors may be accessible for the increased regional glutamate that results from the decrease in glutamate uptake [34] and may contribute to the increase in Aβ afferent fiber evoked and AMPA and NMDA receptor mediated synaptic transmission in the dorsal horn after peripheral nerve injury [35]. Thus, it is interesting to see whether these changes could alter AMPA receptor composition at the synapses in the spinal laminae and contribute to the processing of neuropathic pain.

The changes in inhibitory systems in the spinal dorsal horn appear to be more complicated. The array study shows upregulation of $GABA_A$ receptor $\alpha 5$ and glycine receptor $\alpha 2$ in the dorsal horn, which may counteract the reduction of GABA released from the dorsal horn neurons after peripheral nerve injury [21]. However, κ-opioid receptor and opioid receptor like orphan receptor are downregulated, suggesting that opioid analgesic effects mediated by these receptors are likely reduced.

Furthermore, cDNA array analysis proves the early finding that TrkB receptor is markedly upregulated in the spinal dorsal horn after peripheral nerve injury [30], in parallel with the upregulation of BDNF in DRG neurons [5,36]. The BDNF heterozygous knockout mice exhibit a significant suppression of nerve injury induced pain responses [37]. These data suggested that BDNF plays an important role in pain hypersensitivity.

4.2.3
Signal Transduction Molecules

It is interesting that signal transduction molecules are differentially regulated in neurons and glial cells in the spinal dorsal horn after peripheral nerve injury (Tables 4.3 and 4.4). The cDNA array shows that peripheral nerve injury results in strong upregulation of PKC α and βI in the neurons in laminae I–IV of the spinal cord. Upregulation of JNK1–3, ERK2 and 3, and p38 MAPK in the dorsal horn is consistent with the reports that peripheral nerve injury activates extracellular signal regulated kinase (ERK) and c-Jun N-terminal kinase (JNK) [38] in astrocytes, and p38 mitogen activated protein kinase [39] in microglial cells. Thus, the changes in PKC signaling occur in neurons, while p38 MAPK and ERK pathways are modified in glial cells.

4.3
Potential Pharmacological Impact of the Regulated Molecules

The Ca^{2+} channel $\alpha 2/\delta 1$ and $GABA_A$ receptor $\alpha 5$ subunit [5,30,40] are found in the list of only a few genes that are concurrently regulated in both DRG and the spinal dorsal horn after peripheral nerve injury. The Ca^{2+} channel $\alpha 2/\delta 1$ subunit is the binding site of gabapentin [41], which is an anticonvulsant drug used for neuropathic pain [42]. $GABA_A$ receptor $\alpha 5$ subunit is involved in producing high-affinity binding sites for GABA agonists and BDZs [43]. The increased expression of Ca^{2+} channel $\alpha 2/\delta 1$ subunit and $GABA_A$ receptor $\alpha 5$ subunit indicates that gabapentin and GABA analogs can act on both dorsal horn neurons and DRG neurons. Especially in the dorsal horn, the expression of Ca^{2+} channel $\alpha 2/\delta 1$ is consistently upregulated during the time course of 28 days after peripheral nerve injury, while it is only transiently increased within 14 days in DRG neurons, suggesting that increased Ca^{2+} channel $\alpha2/\delta1$ subunit in the dorsal horn may be the target for long-term treatment of gabapentin.

Moreover, antidepressants such as amitriptyline, antianxiety drugs such as diazepam and midazolam, and anticonvulsants such as gabapentin and carbamazepine represent useful therapies for certain types of neuropathic pain [44]. Pharmacological studies show that amitriptyline acts at Na^+ channel, diazepam and midazolam at BDZ receptors, and carbamazepine at Na^+ channel [45]. Midazolam reduces C fiber evoked firing after nerve injury [46]. The gene array studies demonstrate that multiple tetrodotoxin-sensitive Na^+ channels are increased at spinal level, supporting the notion that Na^+ channels are potential drug targets for neuropathic pain [47]. Upregulation of nACh receptor $\alpha7$ also suggests a potential drug target, since $\alpha7$ subunits are thought to form homomeric nACh receptor in peripheral nervous system and may mediate antinociception [48]. Further studies on the functions of the markedly regulated molecules, especially the receptors and ion channels, would finally lead to the development of the drugs that are designed to act specifically at the regulated subunits of the receptors and ion channels.

4.4
Future Application of Gene Array

The molecular dissection of the mechanism for both acute and chronic pain is still in the early phase. The cDNA array is a sensitive approach for the future studies in several research directions, including the identification of DRG neuron subset-specific genes and their changes in chronic pain states, the analysis of the mechanisms for regulating the gene expression in DRG neurons and spinal cord neurons, and the pharmacological effects of the analgesics on the molecular phenotypic modification in chronic pain states. Moreover, the high-quality array studies are mainly carried out in the nerve injury induced neuropathic pain models. Its application should be extended into the studies on the mechanisms of the chronic inflammatory pain and the cancer pain. The experimental array studies should be combined with the advanced computational/bioinformative analysis. These studies might provide the relatively complete molecular networks that are involved in pain generation and maintenance. Furthermore, the current array studies suggest that the modification of gene expression could occur at all levels of the pain pathways. Therefore, it is necessary to analyze the molecular changes in the brain with gene array. This could be an important step for investigating the structural and functional modification in the critical brain regions for pain sensation. Importantly, the studies on the modification of gene expression in the primates should be carried out, because the current studies have revealed that both gene regulation and structural modification in the primates could be different from these in the rodents. The data from the primate study could be more relevant to the understanding of human pain. Thus, application of cDNA array in pain study is just at the beginning stage. It has a great opportunity in unraveling the mechanisms of acute and chronic pain and in the development of pain therapies.

Acknowledgments

Grants from NNSFC 30621062, 30630029, and 30325024, MSBRPC 973 program 2006CB806604, and CAS grant KSCX2-YW-R-31.

References

1 Hökfelt, T., Zhang, X. and Wiesenfeld-Hallin, Z. (1994) Messenger plasticity in primary sensory neurons following axotomy and its functional implications. *Trends in Neurosciences*, **17**, 22–30.

2 Woolf, C.J. and Salter, M.W. (2000) Neuronal plasticity: increasing the gain in pain. *Science*, **288**, 1765–1769.

3 Reilly, S.C., Cossins, A.R., Quinn, J.P. and Sneddon, L.U. (2004) Discovering genes: the use of microarrays and laser capture microdissection in pain research. *Brain Research. Brain Research Reviews*, **46**, 225–233.

4 Zhang, X. and Xiao, H.S. (2005) Gene array analysis to determine the components of neuropathic pain signaling. *Current Opinion in Molecular Therapeutics*, **7**, 532–537.

5 Xiao, H.S., Huang, Q.H., Zhang, F.X., Bao, L., Lu, Y.J., Guo, C., Yang, L., Huang, W.J., Fu, G., Xu, S.H., Cheng, X.P., Yan, Q., Zhu, Z.D., Zhang, X., Chen, Z., Han, Z.G. and Zhang, X. (2002) Identification of gene expression profile of dorsal root ganglion in the rat peripheral axotomy model of neuropathic pain. *Proceedings of the National Academy of Sciences of the United States of America*, **99**, 8360–8365.

6 Nilsson, A., Moller, K., Dahlin, L., Lundborg, G. and Kanje, M. (2005) Early changes in gene expression in the dorsal root ganglia after transection of the sciatic nerve; effects of amphiregulin and PAI-1 on regeneration. *Brain Research. Molecular Brain Research*, **136**, 65–74.

7 Costigan, M., Befort, K., Karchewski, L., Griffin, R.S., D'Urso, D., Allchorne, A., Sitarski, J., Mannion, J.W., Pratt, R.E. and Woolf, C.J. (2002) Replicate high-density rat genome oligonucleotide microarrays reveal hundreds of regulated genes in the dorsal root ganglion after peripheral nerve injury. *BMC Neuroscience*, **3**, 16.

8 Wang, H., Sun, H., Della Penna, K., Benz, R.J., Xu, J., Gerhold, D.L., Holder, D.J. and Koblan, K.S. (2002) Chronic neuropathic pain is accompanied by global changes in gene expression and shares pathobiology with neurodegenerative diseases. *Neuroscience*, **114**, 529–546.

9 Valder, C.R., Liu, J.J., Song, Y.H. and Luo, Z.D. (2003) Coupling gene chip analyses and rat genetic variances in identifying potential target genes that may contribute to neuropathic allodynia development. *Journal of Neurochemistry*, **87**, 560–573.

10 Hökfelt, T., Wiesenfeld-Hallin, Z., Villar, M. and Melander, T. (1987) Increase of galanin-like immunoreactivity in rat dorsal root ganglion cells after peripheral axotomy. *Neuroscience Letters*, **83**, 217–220.

11 Zhang, X., Ju, G., Elde, R. and Hökfelt, T. (1993) Effect of peripheral nerve cut on neuropeptides in dorsal root ganglia and the spinal cord of monkey with special reference to galanin. *Journal of Neurocytology*, **22**, 342–381.

12 Wang, L.H., Lu, Y.J., Bao, L. and Zhang, X. (2007) Peripheral nerve injury induces reorganization of galanin-containing afferents in the superficial dorsal horn of monkey spinal cord. *The European Journal of Neuroscience*, **25**, 1087–1096.

13 Suarez, V., Guntinas-Lichius, O., Streppel, M., Ingorokva, S., Grosheva, M., Neiss, W.F., Angelov, D.N. and Klimaschewski, L. (2006) The axotomy-induced neuropeptides galanin and pituitary adenylate cyclase-activating peptide promote axonal sprouting of primary afferent and cranial motor neurons. *The European Journal of Neuroscience*, **24**, 1555–1564.

14 Holmes, F.E., Mahoney, S., King, V.R., Bacon, A., Kerr, N.C., Pachnis, V., Curtis, R., Priestley, J.V. and Wynick, D. (2000) Targeted disruption of the galanin gene reduces the number of sensory neurons and their regenerative capacity. *Proceedings of the National Academy of Sciences of the United States of America*, **97**, 11563–11568.

15 Liu, H.X. and Hökfelt, T. (2002) The participation of galanin in pain processing at the spinal level. *Trends in Pharmacological Sciences*, **23**, 468–474.

16 Wiesenfeld-Hallin, Z., Xu, X.J., Crawley, J.N. and Hökfelt, T. (2005) Galanin and spinal nociceptive mechanisms: recent results from transgenic and knock-out models. *Neuropeptides*, **39**, 207–210.

17 Abdulla, F.A. and Smith, P.A. (1999) Nerve injury increases an excitatory action of neuropeptide Y and Y2-agonists on dorsal root ganglion neurons. *Neuroscience*, **89**, 43–60.

18 Antunes Bras, J.M., Laporte, A.M., Benoliel, J.J., Bourgoin, S., Mauborgne, A., Hamon, M., Cesselin, F. and Pohl, M. (1999) Effects of peripheral axotomy on cholecystokinin neurotransmission in the rat spinal cord. *Journal of Neurochemistry*, **72**, 858–867.

19 Faris, P.L., Komisaruk, B.R., Watkins, L.R. and Mayer, D.J. (1983) Evidence for the neuropeptide cholecystokinin as an antagonist of opiate analgesia. *Science*, **219**, 310–312.

20 Sun, T., Xiao, H.S., Zhou, P.B., Lu, Y.J., Bao, L. and Zhang, X. (2006) Differential expression of synaptoporin and synaptophysin in primary sensory neurons and up-regulation of synaptoporin after peripheral nerve injury. *Neuroscience*, **141**, 1233–1245.

21 Ibuki, T., Hama, A.T., Wang, X.T., Pappas, G.D. and Sagen, J. (1997) Loss of GABA-immunoreactivity in the spinal dorsal horn of rats with peripheral nerve injury and promotion of recovery by adrenal medullary grafts. *Neuroscience*, **76**, 845–858.

22 Catterall, W.A. (2000) From ionic currents to molecular mechanisms: the structure and function of voltage-gated sodium channels. *Neuron*, **26**, 13–25.

23 Frederickson, R.M., Mushynski, W.E. and Sonenberg, N. (1992) Phosphorylation of translation initiation factor eIF-4E is induced in a ras-dependent manner during nerve growth factor-mediated PC12 cell differentiation. *Molecular and Cellular Biology*, **12**, 1239–1247.

24 Bennett, D.L., Michael, G.J., Ramachandran, N., Munson, J.B., Averill, S., Yan, Q., McMahon, S.B. and Priestley, J.V. (1998) A distinct subgroup of small DRG cells express GDNF receptor components and GDNF is protective for these neurons after nerve injury. *Journal of Neuroscience*, **18**, 3059–3072.

25 Linnarsson, S., Mikaels, A., Baudet, C. and Ernfors, P. (2001) Activation by GDNF of a transcriptional program repressing neurite growth in dorsal root ganglia. *Proceedings of the National Academy of Sciences of the United States of America*, **98**, 14681–14686.

26 Zhang, K.H., Xiao, H.S., Lu, P.H., Shi, J., Li, G.D., Wang, Y.T., Han, S., Zhang, F.X., Lu, Y.J., Zhang, X. and Xu, X.M. (2004) Differential gene expression after complete spinal cord transection in adult rats: an analysis focused on a subchronic post-injury stage. *Neuroscience*, **128**, 375–388.

27 LeDoux, M.S., Xu, L., Xiao, J., Ferrell, B., Menkes, D.L. and Homayouni, R. (2006) Murine central and peripheral nervous system transcriptomes: comparative gene expression. *Brain Research*, **1107**, 24–41.

28 Li, M.Z., Wang, J.S., Jiang, D.J., Xiang, C.X., Wang, F.Y., Zhang, K.H., Williams, P.R. and Chen, Z.F. (2006) Molecular mapping of developing dorsal horn-enriched genes by microarray and dorsal/ventral subtractive screening. *Developmental Biology*, **292**, 555–564.

29 Sun, H., Xu, J., Della Penna, K.B., Benz, R.J., Kinose, F., Holder, D.J., Koblan, K.S., Gerhold, D.L. and Wang, H. (2002) Dorsal horn-enriched genes identified by DNA microarray, in situ hybridization and immunohistochemistry. *BMC Neuroscience*, **3**, 11.

30 Yang, L., Zhang, F.X., Huang, F., Lu, Y.J., Li, G.D., Bao, L., Xiao, H.S. and Zhang, X. (2004) Peripheral nerve injury induces trans-synaptic modification of channels, receptors and signal pathways in rat dorsal spinal cord. *The European Journal of Neuroscience*, **19**, 871–883.

31 Lacroix-Fralish, M.L., Tawfik, V.L., Tanga, F.Y., Spratt, K.F. and DeLeo, J.A. (2006) Differential spinal cord gene expression in rodent models of radicular and neuropathic pain. *Anesthesiology*, **104**, 1283–1292.

32 Nagy, G.G., Al-Ayyan, M., Andrew, D., Fukaya, M., Watanabe, M. and Todd, A.J. (2004) Widespread expression of the AMPA receptor GluR2 subunit at glutamatergic synapses in the rat spinal cord and phosphorylation of GluR1 in response to noxious stimulation revealed with an antigen-unmasking method. *Journal of Neuroscience*, **24**, 5766–5777.

33 Leem, J.W., Choi, E.J., Park, E.S. and Paik, K.S. (1996) N-methyl-D-aspartate (NMDA) and non-NMDA glutamate receptor antagonists differentially suppress dorsal horn neuron responses to mechanical stimuli in rats with peripheral nerve injury. *Neuroscience Letters*, **211**, 37–40.

34 Sung, B., Lim, G. and Mao, J. (2003) Altered expression and uptake activity of spinal glutamate transporters after nerve injury contribute to the pathogenesis of neuropathic pain in rats. *Journal of Neuroscience*, **23**, 2899–2910.

35 Garry, E.M. and Fleetwood-Walker, S.M. (2004) A new view on how AMPA receptors and their interacting proteins mediate neuropathic pain. *Pain*, **109**, 210–213.

36 Obata, K., Yamanaka, H., Kobayashi, K., Dai, Y., Mizushima, T., Katsura, H., Fukuoka, T., Tokunaga, A. and Noguchi, K. (2006) The effect of site and type of nerve injury on the expression of brain-derived neurotrophic factor in the dorsal root ganglion and on neuropathic pain behavior. *Neuroscience*, **137**, 961–970.

37 Yajima, Y., Narita, M., Usui, A., Kaneko, C., Miyatake, M., Yamaguchi, T., Tamaki, H., Wachi, H., Seyama, Y. and Suzuki, T. (2005) Direct evidence for the involvement of brain-derived neurotrophic factor in the development of a neuropathic pain-like state in mice. *Journal of Neurochemistry*, **93**, 584–594.

38 Ma, W. and Quirion, R. (2002) Partial sciatic nerve ligation induces increase in the phosphorylation of extracellular signal-regulated kinase (ERK) and c-Jun N-terminal kinase (JNK) in astrocytes in the lumbar spinal dorsal horn and the gracile nucleus. *Pain*, **99**, 175–184.

39 Jin, S.X., Zhuang, Z.Y., Woolf, C.J. and Ji, R.R. (2003) p38 mitogen-activated protein kinase is activated after a spinal nerve ligation in spinal cord microglia and dorsal root ganglion neurons and contributes to the generation of neuropathic pain. *Journal of Neuroscience*, **23**, 4017–4022.

40 Luo, Z.D., Chaplan, S.R., Higuera, E.S., Sorkin, L.S., Stauderman, K.A., Williams, M.E. and Yaksh, T.L. (2001) Upregulation of dorsal root ganglion $\alpha 2\delta$ calcium

channel subunit and its correlation with allodynia in spinal nerve-injured rats. *Journal of Neuroscience*, **21**, 1868–1875.

41 Gee, N.S., Brown, J.P., Dissanayake, V.U., Offord, J., Thurlow, R. and Woodruff, G.N. (1996) The novel anticonvulsant drug, gabapentin (Neurontin), binds to the α2δ subunit of a calcium channel. *The Journal of Biological Chemistry*, **271**, 5768–5776.

42 Dickenson, A.H., Matthews, E.A. and Suzuki, R. (2002) Neurobiology of neuropathic pain: mode of action of anticonvulsants. *European Journal of Pain*, **6**, 51–60.

43 Pritchett, D.B. and Seeburg, P.H. (1990) γ-Aminobutyric acid A receptor α5-subunit creates novel type II benzodiazepine receptor pharmacology. *Journal of Neurochemistry*, **54**, 1802–1804.

44 Sindrup, S.H. and Jensen, T.S. (1999) Efficacy of pharmacological treatments of neuropathic pain: an update and effect related to mechanism of drug action. *Pain*, **83**, 389–400.

45 Brau, M.E., Dreimann, M., Olschewski, A., Vogel, W. and Hempelmann, G. (2001) Effect of drugs used for neuropathic pain management on tetrodotoxin-resistant Na^+ currents in rat sensory neurons. *Anesthesiology*, **94**, 137–144.

46 Kontinen, V.K. and Dickenson, A.H. (2000) Effects of midazolam in the spinal nerve ligation model of neuropathic pain in rats. *Pain*, **85**, 425–431.

47 Devor, M., Wall, P.D. and Catalan, N. (1992) Systemic lidocaine silences ectopic neuroma and DRG discharge without blocking nerve conduction. *Pain*, **48**, 261–268.

48 Damaj, M.I., Meyer, E.M. and Martin, B.R. (2000) The antinociceptive effects of α7 nicotinic agonists in an acute pain model. *Neuropharmacology*, **39**, 2785–2791.

5

The Role of Gene Expression Dependent Molecular Pathways in Axon Plasticity and Neuron Repair Following Acute CNS Injury

Simone Di Giovanni

5.1
Introduction

Stroke, brain and spinal cord traumatic injuries are common disorders that affect a large number of individuals of both sexes and different ages. They are acute central nervous system (CNS) diseases with long-term functional impairment in patients for years to come. They have a chronic neurodegenerative component that leads to long-term disability and high social costs.

The following charts show striking prevalence data in the United States and include projections up to the year 2010, when over 13 million people will be affected by stroke, brain and spinal cord injuries. Proportionally to the population size, similar prevalence data assumptions can be made for Europe as well.

Chart 29: Traumatic Brain injury Prevalence in the U.S.

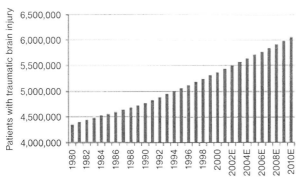

Source. U.S. Census Bureau and UBS Warburg LLC.

Neural Degeneration and Repair: Gene Expression Profiling, Proteomics, and Systems Biology
Edited by Hans Werner Müller
Copyright © 2008 WILEY-VCH Verlag GmbH & Co. KGaA, Weinheim
ISBN: 978-3-527-31707-3

Chart 78: Stroke Prevalence in the U.S.

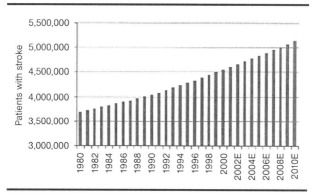

Source. U.S. Census Bureau and UBS Warburg LLC.

Chart 26: Spinal cord injury Prevalence in the U.S.

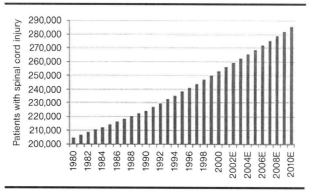

Source. U.S. Census Bureau and UBS Warburg LLC.

Unfortunately, a lack of knowledge of the pathophysiology of tissue damage limits the discovery of effective therapies to cure disability caused by these diseases. Therefore, a better understanding of their pathophysiology is the key to suggest novel and more effective therapeutic strategies.

Acute central nervous system injury leads to sudden cell loss and various degrees of ischemia and hemorrhage at the lesion epicenter. Both necrosis and apoptotic cell death are responsible for the early and subacute stages of tissue damage [1,2]. Inflammation mediated by macrophages that invade the lesion site through the breakage of the blood–brain barrier and by resident microglia is responsible for the majority of the acute and subacute cytotoxic phenomena [3–5].

Importantly, in the hours following the insult, the acute tissual and cellular damage tends to ease and reorganization of the tissue around the lesion epicenter starts. This reorganization includes the reshaping of the vasculature and of the cellular and extracellular environments. Angiogenesis is triggered by increased vascular permeability and endothelial cell division and budding, which lead to a novel vascular tree and new patterns of vascularization [6,7]. Glial cells start both secreting growth factors and providing structural support to neighboring cells including neurons. Importantly, in this early stage, the plasticity of the neuronal and synaptic network is also activated. Neurogenesis and axon sprouting, closely parallel, follow neuronal plasticity, repair lost connections, and partially establish new ones [8–12]. This molecular and structural remodeling is believed to last for weeks and months following the initial insult. The functional outcome of these events results spontaneously in some degree of neuronal reconnectivity and functional recovery in patients affected by stroke, brain and spinal cord injuries. Nevertheless, the recovery of function is in most cases limited and unsatisfactory.

This complex set of events is highly regulated at the molecular level within signaling cascades that influence angiogenesis, neurogenesis, synaptogenesis, axon sprouting, and regeneration.

Molecular mechanisms of axon plasticity and regeneration are largely mediated by *gene expression*. Gene modulation dictates long-term cytoskeleton remodeling that controls axon growth during development and axon sprouting and regeneration following nerve injury [13–18]. Gene expression is mainly regulated by *transcription factors* (TFs) that are in turn modulated at the gene and protein levels by several environmental stimuli, including growth factors.

Overall, a very complex gene expression network is activated following CNS injury, and the classical approach of studying single or several factors at a time has been quite disappointing in terms of providing a more complete picture of the pathogenetic events.

The advent of *microarray technology* at the end of the 1990s opened new avenues to investigate gene expression in an unbiased and high-throughput manner, including the possibility to dissect the temporal and functional profiles of gene changes following acute CNS injury.

Up to now, numerous studies have provided a comprehensive gene expression profiling by using microarrays in several models of stroke, brain and spinal cord injuries in rodents [19–31], allowing discovering the whole picture of gene expression changes from very early to weeks following CNS injuries.

Nevertheless, we are only at the beginning of our understanding of how these transcripts are regulated, and therefore of the role of transcription factors in gene expression.

More recently, chromatin immunoprecipitation (ChIP) combined with microarray analysis of genome-wide promoter regions became a relatively accessible technique [32] that has allowed deciphering the transcriptional cascades downstream specific transcription factors in diverse experimental settings. Therefore, this approach may be an important future application in the study of the pathogenesis of acute neurodegenerative disorders.

5.2

The Mechanisms that Determine Functional Recovery Following Acute CNS Damage

Both loss and recovery of function following acute CNS injury are directly dependent upon the level of functionally appropriate neuronal activity around the damaged area and upon the degree of functional connections with areas distant from the lesion epicenter.

Loss of function following stroke, brain and spinal traumas shares common molecular mechanisms and features of tissue damage, and this has been investigated in particular in the acute and subacute phases.

The epicenter of the ischemic insult or of the trauma is characterized by the interruption of blood flow, massive inflammatory response, cell loss, and tissue disruption. The majority of cellular loss is due to necrosis in the first few hours post injury and to apoptosis in the following days and weeks. Neuronal and oligodendrocyte damage and death are the main immediate and delayed events that contribute to the neurodegenerative and demyelinating phenotype. This determines a functional deficiency due to both local tissue loss and remote uncoupling of neuronal transmission in brain areas connected to the area of tissue damage.

Around the lesion epicenter, within an area of surviving neurons, an inhibitory environment to axon sprouting and growth is soon established [33]. Nevertheless, it is also in this area that the majority of molecular mechanisms can be modulated to promote plasticity and to counteract the inhibitory milieu [34,35].

The tissutal and molecular features that determine recovery of function can be schematically summarized in three main temporally subsequent and partially overlapping phases:

1. repair of tissue damage around the lesion epicenter;
2. plasticity of the neuronal network;
3. reestablishment of long-distance new connections.

The main reason for the failed axon regeneration in the CNS, as opposed to the successful regeneration in the peripheral nerves, is to be found in a complex network of molecules and pathways that are specific of the CNS and limit axon regeneration post injury [33].

Around the injured area, in the so-called injury penumbra, neuronal damage is mediated mainly by oxidative stress and DNA damage that contribute to axon and dendritic collapse and loss of neuronal activity and neurotransmission. In fact, the damaged tissue around the lesion epicenter reacts to injury with proliferation and activation of microglia and macrophages recruited from the bloodstream, and with hypertrophy and hyperplasia of astrocytes. Astrocytes proliferate, become dysmorphic, and together with the production of proteoglycans form the glial scar and limit axon regeneration [36,37]. Interestingly, in physiological conditions, nondysmorphic astrocytes provide neurotrophic factors and play a role in guidance during axon development and remodeling [38–40].

Other critical inhibitors of axon outgrowth and regeneration are proteins derived from disrupted myelin, expressed in oligodendrocytes, and they include the transmembrane proteins NogoA [41,42], myelin-associated glycoprotein (MAG) [43,44], and oligodendrocyte-myelin glycoprotein (OMgp) [33,45,46]. These three proteins signal through a common receptor, the Nogo receptor (NgR). NgR forms a complex with the low-affinity neurotrophin receptor p75 and with LINGO-1 [47–50], and this molecular complex activates the GTPase RhoA, which leads to the recruitment of Rho kinase that in turn mediates cytoskeleton remodeling and inhibits axon outgrowth [51,52].

This inhibitory signaling occurs mainly in the area around the injury epicenter, where tissue that survived the primary insult receives growth promoting signaling that tends to counteract the formation of the inhibitory environment. The best characterized pro-axon growth and sprouting molecules are the so-called regeneration-associated genes (RAGs). They play a role in neurite and axon outgrowth in CNS damage and axon regeneration following peripheral nerve injury. These include transcription factors such as c-jun [53,54] and p53 [55], cytoskeleton-associated proteins such as tubulin-α [56,57], Coronin 1b, and Rab13 [58], microtubule-associated proteins [59], growth-associated proteins (GAP-43 and CAP-23) [60–64], cell adhesion molecules (N-CAM, L1, and TAG1) [65,66], cytokines, and extracellular matrix components (Snap25, Munc13, and cpg15/neuritin, attractin) [67–69]. In some cases, these factors share common molecular pathways. For example, GAP-43 and CAP-23 bind downstream to the cofactor PI[4,5]P[2], at plasmalemmal rafts, contributing to the regulation of actin and modulating neurite outgrowth in neuronal cells [70]. Most of these molecules play a role in nerve regeneration in the peripheral nervous system following nerve injury [71]. As far as their role in promoting axon regeneration *in vivo* and in the CNS is concerned, the only successful example of gain of function was observed by the combined overexpression of the growth cone proteins CAP-23 and GAP-43. In transgenic mice after spinal cord injury (SCI), they triggered regeneration of DRG axons into peripheral nerve grafts transplanted in the thoracic section of the cord [72]. This example holds promise for the enhancement of axon regeneration using a combination of other candidate pro-regeneration factors.

Overall, functional recovery reflects the number of surviving cells and fiber tracts, the extent of neural plasticity, and/or the presence of a permissive environment for regeneration. Importantly, the degree of plasticity of the neuronal network in the area around the lesion epicenter is related to the capacity of surviving neurons to sprout and form functional synapses. Local reestablishment of neuronal connectivity is not sufficient to promote functional recovery. In fact, the highly integrated and hierarchical organization of the CNS requires long-distance connections to be created.

Such processes are substantially regulated by gene expression changes; temporally, these changes follow the acute early phase associated with inflammation, extension of axonal damage, and cell death and loss.

In summary, the success of the reparative processes depends upon factors involved in

a) overcoming the inhibitors of axonal regeneration and limiting the scar formation;
b) facilitating the spontaneous mechanisms of neurite outgrowth and axonal regeneration;
c) protecting and replacing the original cellular environment.

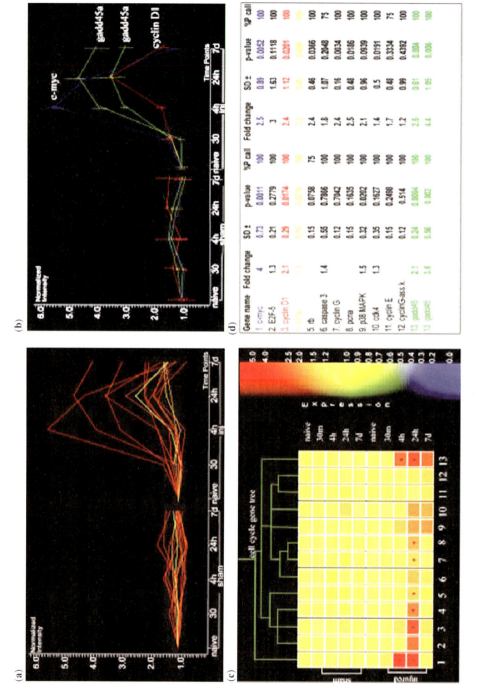

Figure 5.1 (legend see p. 109)

Collectively, these factors likely determine the degree of anatomical and functional recovery after injury.

5.3
Repair and Tissue Plasticity Gene Expression Changes Following Acute CNS Injury

The recent development of microarray technology allowed identifying the expression of thousands of genes following CNS injury in a single experiment. In most studies, rodent models of stroke or traumatic injuries were utilized. Gene expression was mainly measured after dissection of brain and spinal cord tissue at and around the injured brain and spinal cord areas, but in some cases regions connected to the injury epicenter by functionally relevant long-distance projections were also analyzed [19–31,73].

An important common message that emerged from gene expression profiling studies is that gene-mediated neuronal repair mechanisms occur early on, in between minutes and hours following the initial insult. They are mainly genes related to DNA repair such as GADD-45 and PCNA [19,23,24], which are activated by DNA damage triggered by inflammation and oxidative stress.

These genes are likely to rescue partially damaged neurons by repairing their DNA and allow for a reservoir of surviving neurons that can subsequently undergo plasticity and axon sprouting related gene changes, and therefore provide a substrate for partial recovery of function. Importantly, in this early phase, gene-mediated decision making as far as cell fate is concerned, takes place in the tissue around the injury epicenter. This has a double-sided implication by allowing for positive selection of cells that may mediate recovery and elimination of highly damaged or intact cells, and therefore more or less potential for recovery. This picture emerged, for example, by the analysis of functionally related gene clusters that follow a coordinated temporal expression pattern. In fact, by combining microarrays with bioinformatics, we have identified a cluster of genes involved in DNA damage repair, which also mediates cell cycle arrest, transcriptional control, and cell death. These genes were induced in between 4 and 24 hours following spinal cord contusion injury (Figure 5.1). Transcripts include the cell cycle related molecules cyclin D1, CDK4, cyclin G, Rb, and E2F5, which promote cell death in neurons and

Figure 5.1 Functional clustering DNA of damage and cell cycle genes showing high expression 4–24 hours after injury. The genes are clustered on the basis of their involvement in cell cycle progression and apoptosis. Genes of this functional cluster also belong to smaller temporal clusters (gadd45a showed temporal clustering with c-myc, $R^2 = 0.99$, whereas pcna, cyclin D1, cyclin G, Rb, and E2F5 belonged to the same temporal cluster, $R^2 = 0.99$). Data for all cluster members are shown in panels (a), (c), and (d), whereas data with standard deviations for multiple animals are shown in panel (b). Panel (b) shows a self-organizing map graph subcluster applied to the cell cycle gene cluster shown in panel (a). Those genes showing significant *P*-value (<0.05) and fold changes (twofold) between sham and injured time points are indicated with an asterisk in panel (c).

proliferation of microglia and astrocytes, GADD-45 and PCNA, involved in DNA repair and synthesis, and caspase 3, a pro-cell death effector. Therefore, early on after CNS injury, temporally coordinated gene expression patterns seem to influence cell fate toward DNA repair or cell death [23].

Another important chain of events that can favor neuronal repair and plasticity is the one related to angiogenesis. Following CNS injury, an initial increase in blood vessel permeability occurs starting at 24 hours post injury. In this time frame and for one more week, angiopoietin 2, vascular endothelial growth factor (VEGF), and one of its receptors, Flk-1, increase their expression levels around the injured area [7,74,75]. Interestingly, neuropilin-1, integrins, ephrins, and ephrin receptors, which are induced in parallel with VEGF and contribute to vascular remodeling and restoration of collateral circuits, are also expressed on neuronal and glial cells and provide a molecular link between angiogenesis, neural repair, and axon growth [76–82]. In fact, they are essential regulators of axon guidance during development and in the adult after injury. In addition, from hours to days following injury, pro-axon plasticity and specific neuron repair genes such as arc (activity-regulated cytoskeletal-associated protein), NGFI-A (nerve growth factor induced gene-A), and BDNF have been reported to be induced in injured and peri-injured areas following stroke, brain and spinal cord traumas [14,19,23,24,83,84]. Increased expression of VEGF, angiopoietin, and integrins, along with erythropoietin (EPO), also plays a part in the induction of neurogenesis early on after acute CNS damage. Neurogenesis is fueled by neuroblasts, newly born immature neurons, which migrate mainly from the periventricular areas toward the brain parenchyma, and more so following stroke and brain trauma toward areas of ischemic damage. These events can develop as early as 1 day to weeks following brain injury. EPO gene expression and its main regulator, hypoxia inducible factor 1, are induced in the area around the infarct and the epicenter of focal brain trauma starting a few days post injury and are believed to be the main injury-mediated signals to promote neuroblasts formation, migration, and differentiation [85–87]. Administration of EPO increases neurogenesis *in vivo* and EPO receptor null mice display impaired neuroblasts migration following stroke [88,89].

Inflammation accounts for a large part of gene changes in the phase ranging from minutes to several days post injury [90,91]. Even though inflammation leads to a certain degree of cytotoxicity and amplification of tissue damage, it can also serve to clear the environment from too highly damaged cells and release growth factors for neurogenesis and axon sprouting. The best characterized immune system related pro-neuronal survival and axon outgrowth factors, whose expression is triggered from hours to days post injury, are the cell adhesion molecules ICAM, the cytokine IL-6, the transcription factor Stat3, and NFκB [15,19,29,92–95].

Inflammation-related transcripts can also be induced later, days and weeks following CNS injury. An example is a recently identified gene cluster whose activation is highest 1 week following spinal cord contusion [96]. It includes Galectin-3, which is involved in chemotaxis of monocytes [97] and can increase cellular proliferation by enhancing cyclin D1 expression; C1qB, a component of the classical complement pathway that plays a role in debris clearance after injury and increases vascular

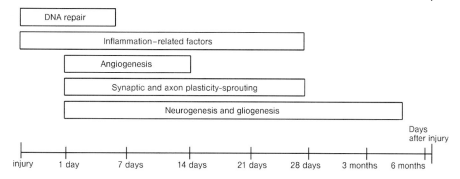

Figure 5.2 Temporal classsification of the major functional classes of transcripts dysregulated following acute CNS injury such as stroke, brain and spinal cord trauma.

permeability, producing NO [98]; and p22^{phox}, which is involved in microglial activation, and can therefore be potentially both beneficial (increase in trophic factors) and detrimental (increase in cytotoxic cytokines) [96].

These factors as a whole induce marked plasticity of the tissue and vasculature around the injury epicenter and have an impact on the long-term functional recovery.

In fact, gene expression in immune cells can also promote the release of neurotrophins and vascular growth factors, leading to increased angiogenesis, and the formation of new vascular circuits that can provide the required oxygen and nutrients for neurogenesis and for preexisting neurons to survive and form new synaptic networks.

Figure 5.2 shows a time line of the main dysregulated gene profiles following acute CNS damage, including transcripts and proteins more specifically involved in neuronal plasticity and cell differentiation.

5.4
Gene Expression Profiles and Gene Clusters Related to Axon Sprouting and Regeneration

The pro-axon growth genetic machinery that is present in the embryonic nervous system and is partially recapitulated in the peripheral nervous system after injury, is largely lost in the adult CNS [17,18,99].

Nevertheless, stroke, brain and spinal cord traumas trigger a limited axon sprouting response.

Functional classification of genes relevant for axon sprouting and potentially for axon regeneration includes different families of genes and proteins: neurotrophic factors, transcription factors, extracellular signaling, membrane-associated, cell adhesion and cytoskeleton-associated molecules.

These genes have often been described individually or grouped in functional classes in microarray experiments in rodents [19–31], but they have been very rarely investigated further for their capacity to belong to functional gene clusters and to affect a coordinated biological outcome such as axon growth or sprouting.

The processes of axon growth, sprouting, and regeneration imply an orchestrated set of events that include the expression of appropriate set of extracellular and cellular signaling proteins and coordinated transcriptional regulation, which together remodel the cytoskeleton to modulate axon and growth cone plasticity.

Stroke as well as brain and spinal cord traumatic injuries induce neuronal growth promoting genes, which are believed to provide a molecular substrate for axon plasticity and sprouting. These events can be schematically subdivided into early, middle, and late sustained responses [100]. In the early phase, ranging from 24 to 72 hours, in the area around the lesion epicenter there is evidence of electrophysiological activity in surviving neurons in the form of neuronal discharges associated with axon sprouting. By 1 week up to 14 days post lesion, there is an intermediate time window within the maintenance phase of the sprouting response. By 4 weeks, the late phase, novel anatomical connections are detected.

The most important transcripts that code for proteins involved in growth cone remodeling expressed in the first few days following brain and spinal traumas and stroke are the small proline-rich protein 1 (SPRR1), GAP-43, CAP-23, and MARCKS, which last for several days during the first wave of the axon sprouting response [72,101–103]. In this time window, the transcription factors c-jun, STAT3, and NFκB are also activated and are believed to trigger the expression of downstream cytoskeleton- and membrane-associated proteins such as GAP-43, galanin, and integrins. In some experimental models of spinal cord and brain trauma, the growth factors VEGF, BDNF, and PDGF were induced from 1 day to weeks following injury [14,24,29]. In the middle phase of the pro-sprouting response, expression of the cell adhesion molecule L1, VCAM, and tubulin Ta1 triggered sprouting [20,22,23,25,29,66,96,104,105]. In the late phase, the most often induced genes are the cytoskeleton remodeling SCG10, neuritin, SCLIP, and GAP-43 [69,106–109].

Interestingly, the number of sprouting-related transcripts induced following CNS acute injury is very limited compared to the long list of genes activated following peripheral nerve injury, where the sprouting response is much stronger and partial regeneration spontaneously occurs. Nevertheless, several of these genes induced in the CNS are also triggered in the peripheral nerve, suggesting partial overlap in the molecular pathways related to sprouting [18,104,105].

Brain and spinal cord injuries also activate gene expression of a family of molecules involved in the limitation of the sprouting and regeneration response that induce growth collapse mainly by binding to the Nogo receptor complex [33]. Importantly, some are induced early within the first days post injury, such as neurocan, ephrins, semaphorin 3A, and its receptor neuroplin-1 [7,14,82,110]. Expression of others is induced only weeks after injury, probably allowing some level of axon plasticity and sprouting in the first period. They include several scar forming molecules such as vimentin and CSPGs [111,112].

A key event for axon sprouting and regeneration, which is also associated with efficient synaptic activity, is the integrity and the plasticity of the growth cone in damaged axons and in axons around the lesioned area. In fact, as injury induces collapse of growth cones in axons and dendrites, the identification of proteins and molecular mechanisms that counteract postinjury growth cone collapse is crucial.

Using a comparative microarray approach, a novel group of genes was recently described as being specifically induced in axotomized neurons and being able to promote growth cone remodeling. These genes include SPRR1, RB3, p21, and s100c [106–109]; importantly, SPRR1 was also shown to allow axon outgrowth over inhibitory substrates [102].

We have recently searched for novel factors involved in neural plasticity by employing high-density oligonucleotide microarrays to examine temporal gene profile changes after spinal cord contusion injury in rats. By comparing mRNA changes that were coordinately regulated over time with genes previously implicated in nerve regeneration or plasticity, we found a gene cluster whose members are involved in cell adhesion processes, synaptic plasticity, and/or cytoskeleton remodeling [58]. This group, which included the small GTPase Rab13 and the actin binding protein Coronin 1b, showed significantly increased mRNA expression from 7 to 28 days after trauma (Figure 5.3).

Overexpression *in vitro* using neuronal like PC12, neuroblastoma, and DRG neurons demonstrated that these genes enhance neurite outgrowth. Moreover, RNAi gene silencing for Coronin 1b or Rab13 in NGF-treated PC12 cells markedly reduced neurite outgrowth. Coronin 1b and Rab13 proteins were expressed in cultured DRG neurons at the cortical cytoskeleton and at growth cones along with the pro-plasticity/regeneration protein GAP-43. Finally, Coronin 1b and Rab13 were induced in the injured spinal cord, where they were also coexpressed with GAP-43 in neurons and axons.

In a similar experimental setting, we employed microarray analysis to identify a subset of genes whose expression patterns were temporally coregulated and correlated to functional recovery after SCI [69]. Steady-state mRNA levels of this synchronously regulated gene cluster were depressed in both ventral and dorsal horn neurons within 24 hours after injury, followed by strong reinduction during the following 2 weeks, which paralleled functional recovery. The identified cluster includes neuritin, attractin, microtubule-associated protein 1a, and myelin oligodendrocyte protein genes (Figure 5.4).

Transcriptional and protein regulation of this novel gene cluster was also evaluated in spinal cord tissue and in single neurons, and shown to play a role in axonal plasticity. Finally, *in vitro* transfection experiments in primary dorsal root ganglion cells showed that cluster members act synergistically to drive neurite outgrowth.

Taken together, these data support a role for these gene clusters in neuronal and axonal plasticity. For most effective regeneration to occur after injury, multiple molecular pathways may need to operate together in a coordinated fashion. These include the ability of the damaged axons to extend the growth cone, make cell contacts with the extracellular matrix (guidance), form connections with nearby

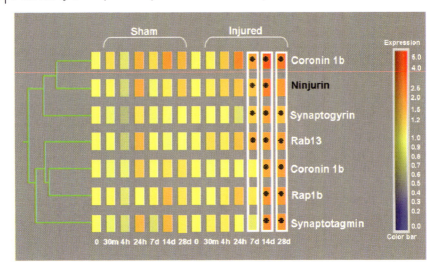

Figure 5.3 Dendogram showing temporally coregulated transcripts induced between 7 and 28 days after SCI. A dendogram (gene tree) obtained using ninjurin as anchor gene to nucleate coregulated transcripts based upon a correlation coefficient $R^2 = 0.99$ (both standard and Pearson correlation) is shown. Expression levels in sham and injured cords at different time points after SCI are represented with a specific color code. Bar graph on the right shows the color code for gene expression level from low (blue) to high (red). These transcripts are upregulated between 7 and 28 days after SCI (asterisk indicates statistical significance).

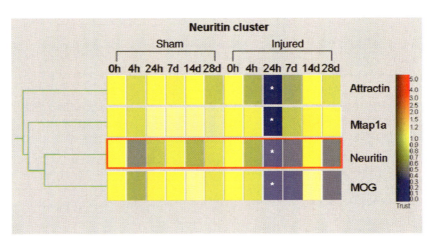

Figure 5.4 Gene tree showing temporally co-ordinated gene profiles obtained by neuritin-nucleated temporal cluster. Neuritin cluster obtained using neuritin as anchor gene (red box) to nucleate transcripts with a similar profile across time point ($R^2 = 0.98$) is shown. All genes show significant downregulation following injury compared to shams at the 24 hour time point (see asterisk, which indicates a Welch t-test P-value <0.05). mRNA expression levels recover to normal levels in 14 days after injury. Gene expression levels in both sham and injured groups were normalized to time point 0 (naïve animals). Bar graph on the right shows the color code for gene expression level (red: high; blue: low).

cells, and achieve functional synapses. These genes and proteins play a known or putative role in several of the above mechanisms; together their coordinated action may induce more effective plasticity and regeneration than that resulting from the expression of a single protein. Therefore, modulation of these clusters of genes and proteins may provide novel targets for facilitating restorative processes after spinal cord injury.

5.5
The Role of Transcription Factors in the Control of Axon Growth and Regeneration

Recently, progress has been made in elucidating the molecular identity of negative cues present in the CNS following injury. Myelin proteins are the major factors responsible for activating intracellular signaling that inhibits regeneration. These myelin-associated inhibitors include Nogo, myelin-associated glycoprotein, and oligodendrocyte-myelin glycoprotein. They all bind to the same Nogo receptor complex and activate the RhoA-dependent pathways that ultimately affect cytoskeleton remodeling, growth cone collapse, and axon growth inhibition [33,46,52,113].

In addition, the intracellular genetic machinery in adult neurons is highly deficient in pro-regeneration genes as compared to the same neurons at an embryonic stage. Embryonic neurons intrinsically have a better potential to grow axons, to regenerate, and are less vigorously inhibited by inhibitory molecules [18,114–116].

Therefore, a potential therapeutic strategy to foster axon regeneration in the adult would be to both inhibit the inhibitory cues and promote a pro-axon growth developmental stage of gene expression.

At the crossroad between pro-axon growth and regeneration and axon inhibition lies a complex family of proteins that drives gene expression: the transcription factors. They contribute to the regulation of both physiological and postinjury axon outgrowth and control cytoskeleton remodeling.

Axonal injury induces biochemical alterations that may induce cell death or tentative regenerative and plasticity responses. Regeneration is largely regulated by gene expression and cytoskeleton remodeling and is therefore under tight transcriptional control. As a consequence, successful axon regeneration very likely requires proper activation of the transcription program in the injured cell.

Partial regeneration occurs spontaneously in the peripheral nervous system following axonal injury. This seems to be due to both intrinsic properties and the lack of strong axon regeneration inhibitory factors such as CNS myelin and astrocytes [71].

A set of transcription factors has been implicated in successful axon regeneration in the peripheral nervous system and a number of possible transcriptional target genes have been identified. Nevertheless, only very rarely was direct DNA binding and transcriptional regulation of specific transcription factors on pro-regeneration promoters reported. In addition, only restricted subsets of these pro-regeneration TFs have been effective in triggering axon regeneration in the CNS.

Most TFs are activated following nerve injury in the context of neurotrophin signaling mediated by Trk receptors and signaling transduced by the IL-6 receptor complex. Their activation is triggered by posttranslational modifications, gene expression changes, and cytoplasm to nucleus translocation.

One of the most important intracellular signaling molecules that influence gene expression in neurite outgrowth relevant pathways is cAMP [46,117]. Its elevation following NGF and BDNF leads to activation of PKA and phosphorylation of the TF cAMP responsive binding element (CREB), which triggers expression of arginase I, and likely other ill-defined gene targets. CREB activation promotes axon growth and regeneration in both the peripheral and CNS, where it is able to overcome myelin inhibition in a model of spinal cord lesion [117–120].

CREB and its signaling pathway represent to date the most promising molecular target to foster regeneration following CNS injury. Other TFs are regulated by Trk receptor signaling and have been variously implicated in axon regeneration.

The TF c-jun, implicated in neuron survival as well as cell death, was recently shown to play an important role in efficient axon regeneration in several models of nerve transection in which c-jun conditional KO mice were employed [53]. c-jun seems to regulate the expression of several cell adhesions and membrane-bound proteins expressed in regenerating axons such as CD44, galanin, and alpha7beta1 integrin. c-jun is required for the expression of these proteins in axon sprouts in CNS locations at the brain stem and the spinal cord following facial and sciatic nerve transections [17,53,121–123]. Another TF, ATF3, seems to synergize with the pro-regeneration features of c-jun, based on coexpression in regenerating neurons and molecular cooperation upon transcription [124–126].

P311 is a TF that is upregulated in the axotomized facial motor neurons. Ectopically expressed P311 localizes in the cytoplasm and the nucleus. Interestingly, adenovirus-mediated P311 gene transfer promotes neurite outgrowth of postnatal dorsal root ganglion neurons and embryonic hippocampal neurons *in vitro* and facilitates nerve regeneration following facial nerve injury *in vivo* [127].

A very important signaling pathway alternative to the neurotrophins is initiated by the binding of two potent and multifunctional cytokines: leukemia inhibiting factor (LIF) and IL-6. Gene expression experiments have shown that transcript levels for both LIF and IL-6 were induced in the brain following ischemia and trauma, and in DRG neurons following sciatic injury [128–139]. Importantly, IL-6 and LIF null mice have impaired axon regeneration following peripheral nerve lesion and lesion of the dorsal columns in the spinal cord [92,140,141]. LIF and IL-6 bind to a receptor complex formed by IL-6 receptor alpha and gp130. Signal is transduced through phosphorylation of Janus kinase (JAK) that phosphorylates the TF STAT3 [142]. Phosphorylation of STAT3 seems a key event in the pro-axon sprouting and regeneration properties of this pathway. In fact, STAT3 phosphorylation is required for sprouting *in vitro* in DRG neurons and *in vivo* following dorsal column transection [93]. Interestingly, in these experimental models it drives the expression of SPRR1, which is able to promote growth cone remodeling in injured axons and prevent myelin-mediated growth cone collapse. Nevertheless, experiments showing promoter occupancy of STAT3 on SPRR1 are still missing.

Using temporal expression profiling to determine genes induced subacutely after experimental spinal cord injury in rats, we recently identified a cluster of temporally correlated genes that promote neuronal plasticity and neurite outgrowth. As mentioned in the previous paragraph, these included genes encoding for Coronin 1b, an actin binding protein, and the GTPase Rab13, which are required for physiological neurite outgrowth in PC12 cells and dorsal root ganglion neurons [58]. The temporally coordinated activation pattern for Coronin 1b and Rab13 suggested that their expression might be regulated by common transcription factor(s). This hypothesis was reinforced by the observation that Coronin 1b and Rab13 have a synergistic role in neuronal plasticity. Thus, concurrent increased or inhibited expression of these two genes in PC12 cells or DRG neurons facilitates or suppresses, respectively, neu- rite outgrowth and differentiation as compared to modulation of either gene alone. To address this hypothesis, we performed an *in silico* computer-based analysis (MatInspector, Genomatix) of the predicted promoters of rat Rab13 and Coronin 1b genes. Results indicated that both genes carry multiple common p53 transcription binding sites (TBSs), which are highly conserved also in the human and mouse genes.

p53 is a tumor suppressor protein and a key determinant of cell fate following exposure to a variety of insults [143,144]. It functions as a DNA-binding, sequence-specific transcription factor that activates expression of multiple genes, causing either reversible cell cycle arrest or apoptosis, but its role in axon growth and regeneration was not defined until recently. In a series of experiments *in vitro* and *in vivo* in a model of facial nerve transection, we have demonstrated that the p53 protein critically regulates the expression of both Coronin 1b and Rab13 by binding to their promoter elements. Moreover, p53 was required for neurite outgrowth of cultured neurons, as well as for axonal regeneration following facial nerve transection. In fact, axon sprouting and expression of Coronin 1b and Rab13 in the CNS, in brain stem facial nuclei, was impaired in p53 null mice (Figure 5.5). Importantly, these actions of p53 were preferentially mediated through specific acetylation at position K320, suggesting that acetylation of specific transcription factors may promote nerve regeneration [55]. This work establishes strong evidence for a novel role of p53 in neurite outgrowth and nerve regeneration and provides the molecular framework for such a function. If this pathway proves to be able to affect regeneration also in CNS injured axons, its modulation may provide a novel therapeutic target for facilitating neuroplasticity and neuroregeneration after injuries to both central and peripheral nervous systems.

Figure 5.6 summarizes the best characterized transcription-dependent signaling pathways in axon growth, sprouting, and regeneration.

5.6
Therapeutic Implications for Neurodegenerative Disorders

It is hard to imagine that modulation of a single component of this complex pathogenetic cascade that follows acute CNS injury can actually lead to efficient anatomical and functional recovery. The understanding of the complexity and the identification of the key factors in this molecular chain of events are necessary to

Rab 13   Coronin 1b

Figure 5.5 p53 is required for axonal regeneration and for Coronin 1b and Rab13 expression in axonal sprouts. (a) FluoroGold fluorescence in the facial nucleus in p53 WT versus p53−/− on the control (ctr) and transected side (trans) 28 days after facial nerve cut. Note the strong reduction in the number of FluoroGold positive neurons in p53−/− compared to p53 WT after nerve cut (trans). (b) Bar graphs showing quantitation of retrograde labeling of facial motor neurons 28 days after facial nerve cut. The overall ratio of labeled neurons in the operated/ unoperated side after sectioning of the entire facial nucleus (five mice per group; *: t-test P-values <0.001) is shown. (c) Immunoperoxidase for Coronin 1b and Rab13 in the facial nucleus in p53 WT versus p53−/− in the control (ctr) and transected side (trans) 28 days after facial nerve cut. Expression of both Coronin 1b and Rab13 is increased in axonal sprouts (arrows) following axotomy in WT (A, B, and E, F), but not in p53 null mice (C, D, and D, H).

design therapies potentially both specific and broad in action. The development of better experimental models of stroke, brain and spinal cord traumas, combined with the extensive use of microarray technology, has helped to improve our understanding of the gene expression machinery post injury and correlate it to physiological, morphological, anatomical, and behavioral outcome measures. We have also learned that it is imperative to go beyond the simple observation of postinjury changes in gene

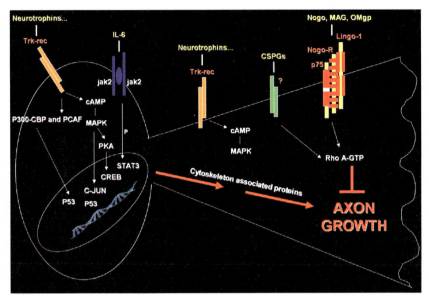

Figure 5.6 Diagram shows the central role of transcription within the pro-growth and inhibitory signaling to axon growth and regeneration.

expression levels to imply function, and that the temporal and spatial pattern of expression of individual transcripts is crucial for their role in postinjury repair.

The observation that clusters of functionally related molecules can be temporally coexpressed and actually cooperate in triggering axon plasticity and axon outgrowth leads us to hypothesize that strategies aimed at enhancing their expression and/or their activity could be valuable to promote recovery following CNS injury.

Possibilities include the identification and modulation of

- proteins such as transcription factors that can control the expression of cluster of genes with synergistic pro-axon sprouting and outgrowth functions, such as in the case of p53, CREB, and STAT3;
- common signaling pathways such as the ones dependent upon neurotrophins, IL-6, and Nogo receptor complex to both foster pro-axon plasticity signals and antagonize the postinjury inhibitory environment to axon regrowth;
- neurogenetic and angiogenetic gene expression program.

Several examples of putative *in vivo* approaches to promote recovery following CNS injury acting on these molecular pathways can be hypothesized.

One possibility would be to increase p53 transcriptional activity by using small molecule compounds that inhibit p53 protein degradation and increase its transcriptional activity by antagonizing its binding with the ubiquitin ligase MDM2, such as Nutlins [145,146]. This would potentially lead to not only the increase in the expression of pro-axon growth target genes, but also to the risk of increasing p53 pro-apoptotic function. Alternatively, increase in p53 acetylation by overexpressing pro-neuronal survival acetyltransferases such as PCAF or CBP using viral vectors would also potentially increase the capacity of p53 to trigger pro-axon growth promoters.

In the case of CREB and STAT3, targeting their phosphorylation status by increasing the expression of specific kinases, respectively, PKA and JAKs, would likely represent a suitable strategy, by using either viral transfer or a pharmacological approach.

Limitations of these strategies include uncertainty regarding efficiency and timing of drug or viral delivery, and lack of a clear picture of the downstream axon growth gene targets, in particular in the case of CREB and STAT3. Finally, the lack of specificity of the action of transcription factors on selected promoters represents both a strength and a risk, as it might not only affect axon regrowth and sprouting powerfully, but also interfere with other cellular events and lead to undesired side effects.

Tackling the upstream signaling at the receptor level has been already performed with very encouraging results, in particular, in the case of the inhibition of Nogo receptor signaling that leads to improvement in axon sprouting and regeneration in experimental models of brain, spinal cord trauma and stroke [147–149]. The most promising approach is the use of NgR antagonist peptides or antibodies. This approach is believed to inhibit the downstream Nogo signaling, including the immediate effects on growth cone collapse and delayed events linked to gene expression, mainly secondary to Rho and Rho kinases' activity. In particular, studies in primates have already shown its safety and efficacy in improving axon regeneration and functional recovery [147] in spinal cord injury, and now clinical trials on humans are under way.

As far as treatment strategies aimed at improving both neurogenesis and angiogenesis are concerned, the use of EPO currently has the highest likelihood of success. In fact, EPO impacts gene expression, redirecting the genetic machinery toward neuroprotective, pro-neurogenic, and angiogenic patterns of gene expression. It was shown to be neuroprotective in animal models of stroke and traumatic brain injury when administered prior to, within the first few hours, and 1 day after injury [88,150]. These studies also showed that EPO leads to significant improvement in several behavioral tests, increases angiogenesis and neurogenesis, and enhances the expression of VEGF and BDNF, which overall could contribute to functional recovery.

5.7
Future Perspectives

ChIP-on-chip assays represent the new frontier to dissect the regulation of biological networks at the gene expression level. It combines chromatin immunoprecipitation with microarrays (chip) [32]. Briefly, DNA and proteins are cross-linked *in vivo* and

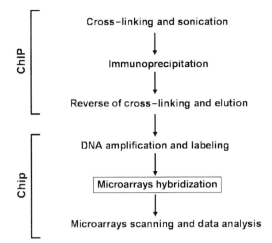

Figure 5.7 Flowchart outlines the ChIP on chip experimental algorithm.

immunoprecipitated with specific antibodies against the protein of interest. DNA bound to the protein is then sheared and fragmented. Fragments are then amplified by PCR and fluorolabeled for detection on microarrays that include whole-genome promoter sequences as in the case of Affymetrix arrays (http://www.affymetrix.com). This allows for unbiased genome-wide identification of gene targets directly regulated by the protein of interest.

Figure 5.7 summarizes the experimental procedure.

Its use in neuroscience is still at the embryonic stage, and it has not been applied in injury paradigms as yet. It would be very useful to perform ChIP on chip, for example, for several known transcription factors such as CREB, c-jun, STAT3, and p53 in various models of injury in purified neuronal populations. Data from ChIP on chip would be even more intriguing if performed *in vivo* in areas around the lesion site or in neuronal populations functionally connected to the lesion epicenter, as supraspinal sites in the case of spinal cord injury. This approach would likely allow unveiling the downstream orchestra of genes involved in TF-mediated axonal plasticity, sprouting, and potential regeneration. In fact, only an effort to understand the role of the single components within the symphony of the cell could lead to a clarification of the genetic machinery that controls such complex molecular networks.

Finally, integration of studies aimed at detecting gene expression patterns with high-throughput protein expression analysis is another very important challenge to clarify the pathogenic mechanisms following CNS injury. The rapid development of proteomics seems to promise a bright future in this regard. In fact, priming of the neuron toward a more plastic phenotype, including its ability to sprout or regenerate, or to differentiate from undifferentiated precursors, is always dependent upon the net balance of protein expression and the pattern of their posttranslational modifications, which will dictate cellular functions at the structural level and influence gene expression.

A better understanding of the reciprocal influence of gene and protein expression will hopefully contribute to improved therapeutic strategies to enhance recovery following CNS injury.

References

1 Yakovlev, A.G. and Faden, A.I. (1995) Molecular biology of CNS injury. *Journal of Neurotrauma*, **12** (5), 767–777.

2 Springer, J.E. (2002) Apoptotic cell death following traumatic injury to the central nervous system. *Journal of Biochemistry and Molecular Biology*, **35** (1), 94–105.

3 Allan, S.M. and Rothwell, N.J. (2003) Inflammation in central nervous system injury. *Philosophical Transactions of the Royal Society of London. Series B Biological Sciences*, **358** (1438), 1669–1677.

4 Murkin, J.M. (2003) Inflammatory responses and CNS injury: implications, prophylaxis, and treatment. *Heart Surgery Forum*, **6** (4), 193–195.

5 Lucas, S.M., Rothwell, N.J. and Gibson, R.N. (2006) The role of inflammation in CNS injury and disease. *British Journal of Pharmacology*, **147** (Suppl. 1), S232–S240.

6 Carmeliet, P. (2000) Mechanisms of angiogenesis and arteriogenesis. *Nature Medicine*, **6** (4), 389–395.

7 Hayashi, T., Noshita, N., Sugawara, T. and Chan, P.H. (2003) Temporal profile of angiogenesis and expression of related genes in the brain after ischemia. *Journal of Cerebral Blood Flow and Metabolism*, **23** (2), 166–180.

8 Arvidsson, A., Collin, T., Kirik, D., Kokaia, Z. and Lindvall, O. (2002) Neuronal replacement from endogenous precursors in the adult brain after stroke. *Nature Medicine*, **8** (9), 963–970.

9 Parent, J.M., Vexler, Z.S., Gong, C., Derugin, N. and Ferriero, D.N. (2002) Rat forebrain neurogenesis and striatal neuron replacement after focal stroke. *Annals of Neurology*, **52** (6), 802–813.

10 Lu, P., Jones, L.L., Snyder, E. Y. and Tuszynski, M.H. (2003) Neural stem cells constitutively secrete neurotrophic factors and promote extensive host axonal growth after spinal cord injury. *Experimental Neurology*, **181** (2), 115–129.

11 Zhang, R.L., Zhang, Z.G. and Chopp, M. (2005) Neurogenesis in the adult ischemic brain: generation, migration, survival, and restorative therapy. *Neuroscientist*, **11** (5), 408–416.

12 Thored, P., Arvidsson, A., Cacci, E., Ahlenius, H., Kallur, T., Darsalia, V., Ekdahl, C.T., Kokaia, Z. and Lindvall, O. (2006) Persistent production of neurons from adult brain stem cells during recovery after stroke. *Stem Cells*, **24** (3), 739–747.

13 Condron, B. (2002) Gene expression is required for correct axon guidance. *Current Biology*, **12** (19), 1665–1669.

14 Bareyre, F.M. and Schwab, M.E. (2003) Inflammation degeneration and regeneration in the injured spinal cord: insights from DNA microarrays. *Trends in Neurosciences*, **26** (10), 555–563.

15 Carmichael, S.T. (2003) Gene expression changes after focal stroke, traumatic brain and spinal cord injuries. *Current Opinion in Neurology*, **16** (6), 699–704.

16 Rossi, F., Gianola, S. and Corvetti, L. (2006) The strange case of Purkinje axon regeneration and plasticity. *Cerebellum*, **5** (2), 174–182.

17 Teng, F.Y. and Tang, B.L. (2006) Axonal regeneration in adult CNS neurons – signaling molecules and pathways. *Journal of Neurochemistry*, **96** (6), 1501–1508.

18 Zhou, F.Q. and Snider, W.D. (2006) Intracellular control of developmental

and regenerative axon growth. *Philosophical Transactions of the Royal Society of London. Series B Biological Sciences*, **361** (1473), 1575–1592.

19 Carmel, J.B., Galante, A., Soteropoulos, P., Tolias, P., Recce, M., Young, W. and Hart, R.P. (2001) Gene expression profiling of acute spinal cord injury reveals spreading inflammatory signals and neuron loss. *Physiological Genomics*, **7** (2), 201–213.

20 Jin, K., Mao, X.O., Eshoo, M.W., Nagayama, T., Minami, M., Simon, R.P. and Greenberg, D.A (2001) Microarray analysis of hippocampal gene expression in global cerebral ischemia. *Annals of Neurology*, **50** (1), 93–103.

21 Song, G., Cechvala, C., Resnick, D.K., Dempsey, R.J. and Rao, V.L. (2001) GeneChip analysis after acute spinal cord injury in rat. *Journal of Neurochemistry*, **79** (4), 804–815.

22 Kim, Y.D., Sohn, N.W., Kang, C. and Soh, Y. (2002) DNA array reveals altered gene expression in response to focal cerebral ischemia. *Brain Research Bulletin*, **58** (5), 491–498.

23 Di Giovanni, S., Knoblach, S.M., Brandoli, C., Aden, S.A., Hoffman, E.P. and Faden, A.I. (2003) Gene profiling in spinal cord injury shows role of cell cycle in neuronal death. *Annals of Neurology*, **53** (4), 454–468.

24 Natale, J.E., Ahmed, F., Cernak, I., Stoica, B. and Faden, A.I. (2003) Gene expression profile changes are commonly modulated across models and species after traumatic brain injury. *Journal of Neurotrauma*, **20** (10), 907–927.

25 Raghavendra Rao, V.L., Dhodda, V.K., Song, G., Bowen, K.K. and Dempsey, R.J. (2003) Traumatic brain injury-induced acute gene expression changes in rat cerebral cortex identified by GeneChip analysis. *Journal of Neuroscience Research*, **71** (2), 208–219.

26 Aimone, J.B., Leasure, J.L., Perreau, V.M. and Thallmair, M. (2004) Spatial and temporal gene expression profiling of the contused rat spinal cord. *Experimental Neurology*, **189** (2), 204–221.

27 Kim, J.B., Piao, C.S., Lee, K.W., Han, P.L., Ahn, J.I., Lee, Y.S. and Lee, J.K. (2004) Delayed genomic responses to transient middle cerebral artery occlusion in the rat. *Journal of Neurochemistry*, **89** (5), 1271–1282.

28 Velardo, M.J., Burger, C., Williams, P.R., Baker, H.V., Lopez, M.C., Mareci, T.H., White, T.E., Muzyczka, N. and Reier, P.J. (2004) Patterns of gene expression reveal a temporally orchestrated wound healing response in the injured spinal cord. *Journal of Neuroscience*, **24** (39), 8562–8576.

29 De Biase, A., Knoblach, S.M. Di Giovanni, S., Fan, C., Molon, A., Hoffman, E.P. and Faden, A.I. (2005) Gene expression profiling of experimental traumatic spinal cord injury as a function of distance from impact site and injury severity. *Physiological Genomics*, **22** (3), 368–381.

30 Penkowa, M., Caceres, M. Borup, R., Nielsen, F.C., Poulsen, C.B., Quintana, A., Molinero, A., Carrasco, J., Florit, S., Giralt, M. and Hidalgo, J. (2006) Novel roles for metallothionein-I II (MT-I II) in defense responses neurogenesis, and tissue restoration after traumatic brain injury: insights from global gene expression profiling in wild-type and MT-I II knockout mice. *Journal of Neuroscience Research*, **84** (7), 1452–1474.

31 Liu, X.S., Zhang, Z.G., Zhang, R.L., Gregg, S., Morris, D.C., Wang, Y. and Chopp, M. (2007) Stroke induces gene profile changes associated with neurogenesis and angiogenesis in adult subventricular zone progenitor cells. *Journal of Cerebral Blood Flow and Metabolism*, **27** (3), 564–574.

32 Wu, J., Smith, L.T., Plass, C. and Huang, T.H. (2006) ChIP-chip comes of age for genome-wide functional analysis. *Cancer Research*, **66** (14), 6899–6902.

33 He, Z. and Koprivica, V. (2004)
The Nogo signaling pathway for
regeneration block. *Annual Review of
Neuroscience*, **27**, 341–368.

34 Ward, N.S. (2004) Functional
reorganization of the cerebral motor
system after stroke. *Current Opinion in
Neurology*, **17** (6), 725–730.

35 Ward, N.S. (2005) Neural plasticity and
recovery of function. *Progress in Brain
Research*, **150**, 527–535.

36 Ribotta, M.G., Menet, V. and Privat, A.
(2004) Glial scar and axonal regeneration
in the CNS: lessons from GFAP and
vimentin transgenic mice. *Acta
Neurochirurgica. Supplement*, **89**, 87–92.

37 Silver, J. and Miller, J.H. (2004)
Regeneration beyond the glial scar. *Nature
Reviews. Neuroscience*, **5** (2), 146–156.

38 Dreyfus, C.F., Dai, X., Lercher, L.D.,
Racey, B.R., Friedman, W.J. and Black,
I.B. (1999) Expression of neurotrophins
in the adult spinal cord *in vivo*. *Journal of
Neuroscience Research*, **56** (1), 1–7.

39 Doucet, G. and Petit, A. (2002) Seeking
axon guidance molecules in the adult rat
CNS. *Progress in Brain Research*, **137**,
453–465.

40 Hsu, J.Y., Stein, S.A. and Xu, X.M.
(2005) Temporal and spatial distribution
of growth-associated molecules and
astroglial cells in the rat corticospinal
tract during development. *Journal of
Neuroscience Research*, **80** (3), 330–340.

41 Chen, M.S., Huber, A.B., van der Haar,
M.E., Frank, M., Schnell, L., Spillmann,
A.A., Christ, F. and Schwab, M.E. (2000)
Nogo-A is a myelin-associated neurite
outgrowth inhibitor and an antigen for
monoclonal antibody IN-1. *Nature*, **403**
(6768), 434–439.

42 GrandPre, T., Nakamura, F., Vartanian,
T. and Strittmatter, S.M. (2000)
Identification of the Nogo inhibitor of
axon regeneration as a Reticulon
protein. *Nature*, **403** (6768), 439–444.

43 Mukhopadhyay, G., Doherty, P., Walsh,
F.S., Crocker, P.R. and Filbin, M.T.
(1994) A novel role for myelin-associated

glycoprotein as an inhibitor of axonal
regeneration. *Neuron*, **13** (3), 757–767.

44 DeBellard, M.E., Tang, S.,
Mukhopadhyay, G., Shen, Y.J. and
Filbin, M.T., (1996) Myelin-associated
glycoprotein inhibits axonal regeneration from a variety of neurons via
interaction with a sialoglycoprotein.
Molecular and Cellular Neurosciences, **7**
(2), 89–101.

45 Yiu, G. and He, Z. (2003) Signaling
mechanisms of the myelin inhibitors of
axon regeneration. *Current Opinion in
Neurobiology*, **13** (5), 545–551.

46 Domeniconi, M. and Filbin, M.T. (2005)
Overcoming inhibitors in myelin to
promote axonal regeneration. *Journal of
Neurochemistry*, **233** (1–2), 43–47.

47 Wang, K.C., Kim, J.A., Sivasankaran, R.,
Segal, R. and He, Z. (2002) P75 interacts
with the Nogo receptor as a co-receptor
for Nogo MAG and OMgp. *Nature*, **420**
(6911), 74–78.

48 Wang, K.C., Koprivica, V., Kim, J.A.,
Sivasankaran, R., Guo, Y., Neve, R.L. and
He, Z. (2002) Oligodendrocyte-myelin
glycoprotein is a Nogo receptor ligand
that inhibits neurite outgrowth. *Nature*,
417 (6892), 941–944.

49 Wong, S.T., Henley, J.R., Kanning, K.C.,
Huang, K.H., Bothwell, M. and Poo,
M.M. (2002) A p75(NTR) and Nogo
receptor complex mediates repulsive
signaling by myelin-associated
glycoprotein. *Nature Neuroscience*, **5** (12),
1302–1308.

50 Mi, S., Lee, X., Shao, Z., Thill, G., Ji, B.,
Relton, J., Levesque, M., Allaire, N.,
Perrin, S., Sands, B., Crowell, T., Cate,
R.L., McCoy, J.M. and Pepinsky, R.B.
(2004) LINGO-1 is a component of the
Nogo-66 receptor/p75 signaling
complex. *Nature Neuroscience*, **7** (3),
221–228.

51 Niederost, B., Oertle, T., Fritsche, J.,
McKinney, R.A. and Bandtlow, C.E.
(2002) Nogo-A and myelin-associated
glycoprotein mediate neurite growth
inhibition by antagonistic regulation of

RhoA and Rac1. *Journal of Neuroscience*, **22** (23), 10368–10376.

52 Alabed, Y.Z., Grados-Munro, E., Ferraro, G.B., Hsieh, S.H. and Fournier, A.E. (2006) Neuronal responses to myelin are mediated by rho kinase. *Journal of Neurochemistry*, **96** (6), 1616–1625.

53 Raivich, G., Bohatschek, M., Da Costa, C., Iwata, O., Galiano, M., Hristova, M., Nateri, A.S., Makwana, M., Riera-Sans, L., Wolfer, D.P., Lipp, H.P., Aguzzi, A., Wagner, E.F. and Behrens, A. (2004) The AP-1 transcription factor c-Jun is required for efficient axonal regeneration. *Neuron*, **43** (1), 57–67.

54 Zhou, F.Q., Walzer, M.A. and Snider, W.D. (2004) Turning on the machine: genetic control of axon regeneration by c-Jun. *Neuron*, **43** (1), 1–2.

55 Di Giovanni, S., Knights, C.D., Rao, M., Yakovlev, A., Beers, J., Catania, J., Avantaggiati, M.L. and Faden, A.I. (2006) The tumor suppressor protein p53 is required for neurite outgrowth and axon regeneration. *The EMBO Journal*, **25** (17), 4084–4096.

56 Gloster, A., Wu, W., Speelman, A., Weiss, S., Causing, C., Pozniak, C., Reynolds, B., Chang, E., Toma, J.G. and Miller, F.D. (1994) The T alpha 1 alpha-tubulin promoter specifies gene expression as a function of neuronal growth and regeneration in transgenic mice. *Journal of Neuroscience*, **14** (12), 7319–7330.

57 Knoops, B. and Octave, J.N. (1997) Alpha 1-tubulin mRNA level is increased during neurite outgrowth of NG 108-15 cells but not during neurite outgrowth inhibition by CNS myelin. *Neuroreport*, **8** (3), 795–798.

58 Di Giovanni, S., De Biase, A., Yakovlev, A., Finn, T., Beers, J., Hoffman, E.P. and Faden, A.I. (2005a) *in vivo* and *in vitro* characterization of novel neuronal plasticity factors identified following spinal cord injury. *The Journal of Biological Chemistry*, **280** (3), 2084–2091.

59 Tucker, R.P. (1990) The roles of micro-tubule-associated proteins in brain morphogenesis: a review. *Brain Research. Brain Research Reviews*, **15** (2), 101–120.

60 Caroni, P. and Grandes, P. (1990) Nerve sprouting in innervated adult skeletal muscle induced by exposure to elevated levels of insulin-like growth factors. *The Journal of Cell Biology*, **110** (4), 1307–1317.

61 Aigner, L. and Caroni, P. (1993) Depletion of 43-kD growth-associated protein in primary sensory neurons leads to diminished formation and spreading of growth cones. *The Journal of Cell Biology*, **123** (2), 417–429.

62 Aigner, L., Arber, S., Kapfhammer, J.P., Laux, T., Schneider, C., Botteri, F., Brenner, H.R. and Caroni, P. (1995) Overexpression of the neural growth-associated protein GAP-43 induces nerve sprouting in the adult nervous system of transgenic mice. *Cell*, **83** (2),269–278.

63 Frey, D., Laux, T., Xu, L., Schneider, C. and Caroni, P. (2000) Shared and unique roles of CAP23 and GAP43 in actin regulation neurite out-growth, and anatomical plasticity. *The Journal of Cell Biology*, **149** (7), 1443–1454.

64 Laux, T., Fukami, K., Thelen, M., Golub, T., Frey, D. and Caroni, P. (2000) GAP43, MARCKS, and CAP23 modulate PI(4,5)P(2) at plasmalemmal rafts, and regulate cell cortex actin dynamics through a common mechanism. *The Journal of Cell Biology*, **149** (7), 1455–1472.

65 Jung, M., Petrausch, B. and Stuermer C.A. (1997) Axon-regenerating retinal ganglion cells in adult rats synthesize the cell adhesion molecule L1 but not TAG-1 or SC-1. *Molecular and Cellular Neurosciences*,**9** (2),116–131.

66 Klocker, N., Jung, M., Stuermer, C.A. and Bahr, M. (2001) BDNF increases the number of axotomized rat retinal

ganglion cells expressing GAP-43, L1, and TAG-1 mRNA – a supportive role for nitric oxide? *Neurobiology of Disease*, **8** (1), 103–113.

67 Naeve, G.S., Ramakrishnan, M., Kramer, R., Hevroni, D., Citri, Y. and Theill, L.E. (1997) Neuritin: a gene induced by neural activity and neurotrophins that promotes neuritogenesis. *Proceedings of the National Academy of Sciences of the United States of America*, **94** (6), 2648–2653.

68 Kimura, K., Mizoguchi, A. and Ide, C. (2003) Regulation of growth cone extension by SNARE proteins. *Journal of Histochemistry & Cytochemistry*, **51** (4), 429–433.

69 Di Giovanni, S., Faden, A.I., Yakovlev, A., Duke-Cohan, J.S., Finn, T., Thouin, M., Knoblach, S., De Biase, A., Bregman, B.S. and Hoffman, E.P. (2005b) Neuronal plasticity after spinal cord injury: identification of a gene cluster driving neurite outgrowth. *FASEB Journal*, **19** (1), 153–154.

70 Caroni, P. (2001) New EMBO members' review: actin cytoskeleton regulation through modulation of PI(4,5)P(2) rafts. *The EMBO Journal*, **20** (16), 4332–4336.

71 Makwana, M. and Raivich, G. (2005) Molecular mechanisms in successful peripheral regeneration. *FEBS Journal*, **272** (11), 2628–2638.

72 Bomze, H.M., Bulsara, K.R. Iskandar, B.J., Caroni, P. and Skene, J.H. (2001) Spinal axon regeneration evoked by replacing two growth cone proteins in adult neurons. *Nature Neuroscience*, **4** (1), 38–43.

73 Kobori, N., Clifton, G.L. and Dash, P. (2002) Altered expression of novel genes in the cerebral cortex following experimental brain injury. *Brain Research. Molecular Brain Research*, **104** (2), 148–158.

74 Lin, T.N., Wang, C.K. Cheung, W.M. and Hsu, C.Y. (2000) Induction of angiopoietin and Tie receptor mRNA expression after cerebral ischemia-reperfusion. *Journal of Cerebral Blood Flow and Metabolism*, **20** (2), 387–395.

75 Zhang, Z.G., Zhang, L., Tsang, W., Soltanian-Zadeh, H., Morris, D., Zhang, R., Goussev, A., Powers, C., Yeich, T. and Chopp, M., (2002) Correlation of VEGF and angiopoietin expression with disruption of blood–brain barrier and angiogenesis after focal cerebral ischemia. *Journal of Cerebral Blood Flow and Metabolism*, **22** (4), 379–392.

76 Varner, J.A., Brooks, P.C. and Cheresh, D.A. (1995) Review: the integrin alpha V beta 3: angiogenesis and apoptosis. *Cell Adhesion and Communication*, **3** (4), 367–374.

77 Adams, R.H. and Klein, R. (2000) Eph receptors and ephrin ligands: essential mediators of vascular development. *Trends in Cardiovascular Medicine*, **10** (5), 183–188.

78 Conover, J.C., Doetsch, F. Garcia-Verdugo, J.M., Gale, N.W., Yancopoulos, G.D. and Alvarez-Buylla, A. (2000) Disruption of Eph/ephrin signaling affects migration and proliferation in the adult subventricular zone. *Nature Neuroscience*, **3** (11), 1091–1097.

79 Zhang, Z.G., Zhang, L., Jiang, Q., Zhang, R., Davies, K., Powers, S., Bruggen, N. and Chopp, M. (2000) VEGF enhances angiogenesis and promotes blood–brain barrier leakage in the ischemic brain. *Journal of Clinical Investigation*, **106** (7), 829–838.

80 Hindges, R., McLaughlin, T., Genoud, N., Henkemeyer, M. and O'Leary, D.D. (2002) EphB forward signaling controls directional branch extension and arborization required for dorsal–ventral retinotopic mapping. *Neuron*, **35** (3), 475–487.

81 Gu, C., Rodriguez, E.R., Reimert, D.V., Shu, T., Fritzsch, B., Richards, L.J., Kolodkin, A.L. and Ginty, D.D. (2003) Neuropilin-1 conveys semaphorin and VEGF signaling during neural and cardiovascular development. *Developmental Cell*, **5** (1), 45–57.

82 Willson, C.A., Miranda, J.D., Foster, R.D., Onifer, S.M. and Whittemore, S.R., (2003) Transection of the adult rat spinal cord upregulates EphB3 receptor and ligand expression. *Cell Transplantation*, **12** (3), 279–290.

83 Kury, P., Schroeter, M. and Jander, S. (2004) Transcriptional response to circumscribed cortical brain ischemia: spatiotemporal patterns in ischemic vs. remote non-ischemic cortex. *The European Journal of Neuroscience*, **19** (7), 1708–1720.

84 Rickhag, M., Wieloch, T., Gido, G., Elmer, E., Krogh, M., Murray, J., Lohr, S., Bitter, H., Chin, D.J., von Schack, D., Shamloo, M. and Nikolich, K. (2006) Comprehensive regional and temporal gene expression profiling of the rat brain during the first 24 h after experimental stroke identifies dynamic ischemia-induced gene expression patterns, and reveals a biphasic activation of genes in surviving tissue. *Journal of Neurochemistry*, **96** (1), 14–29.

85 Studer, L., Csete, M., Lee, S.H., Kabbani, N., Walikonis, J., Wold, B. and McKay, R. (2000) Enhanced proliferation, survival, and dopaminergic differentiation of CNS precursors in lowered oxygen. *Journal of Neuroscience*, **20** (19), 7377–7383.

86 Shingo, T., Sorokan, S.T., Shimazaki, T. and Weiss, S. (2001) Erythropoietin regulates the *in vitro* and *in vivo* production of neuronal progenitors by mammalian forebrain neural stem cells. *Journal of Neuroscience*, **21** (24), 9733–9743.

87 Sun, Y., Jin, K., Xie, L., Childs, J., Mao, X.O., Logvinova, A. and Greenberg, D.A. (2003) VEGF-induced neuroprotection, neurogenesis, and angiogenesis after focal cerebral ischemia. *Journal of Clinical Investigation*, **111** (12), 1843–1851.

88 Lu, D., Mahmood, A., Qu, C., Goussev, A., Schallert, T. and Chopp, M. (2005) Erythropoietin enhances neurogenesis and restores spatial memory in rats after traumatic brain injury. *Journal of Neurotrauma*, **22** (9), 1011–1017.

89 Tsai, P.T., Ohab, J.J., Kertesz, N., Groszer, M., Matter, C., Gao, J., Liu, X., Wu, H. and Carmichael, S.T. (2006) A critical role of erythropoietin receptor in neurogenesis and post-stroke recovery. *Journal of Neuroscience*, **26** (4), 1269–1274.

90 Iadecola, C. and Alexander, M. (2001) Cerebral ischemia and inflammation. *Current Opinion in Neurology*, **14** (1), 89–94.

91 Bethea, J.R. and Dietrich, W.D. (2002) Targeting the host inflammatory response in traumatic spinal cord injury. *Current Opinion in Neurology*, **15** (3), 355–360.

92 Cafferty, W.B., Gardiner, N.J., Das, P., Qui, J., McMahon, S.B. and Thompson, S.W. (2004) Conditioning injury-induced spinal axon regeneration fails in interleukin-6 knock-out mice. *Journal of Neuroscience*, **24** (18), 4432–4443.

93 Qiu, J., Cafferty, W.B., McMahon, S.B. and Thompson, S.W. (2005) Conditioning injury-induced spinal axon regeneration requires signal transducer and activator of transcription 3 activation. *Journal of Neuroscience*, **25** (7), 1645–1653.

94 Cao, Z., Gao, Y. Bryson, J.B., Hou, J., Chaudhry, N., Siddiq, M., Martinez, J., Spencer, T., Carmel, J., Hart, R.B. and Filbin, M.T. (2006) The cytokine interleukin-6 is sufficient but not necessary to mimic the peripheral conditioning lesion effect on axonal growth. *Journal of Neuroscience*, **26** (20), 5565–5573.

95 Memet, S. (2006) NF-kappaB functions in the nervous system: from development to disease. *Biochemical Pharmacology*, **72** (9), 1180–1195.

96 Byrnes, K.R., Garay, J., Di Giovanni, S., De Biase, A., Knoblach, S.M., Hoffman, E.P., Movsesyan, V. and Faden, A.I.,

(2006) Expression of two temporally distinct microglia-related gene clusters after spinal cord injury. *Glia*, **53** (4), 420–433.

97 Sano, H., Hsu, D.K., Yu, L., Apgar, J.R., Kuwabara, I., Yamanaka, T., Hirashima, M. and Liu, F.T., (2000) Human galectin-3 is a novel chemoattractant for monocytes and macrophages. *Journal of Immunology*, **165** (4), 2156–2164.

98 Fonseca, M.I., Zhou, J., Botto, M. and Tenner, A.J. (2004) Absence of C1q leads to less neuropathology in transgenic mouse models of Alzheimer's disease. *Journal of Neuroscience*, **24** (29), 6457–6465.

99 Di Giovanni, S. (2006) Regeneration following spinal cord injury, from experimental models to humans: where are we? *Expert Opinion on Therapeutic Targets*, **10** (3), 363–376.

100 Carmichael, S.T. (2006) Cellular and molecular mechanisms of neural repair after stroke: making waves. *Annals of Neurology*, **59** (5), 735–742.

101 Kapfhammer, J.P. and Schwab, M.E. (1994) Inverse patterns of myelination and GAP-43 expression in the adult CNS: neurite growth inhibitors as regulators of neuronal plasticity? *The Journal of Comparative Neurology*, **340** (2), 194–206.

102 Bonilla, I.E., Tanabe, K. and Strittmatter, S.M. (2002) Small proline-rich repeat protein 1A is expressed by axotomized neurons and promotes axonal outgrowth. *Journal of Neuroscience*, **22** (4), 1303–1315.

103 Carmichael, S.T., Archibeque, I. Luke, L., Nolan, T., Momiy, J. and Li, S. (2005) Growth-associated gene expression after stroke: evidence for a growth-promoting region in peri-infarct cortex. *Experimental Neurology*, **193** (2), 291–311.

104 Farlow, D.N., Vansant, G., Cameron, A.A., Chang, J., Khoh-Reiter, S., Pham, N.L., Wu, W., Sagara, Y., Nicholls, J.G., Carlo, D.J. and Ill, C.R. (2000) Gene expression monitoring for gene

discovery in models of peripheral and central nervous system differentiation regeneration, and trauma. *Journal of Cellular Biochemistry*, **80** (2), 171–180.

105 Schmitt, A.B., Breuer, S., Liman, J., Buss, A., Schlangen, C., Pech, K., Hol, E.M., Brook, G.A., Noth, J. and Schwaiger, F.W. (2003) Identification of regeneration-associated genes after central and peripheral nerve injury in the adult rat. *BMC Neuroscience*, **4**, 8.

106 Iwata, T., Namikawa, K., Honma, M., Mori, N., Yachiku, S. and Kiyama, H. (2002) Increased expression of mRNAs for microtubule disassembly molecules during nerve regeneration. *Brain Research. Molecular Brain Research*, **102** (1–2), 105–109.

107 Mori, N. and Morii, H. (2002) SCG10-related neuronal growth-associated proteins in neural development plasticity, degeneration, and aging. *Journal of Neuroscience Research*, **70** (3), 264–273.

108 Mason, M.R., Lieberman, A.R. and Anderson, P.N. (2003) Corticospinal neurons up-regulate a range of growth-associated genes following intracortical but not spinal, axotomy. *The European Journal of Neuroscience*, **18** (4), 789–802.

109 Suh, L.H., Oster, S.F., Soehrman, S.S., Grenningloh, G. and Sretavan, D.W. (2004) L1/laminin modulation of growth cone response to EphB triggers growth pauses and regulates the microtubule destabilizing protein SCG10. *Journal of Neuroscience*, **24** (8), 1976–1986.

110 De Winter, F., Holtmaat, A.J. and Verhaagen, J. (2002) Neuropilin and class 3 semaphorins in nervous system regeneration. *Advances in Experimental Medicine and Biology*, **515**, 115–139.

111 Schwab, J.M., Beschorner, R., Nguyen, T.D., Meyermann, R. and Schluesener, H.J. (2001) Differential cellular accumulation of connective tissue growth factor defines a subset of reactive

astrocytes, invading fibroblasts, and endothelial cells following central nervous system injury in rats and humans. *Journal of Neurotrauma*, **18** (4), 377–388.

112 Lin, J. and Cai, W. (2004) Effect of vimentin on reactive gliosis: *in vitro* and *in vivo* analysis. *Journal of Neurotrauma*, **21** (11), 1671–1682.

113 Sandvig, A., Berry, M., Barrett, L.B., Butt, A. and Logan, A. (2004) Myelin-, reactive glia-, and scar-derived CNS axon growth inhibitors: expression, receptor signaling, and correlation with axon regeneration. *Glia*, **46** (3), 225–251.

114 Emery, D.L., Royo, N.C., Fischer, I., Saatman, K.E. and McIntosh, T.K. (2003) Plasticity following injury to the adult central nervous system: is recapitulation of a developmental state worth promoting? *Journal of Neurotrauma*, **20** (12), 1271–1292.

115 Gris, P., Murphy, S., Jacob, J.E., Atkinson, I. and Brown, A. (2003) Differential gene expression profiles in embryonic adult-injured and adult-uninjured rat spinal cords. *Molecular and Cellular Neurosciences*, **24** (3), 555–567.

116 Harel, N.Y. and Strittmatter, S.M. (2006) Can regenerating axons recapitulate developmental guidance during recovery from spinal cord injury? *Nature Reviews. Neuroscience*, **7** (8), 603–616.

117 Spencer, T. and Filbin, M.T. (2004) A role for cAMP in regeneration of the adult mammalian CNS. *Journal of Anatomy*, **204** (1), 49–55.

118 Cai, D., Deng, K. Mellado, W., Lee, J., Ratan, R.R. and Filbin, M.T. (2002) Arginase I and polyamines act down-stream from cyclic AMP in over-coming inhibition of axonal growth MAG and myelin *in vitro*. *Neuron*, **35** (4), 711–719.

119 Qiu, J., Cai, D., Dai, H., McAtee, M., Hoffman, P.N., Bregman, B.S. and Filbin, M.T. (2002) Spinal axon regeneration induced by elevation of cyclic AMP. *Neuron*, **34** (6), 895–903.

120 Gao, Y., Deng, K., Hou, J., Bryson, J.B., Barco, A., Nikulina, E., Spencer, T., Mellado, W., Kandel, E.R. and Filbin, M.T. (2004) Activated CREB is sufficient to overcome inhibitors in myelin and promote spinal axon regeneration *in vivo*. *Neuron*, **44** (4), 609–621.

121 Herdegen, T., Skene, P. and Bahr, M. (1997) The c-Jun transcription factor-bipotential mediator of neuronal death survival and regeneration. *Trends in Neurosciences*, **20** (5), 227–231.

122 Lindwall, C., Dahlin, L., Lundborg, G. and Kanje, M. (2004) Inhibition of c-Jun phosphorylation reduces axonal outgrowth of adult rat nodose ganglia and dorsal root ganglia sensory neurons. *Molecular and Cellular Neurosciences*, **27** (3), 267–279.

123 Lindwall, C. and Kanje, M. (2005) The role of p-c-Jun in survival and outgrowth of developing sensory neurons. *Neuroreport*, **16** (15), 1655–1659.

124 Pearson, A.G., Gray, C.W., Pearson, J.F., Greenwood, J.M., During, M.J. and Dragunow, M. (2003) ATF3 enhances c-Jun-mediated neurite sprouting. *Brain Research. Molecular Brain Research*, **120** (1), 38–45.

125 Campbell, G., Hutchins, K., Winterbottom, J., Grenningloh, G., Lieberman, A.R. and Anderson, P.N. (2005) Upregulation of activating transcription factor 3 (ATF3) by intrinsic CNS neurons regenerating axons into peripheral nerve grafts. *Experimental Neurology*, **192** (2), 340–347.

126 Seijffers, R., Allchorne, A.J. and Woolf, C.J. (2006) The transcription factor ATF-3 promotes neurite outgrowth. *Molecular and Cellular Neurosciences*, **32** (1–2), 143–154.

127 Fujitani, M., Yamagishi, S., Che, Y.H., Hata, K., Kubo, T., Ino, H., Tohyama, M. and Yamashita, T. (2004) P311 accelerates nerve regeneration of the

axotomized facial nerve. *Journal of Neurochemistry*, **91** (3), 737–744.

128 Banner, L.R. and Patterson, P.H. (1994) Major changes in the expression of the mRNAs for cholinergic differentiation factor/leukemia inhibitory factor and its receptor after injury to adult peripheral nerves and ganglia. *Proceedings of the National Academy of Sciences of the United States of America*, **91** (15), 7109–7113.

129 Bolin, L.M., Verity, A.N., Silver, J.E., Shooter, E.M. and Abrams, J.S. (1995) Interleukin-6 production by Schwann cells and induction in sciatic nerve injury. *Journal of Neurochemistry*, **64** (2), 850–858.

130 Kurek, J.B., Austin, L., Cheema, S.S., Bartlett, P.F. and Murphy, M. (1996) Up-regulation of leukaemia inhibitory factor and interleukin-6 in transected sciatic nerve and muscle following denervation. *Neuromuscular Disorders*, **6** (2), 105–114.

131 Blesch, A., Uy, H.S., Grill, R.J., Cheng, J.G., Patterson, P.H. and Tuszynski, M.H. (1999) Leukemia inhibitory factor augments neurotrophin expression and corticospinal axon growth after adult CNS injury. *Journal of Neuroscience*, **19** (9), 3556–3566.

132 Guo, X., Chandrasekaran, V., Lein, P., Kaplan, P.L. and Higgins, D. (1999) Leukemia inhibitory factor and ciliary neurotrophic factor cause dendritic retraction in cultured rat sympathetic neurons. *Journal of Neuroscience*, **19** (6), 2113–2121.

133 Raivich, G., Jones, L.L. Werner, A., Bluthmann, H., Doetschmann, T. and Kreutzberg, G.W., (1999) Molecular signals for glial activation: pro- and anti-inflammatory cytokines in the injured brain. *Acta Neurochirurgica. Supplement*, **73**, 21–30.

134 Suzuki, S., Tanaka, K., Nogawa, S., Ito, D., Dembo, T., Kosakai, A. and Fukuuchi, Y. (2000) Immuno-histochemical detection of leukemia inhibitory factor after focal cerebral ischemia in rats. *Journal of Cerebral Blood Flow and Metabolism*, **20** (4), 661–668.

135 Swartz, K.R., Liu, F., Sewell, D., Schochet, T., Campbell, I., Sandor, M. and Fabry, Z. (2001) Interleukin-6 promotes post-traumatic healing in the central nervous system. *Brain Research*, **896** (1–2), 86–95.

136 Naumann, T., Schnell, O. Zhi, Q., Kirsch, M., Schubert, K.O., Sendtner, M. and Hofmann, H.D. (2003) Endogenous ciliary neurotrophic factor protects GABAergic but not cholinergic, septohippocampal neurons following fimbria-fornix transection. *Brain Pathology*, **13** (3), 309–321.

137 Suzuki, S., Yamashita, T., Tanaka, K., Hattori, H., Sawamoto, K., Okano, H. and Suzuki, N. (2005) Activation of cytokine signaling through leukemia inhibitory factor receptor (LIFR)/gp130 attenuates ischemic brain injury in rats. *Journal of Cerebral Blood Flow and Metabolism*, **25** (6), 685–693.

138 Pan, W., Cain, C., Yu, Y. and Kastin, A.J. (2006) Receptor-mediated transport of LIF across blood–spinal cord barrier is upregulated after spinal cord injury. *Journal of Neuroimmunology*, **174** (1–2), 119–125.

139 Hakkoum, D., Stoppini, L. and Muller, D. (2007) Interleukin-6 promotes sprouting and functional recovery in lesioned organotypic hippocampal slice cultures. *Journal of Neurochemistry*, **100** (3), 747–757.

140 Klein, M.A., Moller, J.C., Jones, L.L., Bluethmann, H., Kreutzberg, G.W. and Raivich, G. (1997) Impaired neuroglial activation in interleukin-6 deficient mice. *Glia*, **19** (3), 227–233.

141 Cafferty, W.B., Gardiner, N.J., Gavazzi, I., Powell, J., McMahon, S.B., Heath, J.K., Munson, J., Cohen, J. and Thompson, S.W. (2001) Leukemia inhibitory factor determines the growth status of injured adult sensory neurons. *Journal of Neuroscience*, **21** (18), 7161–7170.

142 Taga, T. (1996) Gp130, a shared signal transducing receptor component for hematopoietic and neuropoietic cytokines. *Journal of Neurochemistry*, **67** (1), 1–10.

143 Xu, Y. (2003) Regulation of p53 responses by post-translational modifications. *Cell Death and Differentiation*, **10** (4), 400–403.

144 Helton, E.S. and Chen, X. (2007) p53 modulation of the DNA damage response. *Journal of Cellular Biochemistry*, **100** (4), 883–896.

145 Klein, C. and Vassilev, L.T. (2004) Targeting the p53–MDM2 interaction to treat cancer. *British Journal of Cancer*, **91** (8), 1415–1419.

146 Vassilev, L.T. (2004) Small-molecule antagonists of p53–MDM2 binding: research tools and potential thera-peutics. *Cell Cycle*, **3** (4), 419–421.

147 Fouad, K., Klusman, I. and Schwab, M.E. (2004) Regenerating corticospinal fibers in the Marmoset (*Callitrix jacchus*) after spinal cord lesion and treatment with the anti-Nogo-A antibody IN-1. *The European Journal of Neuroscience*, **20** (9), 2479–2482.

148 Lee, J.K., Kim, J.E., Sivula, M. and Strittmatter, S.M. (2004) Nogo receptor antagonism promotes stroke recovery by enhancing axonal plasticity. *Journal of Neuroscience*, **24** (27), 6209–6217.

149 Buchli, A.D. and Schwab, M.E. (2005) Inhibition of Nogo: a key strategy to increase regeneration plasticity and functional recovery of the lesioned central nervous system. *Annals of Medicine*, **37** (8), 556–567.

150 Wang, L., Zhang, Z., Wang, Y., Zhang, R. and Chopp, M. (2004) Treatment of stroke with erythropoietin enhances neurogenesis and angiogenesis and improves neurological function in rats. *Stroke*, **35** (7), 1732–1737.

6
Axonal mRNA in Regeneration

Christina F. Vogelaar and James W. Fawcett

6.1
Introduction

Neurons are highly polarized cells. Especially, their axons can be very long, up to 1 m in humans. It would, therefore, not be surprising if specific axonal functions would be performed and regulated locally rather than back in the cell body. In fact, the axon volume is some hundred times larger than the volume of the cell body, and about 99% of the cell content of proteins is located in the axon. Proteins transported by slow transport may not be able to reach the axon terminal because their half-life may be too short [1,2]. It was therefore proposed that long axons may have a local source of newly synthesized proteins, possibly from a local pool of mRNA. Axonal mRNA localization was reported as early as 1962. The field remained relatively unexplored, however, because of the lack of evidence for functional translation machinery in axons [2]. In contrast, the field of mRNA localization and local protein synthesis in dendrites has recently flourished. Hundreds of dendritically localized mRNAs have been identified and implicated in processes such as synaptic plasticity [2–4]. Most mammalian central nervous system (CNS) neurons appear to transport mRNA exclusively to their dendrites but not to their axons [5,6]. However, it has now become clear that axons in the peripheral nervous system (PNS) and also some particular CNS axons do contain mRNA (see Section 6.3). It has also been established that axonal mRNA molecules contain a variety of targeting sequences in their 3′ UTR that enable RNA-binding proteins to bind and transport them into the axon. The axonal transport of these so-called RNP granules that also contain ribosomes is tubulin dependent and exerted by kinesin motor proteins [7,8]. There is still much to be done on the identification of mRNAs, on the local control of translation, and on the functions of local protein synthesis from axonal mRNA. Here, we review recent progress made in this area, with a particular emphasis on the role of local protein synthesis in axon regeneration.

6.2
A Link Between Axon Regeneration and Local Protein Synthesis

In mammals, PNS neurons are able to regenerate their axons after injury. Severed axons in the proximal nerve stump sprout and regenerate into the permissive environment created by Schwann cells forming endoneurial tubes. Axons reinnervate their target organs leading to complete functional recovery depending on the type of lesion made [9]. In contrast, CNS axons mostly fail to regenerate. After spinal cord injury, for instance, regeneration of CNS axons is impaired due to the formation of a scar containing inhibitory molecules, such as proteoglycans, myelin proteins, Nogo, and semaphorins [10,11]. However, it has amply been demonstrated that, apart from encountering an inhibitory environment, CNS axons lack the intrinsic capacity to regenerate, particularly if they are cut far from the cell body [12–14]. Using an *in vitro* transection paradigm, we recently showed that dorsal root ganglion (DRG) axons (i.e., PNS) were more capable of regenerating a new growth cone than retinal axons (i.e., CNS) [15,16]. Even after the removal of the DRG, axons were still capable of regenerating a growth cone, indicating that this process was independent of the cell body. The treatment of axons with protein synthesis inhibitors decreased the regenerative capacity of the PNS axons to the CNS axon levels. Quantifications of ribosomes and phosphorylated translation elongation factors showed that peripheral axons contain ribosomes and translation machinery, while ribosomes were undetectable in mature central axons [16]. These data suggest that PNS axons possess a higher intrinsic capacity to regenerate, in part because of their ability to synthesize proteins locally within the axon. It is, however, not clear yet which mRNAs are translated in response to injury. The following section will summarize what is known to date about mRNA molecules that are localized in axons.

6.3
Axonal mRNA Update

There are numerous studies identifying axonally localized mRNA molecules. A variety of techniques have been used both *in vitro* and *in vivo*, showing selective localization of relatively few mRNAs. This suggests that the axonal transport of mRNA is highly selective and that the function of mRNA translation in axons may be confined to very specific axonal processes. Table 6.1 summarizes studies performed on invertebrate species, such as squid and snails, with well-defined nervous systems consisting of a limited number of neurons, whose processes are generally referred to as axons. The squid giant axon is the classic model for studying axonal physiology. Striking from these studies on invertebrate axons is the presence of cytoskeletal mRNAs, such as β-*actin, actin depolymerizing factor* (*cofilin*), and β-*tubulin* [17–20]. This suggests that the cytoskeletal building blocks for axon growth can be locally synthesized. The presence of mRNAs for ribosomal proteins and translation elongation factors suggests that the local protein synthesis machinery at least partly maintains itself [17–19]. mRNAs encoding metabolic proteins again support the view that the axon is, at least in

Table 6.1 mRNA molecules localized in invertebrate axons.

Species/references	Tissue preparation	Gene group	mRNA
Aplysia [19,21]	Pedal pleural ganglia	Protein synthesis	Ribosomal proteins L8, L18, L31, S6, S15, S16, elongation factor 1α, Cytoplasmic polyadenylation element binding protein (CPEB)
	Cell culture	Cytoskeletal	Tα1-tubulin, β-thymosin
		Neuropeptides	Sensorin
		Others	Fasciclin-like, ubiquitin
Lymnaea stagnalis [20,22]	Pedal A neurons/CNS	Cytoskeletal	β-Thymosin, β-actin
	Cell culture/tissue	Neuropeptides	Ala-Pro-Gly-Trp(APGW)-amide, egg laying hormone, Phe-Met-Arg-Phe(FMRF)-amide Light yellow cell mRNA. Moluscan insulin-related peptide 1 and III
Squid [17,18]	Giant axon	Protein synthesis	Ribosomal proteins L7, L7A, L8, L9, L27A, S5, S8, S25, S27A, elongation factor 2
	Axoplasm/synaptosomes	Cytoskeletal	β-Actin, α-tubulin, β-tubulin, β-spectrin, kinesin (transport), neurofilament proteins
		Metabolism	Enolase, fructose PTS enzyme III
		Mitochondrial (nuclear encoded)	Cytochrome oxidase assembly protein, cytochrome c oxidase subunit Vb and XVII, dihydrolipamine dehydrogenase, ubiquinone biosynthesis protein CoQ7
		Others	Heat shock protein 70 (HSP70), selenoprotein W, protein phosphatase 2C, ubiquitin C LDL receptor adaptor protein, nucleoside diphosphate kinase

Table 6.2 mRNA molecules localized in vertebrate axons.

Species and tissue/references	Age	Preparation technique	Gene group	Axonally localized mRNA molecules
Xenopus retina [39,40]	E	Cell culture FISH, reporter gene	Cytoskeletal Metabolism	β-Actin, cofilin Enolase
Goldfish Mauthner neurons [7,55,56]	A	Axoplasm/PARPs ISH, reporter gene	Cytoskeletal	β-Actin, neurofilament-M
			Others	BC1
Chicken sympathetic neurons [26]	E	Cell/explant culture ISH, metabolic labeling	Cytoskeletal	β-Actin, actin-depolymerizing factor (cofilin), neurofilament-L
Rat sympathetic neurons [23]	N	Cell culture (comp.) Metabolic labeling	Cytoskeletal	β-Actin, β-tubulin
Rat hippocampal neurons [5,57]	E	Cell culture ISH	Cytoskeletal	β-Actin, microtubule-associated protein 1B
Rat olfactory bulb [28]	E	Tissue sections *In situ* EM	Neuropeptides	Calcitonin gene-related peptide (CGRP)
Rat olfactory bulb [29,30]	A	Tissue sections ISH	Others	Olfactory marker protein, odorant receptors
Mouse motor neurons [58]	E	Cell culture ISH	Cytoskeletal	β-Actin
Rat hypothalamic neurons ([31,32]; review)	A	Tissue sections ISH	Cytoskeletal Neuropeptides Other	Neurofilament Vasopressin, oxytocin, galanin, dynorphin BC1
Rat dorsal root ganglion [42]	E	Cell/explant culture (comp.)/FISH, PCR	Signaling	RhoA

Rat dorsal root ganglion [24,25,49]	ACL	Cell culture (comp.) Microarrays, PCR, proteomics	Protein synthesis	Calreticulin, endoplasmic reticulum p29, cyclophilin A
			Cytoskeletal	β-Actin, peripherin, vimentin, neurofilament-L, γ-tropomyosin-3, cofilin 1
			Metabolism	Phosphoglycerate kinase1, α enolase1, aldolase C, GAPDH
			Chaperones	HSP27, -60, and -79, glucose-regulated protein (grp) 75 and 78, aB crystallin
			Others	γ-Synuclein, ubiquitin C-terminal hydrolase L1, peroxiredoxin 1 and 6 Superoxide dismutase 1, dimethylarginine dimethylaminohydrolase 2 Sperm protein 22 (homologue of human Park7), importin-β, hnRNPH'

E=embryonic, N=neonatal, A=adult, ACL=adult conditioning lesioned, comp.=compartmented, EM=electron microscopy, ISH=*in situ* hybridization, FISH=fluorescent *in situ* hybridization, PARPS=periaxoplasmic ribosomal plaques, PCR=polymerase chain reaction.

part, independent of the cell body. The presence of neuropeptide mRNAs suggests a functional role for axonal mRNA in synaptic transmission [21,22].

Studies of mRNA localization in vertebrate axons – summarized in Table 6.2 – have been somewhat limited due to the difficulty of obtaining axon-only preparations. In many studies (fluorescent), *in situ* hybridization was used to show the presence of selected target genes. Studies using metabolic labeling, in general, have lead to the identification of only a couple of newly synthesized proteins, due to a lack of sensitivity. These studies show that mRNAs encoding cytoskeletal proteins, such as β-*actin* and β-*tubulin*, are localized and translated in axons. The development of compartmented cultures, such as Campenot chambers and filter inserts, provided tools for more generalized techniques [23,24]. A recent study on conditioning-lesioned DRG axons shows the presence of numerous mRNAs in various functional classes, the main ones encoding, again, cytoskeletal and metabolic proteins, as well as chaperones and proteins involved in protein synthesis [25]. These axons are regarded as regenerating axons, since they underwent a conditioning-lesion some days before the DRG isolation for axon culture was conducted. Generally lacking are the data on adult axons that have not been stimulated by a conditioning lesion. In order that they can response to injury, we think that mRNA should be present in uninjured adult axons. We are currently working on embryonic, neonatal, and adult axons, for which we have developed a new culture model. Using real-time quantitative PCR, we are in the process of identifying additional axonal mRNAs and quantifying their levels during axon maturation (unpublished data).

PNS axons in general are capable of regeneration, and not only DRG axons but also sympathetic axons and motor axons have been shown to contain mRNA [23,26,27]. Mammalian CNS axons, in contrast, contain mRNA only at embryonic stages and lose their capacity to transport mRNA upon maturation [5,6,26]. There are, however, two types of mammalian CNS axons that do contain mRNA in adulthood: olfactory axons [28–30] and hypothalamic axons [31,32]. Since these are among the rare CNS axons capable of regeneration [33–35], it is very tempting to speculate that their ability to transport mRNA in their axons is involved. Although mainly mRNAs encoding neuropeptides were identified, this was done by means of *in situ* hybridization; therefore, other mRNAs have not been searched for in these axons.

The various experiments described above show that there is a good correlation between the presence of mRNA and their ability to regenerate. These experiments, however, do not prove that local protein synthesis really plays a role in axon regeneration. In the following sections, we will review studies that point more directly to a role of axonal protein synthesis in growth cone function and regeneration.

6.4
Axonal RNA Transport and Translation in Axon Guidance

6.4.1
Growth Cone Guidance of *Xenopus* Retinal Axons is Dependent on Axonal Protein Synthesis

In the laboratory of Christine Holt, the dependence of axon growth and guidance on local translation has been investigated using *Xenopus* retinal axons. For this purpose, the guidance molecules netrin-1, semaphorin 3A (Sema3A), and BDNF were added to the axon cultures in a gradient in order to assess the turning of the growth cone away from the repellent or toward the attractant. The axon acted independently of the cell body, as the growth cone turning response still occurred even after the cell body was removed from the culture. Inhibition of local protein synthesis abolished the normal turning responses to Sema3A (repellent), netrin-1 (attractant or repellent, depending on the substrate), and BDNF (attractant) [36]. Axon extension, however, was not affected, indicating that local protein synthesis is not required for normal growth. The authors then showed that addition of the guidance cues resulted in activation of the translation initiation factor eIF-4E by release from its binding partner eIF-4EBP1 through phosphorylation by target of rapamycin (TOR). Incorporation of ^{3}H-leucine into newly synthesized proteins was assayed, showing an increase of local protein synthesis after the addition of guidance molecules [36].

A very interesting new guidance cue is provided by the homeodomain transcription factor engrailed-2 (En-2), internalized by *Xenopus* retinal axons, which elicited differential responses in turning of nasal and temporal axons. En-2 induced these responses in a transcription-independent manner, as the responses occurred in axons after cell body removal and were abolished by protein synthesis inhibitors. En-2 induced the incorporation of ^{3}H-leucine and the phosphorylation of eIF-4E and eIF-4EBP1 [37]. Slit2-induced growth cone collapse and turning also depend on local protein synthesis through phosphorylation of the translation factor and its inhibitor. A correlated decline in filamentous (F)-actin and increase in cofilin immunoreactivity was observed. The authors showed that *cofilin* mRNA was present in axons and that local synthesis of cofilin protein was increased as fast as 5 minutes after incubation with Slit2. Sema3A, another collapsing agent, elicited the same increase in cofilin synthesis. Since cofilin is an actin-depolymerizing protein, it was concluded that the decline in F-actin was likely to be mediated by newly synthesized cofilin [38].

6.4.2
Growth Cone Guidance is Mediated by Asymmetrical Transport and Translation of Selective mRNA Molecules

The Holt laboratory then moved on to investigate in more detail the mechanisms of local protein synthesis dependent netrin-1 attraction. They demonstrated the binding of β-*actin* mRNA to the RNA-binding protein Vg1RBP, the *Xenopus* homologue of zip-code binding protein 1 (ZBP1), which had been shown to bind to and

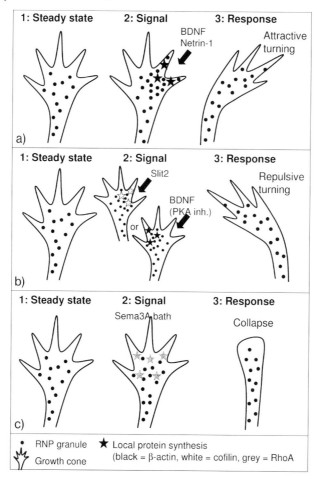

Figure 6.1 Model describing the local translation events immediately after exposure to guidance molecules. (a) Local transport and translation of β-*actin* mRNA in response to a gradient of BDNF or netrin-1, causing attractive turning [39,40]. (b) Repellent Slit2 elicits local synthesis of cofilin in the near side of the growth cone, causing actin depolymerization and repulsive turning [38]. In contrast, BDNF under repulsive conditions (using a PKA inhibitor) causes translation of β-*actin* at the far side of the growth cone, causing repulsive turning [40]. (c) Bath application of Sema3A induces the translation of *RhoA* mRNA, required for growth cone collapse [42].

transport β-*actin* mRNA in axons. Vg1RBP immunoreactivity colocalized with β-*actin* mRNA in growth cones and filopodia in a punctuate pattern. A netrin-1 gradient induced rapid translocation of Vg1RBP/β-*actin* RNA granules to the near side of the growth cone and to the filopodia closest to the (attracting) netrin-1 [39]. Asymmetrical phosphorylation of eIF-4EBP1 was also observed. Newly synthesized β-actin protein at the near side of the growth cone was shown as early as 5 minutes after incubation with netrin-1, prior to turning (Figure 6.1a). Downregulation of β-*actin* mRNA using morpholinos abolished the growth cone turning response. A very important observation made in this study was that other localized mRNAs – *enolase* and *cofilin* – were not translated in response to netrin-1, indicating that the regulation of local protein synthesis by guidance molecules is selective and specific [39].

At the same time, Gary Bassell and coworkers looked at the guidance of *Xenopus* spinal neurons, showing the BDNF-induced bidirectional turning (normally attractive but becoming repulsive through PKA inhibition) to depend on local protein synthesis. The BDNF treatment increased the number of ZBP1 granules colocalizing with β-*actin* mRNA, while a gradient of BDNF induced a local increase of ZBP1/β-*actin* mRNA granules on the near side of the attracted growth cone [40]. The application of antisense oligonucleotides directed against β-*actin* abolished the increase in ZBP1/β-*actin* mRNA colocalization and abolished the BDNF-induced turning. Asymmetrical synthesis of β-actin protein took place in response to BDNF under both attractive and repulsive conditions, blocked by the oligos (Figure 6.1a and b). Notably, the β-actin increase under repulsive conditions was seen in the far side of the growth cone (Figure 6.1b), accompanied by a decrease on the side close to the repulsive signal. The authors termed this phenomenon as reverse asymmetry. The same observations were made using local photolysis of caged Ca^{2+} compounds instead of BDNF, suggesting that the turning response to BDNF is mediated by a local rise in Ca^{2+}. In conclusion, both the attraction and the repulsion of growth cones were mediated by ZBP1-dependent translocation and translation of β-*actin* mRNA in a Ca^{2+}-dependent manner [40].

The above-described data are summarized in Table 6.3. However, there appears to be a discrepancy between the data of Holt's group and those of Bassell's with respect to repulsive turning, as the attraction and repulsion responses were studied using either different guidance molecules – netrin-1/BDNF versus Sema3A/Slit2 – under the same conditions, or using only one guidance molecule – BDNF (and Ca^{2+}) – under different conditions. This might indicate that the mRNA(s) involved is (are) specified by the guidance molecule rather than the modality of the turning response. If attraction to a guidance molecule under standard conditions is mediated by β-*actin* translation, the repulsion by the same molecule seems to be so, too. Molecules that are repulsive under standard conditions, though, seem to be acting through the translation of mRNA molecules different from β-*actin*, for Sema3A and Slit that

Table 6.3 Differential regulation of mRNA translation in response to guidance cues.

Guidance molecule	Turning response	mRNA translated	mRNA not translated
BDNF	Attraction	β-*actin*	n.d.
BDNF + PKA inh.	Repulsion	β-*actin*	n.d.
Netrin-1	Attraction	β-*actin*	*enolase, cofilin*
Netrin-1on laminin	Repulsion	n.d.	n.d.
Sema3A	Repulsion/collapse	*cofilin/RhoA*	β-*actin*
Slit2	Repulsion/collapse	*cofilin*	n.d.

Local synthesis of specific proteins precedes and is required for the growth cone turning response [38–40,42].

molecule is *cofilin*. It would be interesting to test this hypothesis using netrin-1 under repulsive conditions.

These studies provided a wealth of important information: (1) guidance cues stimulate selective asymmetrical localization and translation of specific mRNAs, (2) this response is rapid and precedes the turning response of the growth cone, (3) local protein synthesis is essential for turning, and (4) normal axon extension does not depend on local protein synthesis. This work, however, was done on embryonic *Xenopus* axons, which are capable of growth and regeneration [41]. In the next section, we will describe the data on axonal translation machinery and functions in mammalian axons.

6.5
Axonal RNA in Mammalian Axons

6.5.1
Axon Guidance in Rat Dorsal Root Ganglion Axons

Using embryonic DRG neurons, Wu *et al.* [42] were able to show that Sema3A-induced growth cone collapse was, as in *Xenopus*, blocked by inhibiting local protein synthesis. The axonal localization of *RhoA* mRNA was shown using *in situ* hybridization as well as RT-PCR on cultured axons isolated by using compartmented cultures. RhoA is known to be essential for Sema3A-induced growth cone collapse. However, mRNAs for other members of the Rho family of small GTPases, *cdc42* and *rac1* were absent in axons, and *ROCK1* (Rho kinase 1) mRNA was also not observed. Treatment of axons with Sema3A resulted in an increase of RhoA immunofluorescence in growth cones prior to collapse (Figure 6.1c), which was blocked by applying protein synthesis inhibitors. Infection of DRG neurons with viral vectors containing the 3' UTR of RhoA linked to EGFP showed localization of EGFP mRNA in axons. Using *RhoA* 3' UTR linked to destabilized EGFP (with a half-life of 1 hour) newly synthesized EGFP in the axon after treatment with Sema3A was observed. siRNA directed against *RhoA* mRNA abolished Sema3A-induced growth cone collapse [42].

Similarly, cultured adult DRG axons have been shown to respond to Sema3A by rapid phosphorylation of eIF-4E and inhibition of local protein synthesis inhibited Sema3A-induced growth cone collapse. Low levels of Sema3A were observed to increase anterograde and retrograde axonal transports, which were also inhibited by protein synthesis inhibitors. In addition, these responses were also seen in axons isolated from their cell bodies and were mediated by Fyn and cdk5 [43].

6.5.2
RNA Binding Proteins: A Link Between Axonal RNA and Axon Maintenance

Transport of mRNA into axons (and dendrites) is mediated by RNA-binding proteins in structures called RNP granules. These stabilize the mRNA molecules and some also regulate translation. One of the best characterized axonal RNA-binding proteins is survival motoneuron 1 (SMN1). Mutations in the SMN1 gene lead to spinal motor atrophy (SMA), a disease characterized by motor neuron death. Mice homozygous for SMN1 disruption die, but can be rescued by introducing human SMN2, a close homologue in humans, known to compensate for SMN1 deficiency. SMN1−/−; SMN2 mice survive, but develop SMA-type phenotypes [27]. Cultured embryonic primary motor neurons from these mice exhibited decreased axon growth and a reduction in growth cone size. *In situ* hybridization revealed absence of axonal and growth cone β-*actin* mRNA in the SMN1−/−;SMN2 motor neurons, accompanied by decreased axonal levels of β-actin protein. This is the first study showing that the transport of β-*actin* mRNA is essential for the expression of β-actin protein in motor neuron axons. Although SMN1 also plays a role in assembly of spliceosomal small nuclear ribonucleoproteins (snRNPs), these data suggest that the motor neuron loss in SMA patients may be due to a lack of axon growth and maintenance [27]. Similarly, Fragile X mental retardation protein (FRMP), an RNA-binding protein predominantly studied in dendrites in association with Fragile X syndrome, was localized to cultured embryonic hippocampal axons. *FMR1* knock-out neurons displayed reduced growth cone motility and excess filopodia. These data suggest that, apart from the well-studied dendritic phenotype, Fragile X syndrome may also have a developmental axonal phenotype, which merits further attention [44]. Finally, the RNA-binding protein HuD is colocalized with ribosomes and with *GAP-43* mRNA in dendrites of PC12 cells [45]. HuD, as shown before, stabilizes GAP-43 mRNA in cell bodies and is upregulated after injury [46]. HuD knockout mice displayed an aberrant hind limb reflex and reduced rotarod performance but without the loss of motoneurons [47].

6.5.3
Conditioning Lesioned Adult Rat DRG Axons

After a conditioning axonal crush lesion, cultured adult sensory neurons rapidly extend long axons. In the laboratory of Jeffery Twiss, cultures were made of these regenerating DRG neurons on porous membranes. The axons growing through the pores were harvested for isolation of pure axonal RNA. Using RT-PCR, several cytoskeletal, injury-response, metabolic, and neurodegeneration protein mRNAs were found (see Table 6.2). A proteomic approach, using [^{35}S]methionine/cysteine proved that these mRNAs were indeed locally translated. Local treatment of axons with NGF and BDNF leads to an increase in axonal levels of β-*actin*, *peripherin*, and *vimentin* mRNA, indicating that the transport of specific mRNAs is regulated by neurotrophic factors [25,47]. In collaboration with the Twiss laboratory, Mike Fainzilber and coworkers showed that β-*importin* mRNA was present in these axon preparations. β-Importin, through heterodimers with α-importin, mediates nuclear import of proteins with a nuclear localization signal (NLS) [47,48]. α-Importin was constitutively present in axons, whereas β-importin protein was only expressed after nerve injury. The authors showed that nerve injury induces local synthesis of β-importin, which then dimerizes with α-importin and is transported retrogradely by dynein [49]. This complex was shown to carry synthetic biotin-NLS, suggesting that injury induces the formation of a nuclear import complex in the axon, through local synthesis of β-importin, and that the retrograde transport of this complex mediates the transcriptional cell body reaction to injury. Indeed, a competitive NLS peptide inhibited regeneration of adult DRG neurons [49]. The Fainzilber group then moved on to show that locally synthesized vimentin binds to β-importin and is responsible for the retrograde transport of phosphorylated Erk to the cell body. Axon regeneration was shown to be delayed in *vimentin* null mutant mice [50].

6.6
Summary and Conclusions

The evidence for the localization of a subset of mRNAs in some classes of axon is now overwhelming. The presence of many cytoskeletal mRNAs suggests a role for local protein synthesis in axonal maintenance and growth. It is striking that axonal RNA is mostly found in axons that are capable of regeneration. Axon regeneration

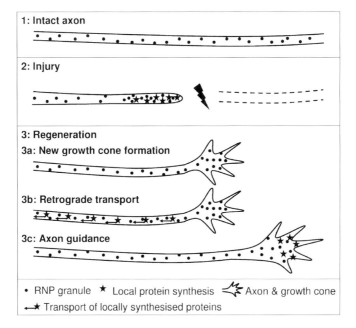

Figure 6.2 Model describing the local translation events immediately after axonal injury. (1) The intact axon is likely to contain RNA granules, scattered over its whole length, traveling in both directions. (2) Upon injury, RNP granules may accumulate in (or be actively transported to) the proximal nerve stump, where local translation will take place. (3a) The formation of a new growth cone depends on local synthesis of presumably cytoskeletal proteins [16]. (3b) Newly synthesized β-importin forms a complex with α-importin and is retrogradely transported by dynein, carrying target proteins that may elicit the cell body gene expression changes [49,54]. (3c) Guidance of molecules to their denervated targets is likely to be regulated by local protein synthesis (extrapolation from Figure 6.1).

is a complex process, whose first step is the formation of a new growth cone, followed by axon elongation and pathfinding. In response to retrograde signals, the cell bodies of axons that project peripherally undergo a wide variety of gene expression changes enabling them to regenerate (reviewed in [51]). Current evidence suggests that local protein synthesis is required for these three processes (Figure 6.2): new growth cone formation, retrograde signaling, and axon guidance [16,39,40,52]. In *in vitro* models, axon elongation does not require local protein synthesis [16,39]. The bulk of evidence suggests that the translation of local mRNA is necessary for the initiation of regeneration, whereas subsequent growth can probably be provided by proteins transported from the cell body. Since adult mammalian CNS axons seem to lack axonal RNA, they are presumably impaired in the initiation of the regenerative process. A second event that occurs shortly after axon injury is the change in gene expression profile in the neuronal cell bodies that facilitates regeneration. The retrograde signal that initiates this process relies on axonally produced β-importin [49]. The ability of CNS neurons to activate a regeneration-associated gene profile after injury is unclear. Corticospinal neurons failed to induce regeneration genes such as c-jun, ATF3, GAP-43, and SCG10 after injury far away from the cell bodies, whereas injury close to the cell bodies did induce growth-related genes [13].

The various studies discussed in this review suggest that the poor regeneration of CNS axons can be partly explained by the absence or very low levels of protein translation within them. This may lead to a slow or an absent regenerative response to injury. However, many CNS axons do attempt to regenerate, presumably relying on the protein transport system in the axons that still enables some of them to make a new growth cone and grow, particularly when the lesion is close to the cell body. This regenerative effort can be stimulated by growth factors or by the removal of inhibitory molecules [53]. The challenge in the future lies in the elucidation of the axonal transport mechanisms and in finding ways to stimulate or re-induce adult CNS axonal RNA transport.

References

1 Alvarez, J., Giuditta, A. and Koenig, E. (2000) Protein synthesis in axons and terminals: significance for maintenance, plasticity and regulation of phenotype – with a critique of slow transport theory. *Progress in Neurobiology* **62**, 1–62.

2 Twiss, J.L. and van Minnen, J. (2006) New insights into neuronal regeneration: the role of axonal protein synthesis in pathfinding and axonal extension. *Journal of Neurotrauma*, **23**, 295–308.

3 Eberwine, J., Belt, B., Kacharmina, J.E. and Miyashiro, K. (2002) Analysis of subcellularly localized mRNAs using *in situ* hybridization mRNA amplification, and expression profiling. *Neurochemical Research*, **27**, 1065–1077.

4 Martin, K.C. (2004) Local protein synthesis during axon guidance and synaptic plasticity. *Current Opinion in Neurobiology*, **14**, 305–310.

5 Bassell, G.J., Zhang, H.L., Byrd, A.L., Femino, A.M., Singer, R.H., Taneja, K.L., Lifshitz, L.M., Herman, I.M. and Kosik, K.S. (1998) Sorting of beta-actin mRNA and protein to neurites and growth cones in culture. *Journal of Neuroscience*, **18**, 251–265.

6 Sossin, W.S. and DesGroseillers, L. (2006) Intracellular trafficking of RNA in neurons. *Traffic*, **7**, 1581–1589.

7 Sotelo-Silveira, J.R., Calliari, A., Kun, A., Koenig, E. and Sotelo, J.R. (2006) RNA trafficking in axons. *Traffic*, **7**, 508–515.

8 Zhang, H.L., Oleynikov, Y., Singer, R.H. and Bassell, G.J. (1998) Involvement of 3′ UTR sequences and RNA binding proteins in beta-actin protein localization to growth cones. *Molecular Biology of the Cell*, **9**, 189A.

9 Vogelaar, C.F., Vrinten, D.H., Hoekman, M.F., Brakkee, J.H., Burbach, J.P. and Hamers, F.P. (2004) Sciatic nerve regeneration in mice and rats: recovery of sensory innervation is followed by a slowly retreating neuropathic pain-like syndrome. *Brain Research*, **1027**, 67–72.

10 Fawcett, J. (2002) Repair of spinal cord injuries: where are we, where are we going? *Spinal Cord*, **40**, 615–623.

11 Pasterkamp, R.J. and Verhaagen, J. (2001) Emerging roles for semaphorins in neural regeneration. *Brain Research. Brain Research Reviews*, **35**, 36–54.

12 Fernandes, K.J., Fan, D.P., Tsui, B.J., Cassar, S.L. and Tetzlaff, W. (1999) Influence of the axotomy to cell body distance in rat rubrospinal and spinal motoneurons: differential regulation of GAP-43 tubulins, and neurofilament-M. *The Journal of Comparative Neurology*, **414**, 495–510.

13 Mason, M.R., Lieberman, A.R. and Anderson, P.N. (2003) Corticospinal neurons up-regulate a range of growth-associated genes following intracortical but not spinal, axotomy. *European Journal of Neuroscience*, **18**, 789–802.

14 Richardson, P.M., Issa, V.M. and Aguayo, A.J. (1984) Regeneration of long spinal axons in the rat. *Journal of Neurocytology*, **13**, 165–182.

15 Chierzi, S., Ratto, G.M., Verma, P. and Fawcett, J.W. (2005) The ability of axons to regenerate their growth cones depends on axonal type and age, and is regulated by calcium, cAMP and ERK. *European Journal of Neuroscience*, **21**, 2051–2062.

16 Verma, P., Chierzi, S., Codd, A.M., Campbell, D.S., Meyer, R.L., Holt, C.E. and Fawcett, J.W. (2005) Axonal protein synthesis and degradation are necessary for efficient growth cone regeneration. *Journal of Neuroscience*, **25**, 331–342.

17 Gioio, A.E., Eyman, M., Zhang, H.S., Lavina, Z.S., Giuditta, A. and Kaplan, B.B. (2001) Local synthesis of nuclear-encoded mitochondrial proteins in the presynaptic nerve terminal. *Journal of Neuroscience Research*, **64**, 447–453.

18 Gioio, A.E., Lavina, Z.S., Jurkovicova, D., Zhang, H., Eyman, M., Giuditta, A. and Kaplan, B.B. (2004) Nerve terminals of squid photoreceptor neurons contain a heterogeneous population of mRNAs and translate a transfected reporter mRNA. *European Journal of Neuroscience*, **20**, 865–872.

19 Moccia, R., Chen, D., Lyles, V., Kapuya, E., Yaping, E., Kalachikov, S., Spahn, C.M.T., Frank, J., Kandel, E.R., Barad, M. and Martin, K.C. (2003) An unbiased cDNA library prepared from isolated *Aplysia* sensory neuron processes is enriched for cytoskeletal and translational mRNAs. *Journal of Neuroscience*, **23**, 9409–9417.

20 van Kesteren, R.E., Carter, C., Dissel, H.M.G., van Minnen, J., Gouwenberg, Y., Syed, N.I., Spencer, G.E. and Smit, A.B. (2006) Local synthesis of actin-binding protein beta-thymosin regulates neurite outgrowth. *Journal of Neuroscience*, **26**, 152–157.

21 Schacher, S., Wu, F., Panyko, J.D., Sun, Z.Y. and Wang, D.N. (1999) Expression and branch-specific export of mRNA are regulated by synapse formation and interaction with specific postsynaptic targets. *Journal of Neuroscience*, **19**, 6338–6347.

22 van Minnen, J. (1994) Axonal localization of neuropeptide-encoding messenger-RNA in identified neurons of the snail

Lymnaea stagnalis. Cell and Tissue Research, **276**, 155–161.

23 Eng, H., Lund, K. and Campenot, R.B. (1999) Synthesis of beta-tubulin actin, and other proteins in axons of sympathetic neurons in compartmented cultures. *Journal of Neuroscience*, **19**, 1–9.

24 Zheng, J.Q., Kelly, T.K., Chang, B.S., Ryazantsev, S., Rajasekaran, A.K., Martin, K.C. and Twiss, J.L. (2001) A functional role for intra-axonal protein synthesis during axonal regeneration from adult sensory neurons. *Journal of Neuroscience*, **21**, 9291–9303.

25 Willis, D., Li, K.W., Zheng, J.Q., Chang, J.H., Smit, A., Kelly, T., Merianda, T.T., Sylvester, J., van Minnen, J. and Twiss, J.L. (2005) Differential transport and local translation of cytoskeletal injury-response, and neurodegeneration protein mRNAs in axons. *Journal of Neuroscience*, **25**, 778–791.

26 Lee, S.K. and Hollenbeck, P.J. (2003) Organization and translation of mRNA in sympathetic axons. *Journal of Cell Science*, **116**, 4467–4478.

27 Rossoll, W., Jablonka, S., Andreassi, C., Kroning, A.K., Karle, K., Monani, U.R. and Sendtner, M. (2003) Smn, the spinal muscular atrophy-determining gene product, modulates axon growth and localization of beta-actin mRNA in growth cones of motoneurons. *Journal of Cell Biology*, **163**, 801–812.

28 Denis-Donini, S., Branduardi, P., Campiglio, S. and Carnevali, M.D.C. (1998) Localization of calcitonin gene-related peptide mRNA in developing olfactory axons. *Cell and Tissue Research*, **294**, 81–91.

29 Vassar, R., Chao, S.K., Sitcheran, R., Nunez, J.M., Vosshall, L.B. and Axel, R. (1994) Topographic organization of sensory projections to the olfactory-bulb. *Cell*, **79**, 981–991.

30 Wensley, C.H., Stone, D.M., Baker, H., Kauer, J.S., Margolis, F.L. and Chikaraishi, D.M. (1995) Olfactory marker protein messenger-RNA is found in axons of olfactory receptor neurons. *Journal of Neuroscience*, **15**, 4827–4837.

31 Landry, M. and Hokfelt, T. (1998) Subcellular localization of preprogalanin messenger RNA in perikarya and axons of hypothalamo-posthypophyseal magnocellular neurons: an *in situ* hybridization study. *Neuroscience*, **84**, 897–912.

32 Mohr, E. and Richter, D. (2000) Axonal mRNAs: functional significance in vertebrates and invertebrates. *Journal of Neurocytology*, **29**, 783–791.

33 Alonso, G., Oestreicher, A.B., Gispen, W.H. and Privat, A. (1995) Immuno-localization of B-50 (Gap-43) in intact and lesioned neurohypophysis of adult-rats. *Experimental Neurology*, **131**, 93–107.

34 Astic, L. and Saucier, D. (2001) Neuronal plasticity and regeneration in the olfactory system of mammals: morphological and functional recovery following olfactory bulb deafferentation. *Cellular and Molecular Life Sciences*, **58**, 538–545.

35 Schwob, J.E. (2002) Neural regeneration and the peripheral olfactory system. *The Anatomical Record*, **269**, 33–49.

36 Campbell, D.S. and Holt, C.E. (2001) Chemotropic responses of retinal growth cones mediated by rapid local protein synthesis and degradation. *Neuron*, **32**, 1013–1026.

37 Brunet, I., Weinl, C., Piper, M., Trembleau, A., Volovitch, M., Harris, W., Prochiantz, A. and Holt, C. (2005) The transcription factor Engrailed-2 guides retinal axons. *Nature*, **438**, 94–98.

38 Piper, M., Anderson, R., Dwivedy, A., Weinl, C., van Horck, F., Leung, K.M., Cogill, E. and Holt, C. (2006) Signaling mechanisms underlying Slit2-induced collapse of *Xenopus* retinal growth cones. *Neuron*, **49**, 215–228.

39 Leung, K.M., van Horck, F.P.G., Lin, A.C., Allison, R., Standart, N. and Holt, C.E. (2006) Asymmetrical beta-actin mRNA translation in growth cones mediates attractive turning

to netrin-1. *Nature Neuroscience*, **9**, 1247–1256.

40 Yao, J.Q., Sasaki, Y., Wen, Z.X., Bassell, G.J. and Zheng, J.Q. (2006) An essential role for beta-actin mRNA localization and translation in Ca2+-dependent growth cone guidance. *Nature Neuroscience*, **9**, 1265–1273.

41 Piper, M. and Holt, C. (2004) RNA translation in axons. *Annual Review of Cell and Developmental Biology*, **20**, 505–523.

42 Wu, K.Y., Hengst, U., Cox, L.J., Macosko, E.Z., Jeromin, A., Urquhart, E.R. and Jaffrey, S.R. (2005) Local translation of RhoA regulates growth cone collapse. *Nature*, **436**, 1020–1024.

43 Li, C., Sasaki, Y., Takei, K., Yamamoto, H., Shouji, M., Sugiyama, Y., Kawakami, T., Nakamura, F., Yagi, T., Ohshima, T. and Goshima, Y. (2004) Correlation between semaphorin3A-induced facilitation of axonal transport and local activation of a translation initiation factor eukaryotic translation initiation factor 4E. *Journal of Neuroscience*, **24**, 6161–6170.

44 Antar, L.N. and Bassell, G.J. (2003) Sunrise at the synapse: the FMRP mRNP shaping the synaptic interface. *Neuron*, **37**, 555–558.

45 Smith, C.L., Afroz, R., Bassell, G.J., Furneaux, H.M., Perrone-Bizzozero, N.I. and Burry, R.W. (2004) GAP-43 mRNA in growth cones is associated with HuD and ribosomes. *Journal of Neurobiology*, **61**, 222–235.

46 Anderson, K.D., Merhege, M.A., Morin, M., Bolognani, F. and Perrone-Bizzozero, N.I. (2003) Increased expression and localization of the RNA-binding protein HuD and GAP-43 mRNA to cytoplasmic granules in DRG neurons during nerve regeneration. *Experimental Neurology*, **183**, 100–108.

47 Akamatsu, W., Fujihara, H., Mitsuhashi, T., Yano, M., Shibata, S., Hayakawa, Y., Okano, H.J., Sakakibara, S., Takano, H., Takano, T., Takahashi, T., Noda, T. and Okano, H. (2005) The RNA-binding protein HuD regulates neuronal cell identity and maturation. *Proceedings of the National Academy of Sciences of the United States of America*, **102**, 4625–4630.

48 Hanz, S. and Fainzilber, M. (2004) Integration of retrograde axonal and nuclear transport mechanisms in neurons: implications for therapeutics. *Neuroscientist*, **10**, 404–408.

49 Hanz, S., Perlson, E., Willis, D., Zheng, J.Q., Massarwa, R., Huerta, J.J., Koltzenburg, M., Kohler, M., van Minnen, J., Twiss, J.L. and Fainzilber, M. (2003) Axoplasmic importins enable retrograde injury signaling in lesioned nerve. *Neuron*, **40**, 1095–1104.

50 Perlson, E., Hanz, S., Ben Yaakov, K., Segal-Ruder, Y., Seger, R. and Fainzilber, M. (2005) Vimentin-dependent spatial translocation of an activated MAP kinase in injured nerve. *Neuron*, **45**, 715–726.

51 Vogelaar, C.F., Hoekman, M.F., Gispen, W.H. and Burbach, J.P. (2003) Homeobox gene expression in adult dorsal root ganglia during sciatic nerve regeneration: is regeneration a recapitulation of development? *European Journal of Pharmacology*, **480**, 233–250.

52 Wu, C.W.K., Zeng, F.Y. and Eberwine, J. (2007) mRNA transport to and translation in neuronal dendrites. *Analytical and Bioanalytical Chemistry*, **387**, 59–62.

53 Fawcett, J.W. (2006) Overcoming inhibition in the damaged spinal cord. *Journal of Neurotrauma*, **23**, 371–383.

54 Hanz, S. and Fainzilber, M. (2006) Retrograde signaling in injured nerve – the axon reaction revisited. *Journal of Neurochemistry*, **99**, 13–19.

55 Weiner, O.D., Zorn, A.M., Krieg, P.A. and Bittner, G.D. (1996) Medium weight neurofilament mRNA in goldfish Mauthner axoplasm. *Neuroscience Letter* **213**, 83–86.

56 Muslimov, I.A., Titmus, M., Koenig, E. and Tiedge, H. (2002) Transport of Neuronal BC1 RNA in Mauthner Axons. *Journal of Neuroscience*, **22**, 4293–4301.

57 Antar, L.N., Li, C., Zhang, H., Carroll, R.C. and Bassell, G.J. (2006) Local functions for FMRP in axon growth cone motility and activity-dependent regulation of filopodia and spine synapses. *Molecular and Cellular Neuroscience*, **32**, 37–48.

58 Rossoll, W., Jablonka, S., Andreassi, C., Kröning, A.K., Karle, K., Monani, U.R. and Sendtner, M. (2003) Smn, the spinal muscular atrophy-determining gene product, modulates axon growth and localization of beta-actin mRNA in growth cones of motoneurons. *Journal of Cell Biology*, **163**, 801–812.

7
Proteomic Approaches to Axon Injury –
Postgenomic Approaches to a Posttranscriptional Process

Izhak Michaelevski and Mike Fainzilber

Axonal injury to peripheral neurons elicits a sequence of molecular, ultrastructural, and cellular responses that are required for a successful regenerative response. Injured nerve fibers must overcome inhibitory influences in the environment [1] and mobilize intrinsic capacity for neurite outgrowth [2,3] to achieve functional regeneration. In the injured neurons, arrival of signals for cellular injury and stress is followed by the induction of transcription factors, adhesion molecules, growth-associated proteins, and structural components needed for axonal elongation. These molecular changes are accompanied by shifts in cellular organization such as the appearance of growth cones at the proximal tip of the lesioned axons and a strong increase in cellular metabolism and protein synthesis. Strikingly, this entire battery of early changes in the axon after injury must occur in the absence of transcriptional processes, due to the distance between axonal lesion sites and the cell body and nucleus of the injured cell. We will first set the stage by briefly describing the main events that take place within an axon following a lesion event.

7.1
Rapid Responses to Injury

Rapid ion fluxes at the lesion site are likely to be the first indication of breach of axonal integrity upon injury. Axotomy of *Aplysia* neurons in culture elevates intra-axonal calcium concentrations and elicits a wave of increased calcium that propagates from the point of transection toward the intact portions of the cell. Calcium recovery in these invertebrate neurons occurs within minutes once the cut ends are resealed, and calcium levels recover as a retreating front traveling back toward the lesion site [4,5]. Such increases in calcium are likely to be important for cytoskeletal rearrangement and growth cone formation (see below), as well as potentially acting as a retrograde signal. In mammalian systems, axotomy of postnatal cortical neurons induces an increase in axonal calcium, followed by vigorous spiking activity that causes a sodium load. Subsequent inversion of the sodium–calcium exchange pump

Neural Degeneration and Repair: Gene Expression Profiling, Proteomics, and Systems Biology
Edited by Hans Werner Müller
Copyright © 2008 WILEY-VCH Verlag GmbH & Co. KGaA, Weinheim
ISBN: 978-3-527-31707-3

provides an additional and sustained means of entry for calcium [6]. Similar observations have been reported in studies of stretch-induced injuries, where propagation of signal is facilitated by calcium-dependent proteolysis of an intra-axonal domain in tetrodotoxin-sensitive sodium channels [7,8]. *In vivo* resealing of lesioned mammalian axons can take hours and is dependent on axon diameter and calcium in the extracellular environment [9]; thus, the rapid changes in axonal calcium levels following injury may be sustained over time to a degree that is proportional to severity of the injury and the resealing capacity of the axon. These studies highlight the potential importance of calcium-regulated processes in the axonal injury response.

7.2
Retrograde Injury Signaling via Molecular Motors

Some time after the ion flux driven processes described above, signals dependent on motor-driven transport systems start to affect the cell body. This phase includes both an interruption of the normal supply of retrogradely transported molecules such as trophic factor signals and arrival of new signals elicited at the injury site [10–12]. Early studies on retrogradely transported injury signals in *Aplysia* demonstrated that a cross-linked nuclear localization signal (NLS) peptide conveys microtubule-dependent retrograde transport of heterologous proteins [13]. Rhodamine-labeled axoplasm protein fractions were shown to undergo retrograde transport, and microinjection of ligature-concentrated axoplasm from lesioned nerve into cell bodies of uninjured neurons *in vitro* elicited both growth and survival responses [14,15]. The signaling components involved in *Aplysia* include MAP kinases and protein kinase G [16,17].

In mammals, conditioning lesion of the sciatic nerve switches L4/L5 dorsal root ganglia (DRG) neurons from arborizing to elongating axonal growth if the lesion is carried out several days prior to the culture [18]. This phenomenon is thought to be due to retrograde signals transported in the axon (reviewed in [11]). The evidence from *Aplysia* that NLS sequences might target injury-signaling proteins to the retrograde transport system suggested that importins, nuclear import proteins from the karyopherin superfamily, might be involved in retrograde transport in axons. A number of importin αs were found in axons of both control and injured sciatic nerve in constitutive association with dynein, while importin β protein was present only after injury [19]. Interestingly, mRNA for importin β was found in axons, and the upregulation of importin β protein after injury was attributed to local translation in the axon [19]. This leads to the formation of importin α/β heterodimers bound to the retrograde motor dynein, which enables transport of signaling cargos that bind to the importins. Identification of signaling molecules transported by this complex has been highly dependent on proteomics (see Figure 7.1a and text below). In addition to importins, other adaptor proteins such as Sunday driver (Syd) may link signaling molecules to retrograde transport. Both Syd and activated Jnk3 are present on vesicular structures in axons and are transported in both anterograde and retrograde

a)

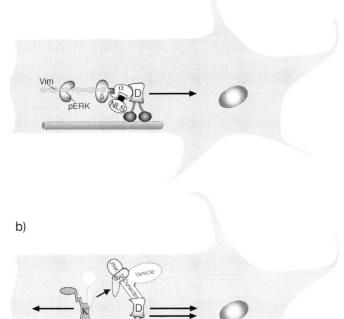

b)

Figure 7.1 (a) Retrograde injury signals link to the dynein motor complex via binding of importin α with dynein. Complexation of importin β with importin α provides a high-affinity site for as yet unidentified cargo molecules binding via nuclear localization signals. Phosphorylated Erk can hitchhike on the complex via a direct interaction with vimentin that binds to importin β. For more details on this mechanism, see Hanz *et al.* [19] and Perlson *et al.* [20].

(b) An alternative or complementary mechanism for retrograde injury signaling is exemplified by Jnk binding to the dynein complex via Syd in a dynactin-dependent manner. Since the Syd–Jnk complex may also link to anterograde transport on kinesin, translocation of Syd from kinesins to dynein may determine directionality of signaling by this mechanism [21].

directions (Figure 7.1b). Nerve injury induces axonal activation of Jnk3, following which the activated Jnk is transported together with Syd, predominantly in the retrograde direction, most likely due to an enhanced interaction between Syd and dynactin after injury [21]. Cavalli *et al.* [21] propose that the Jnk–Syd complex acts as a damage surveillance system and that the direction switch after injury provides a rapid response mechanism for the propagation of retrograde injury signals (Figure 7.1b).

7.3
Posttranscriptional Mechanisms in Axon Maintenance or Regrowth After Injury

Under normal conditions, the distal segment of a lesioned axon undergoes rapid Wallerian degeneration after a short latent phase following the injury [22]. Thus, axonal regrowth for repair after injury must cover significant distances in large mammals, and this mode of repair requires elongating growth mechanisms, which likely differ from the interstitial axonal growth seen in the development after growth cones connect to their target tissues [3,23]. Elongating growth over lengthy distances in a nonembryonic environment is likely to be a daunting challenge for the injured neuron. The first step in elongating growth is formation of a new growth cone at the injury site. This process has been studied extensively in *Aplysia*, revealing that the calcium-activated protease calpain is required for growth cone formation [24]. Calpain activation restructures the axonal cytoskeleton near the injury site, forming microtubule-enclosed compartments that trap vesicles transported by molecular motors [25,26]. These specialized structures seem to facilitate the fusion of vesicles with the plasma membrane, promoting the extension of the growth cone. Similar cytoskeletal transformations have been described in vertebrates [27,28]; however, it should be noted that overactivation of proteolysis in axons may underlie pathological aspects of nerve injury [29]. Growth cone formation can proceed solely by posttranscriptional events, since adult DRG axons maintained a capacity to form new growth cones even after disconnection from their cell bodies [30]. This ability was shown to depend on local protein synthesis and degradation within the axon. Indeed, local protein synthesis within axons has been shown to be important for growth of adult DRG axons *in vitro* [31], whereas adult retinal axons seem to be deficient in local synthesis capacity [30]. Thus, deficiency in local translation mechanisms might account for part of the poor regenerative capacity in central neuronal populations [32].

In contrast to the long distance regrowth challenge posed by rapid Wallerian degeneration of wild-type injured axons, a mutant mouse termed Wlds (for Wallerian degeneration slow) has the remarkable phenotype of extremely delayed degeneration in distal nerve projections after injury [33]. The Wlds gene product is an in-frame fusion protein combining the 70 N-terminal amino acids of a ubiquitination assembly factor (Ube4b/Uf2a) with the entire coding sequence of nicotinamide mononucleotide adenyltransferase-1 (Nmnat-1), an essential enzyme in the biosynthesis pathway of nicotinamide adenine dinucleotide (NAD). Transgenic expression of Wlds in diverse genetic backgrounds in both rat and mouse slows Wallerian degeneration after injury and in various models of neurodegeneration [22]. The fact that Wlds is a fusion of two gene products suggests two possibilities for its mode of action: on the one hand, a putative dominant negative effect of the ubiquitination factor fragment, and on the other hand, activity of Nmnat1 via NAD biosynthesis [34]. An interesting twist on the latter possibility was recently raised by Bellen and colleagues, who showed that *Drosophila* Nmnat maintains neuronal integrity independently of its NAD synthesis activity [35]. Perplexingly however, neither the Ube4b nor the Nmnat1 domains of Wlds can recapitulate Wlds-like protection in transgenic rodents beyond the first few hours after injury [36], suggesting a novel role for the combined molecule, or targeting or modulatory functions of the 18 amino acid linker region or 3′ or 5′ untranslated sequences [34]. If the Wlds transcript contains axon-targeting sequences, translation upon injury might upregulate Nmnat1 locally at the lesion site. On the contrary, different studies have localized Wlds in the nucleus, suggesting that it might indirectly prime axons for greater resistance to degeneration by inducing changes in neuronal gene expression or differential acetylation of axoplasmic proteins shipped out from the cell body. Finally, very recent studies in *Drosophila* suggest that Wlds might act in part by modulating surface expression of signals on damaged axons that induce their clearance by activated glia [37,38]. Pinpointing the critical features underlying resistance to degeneration in Wlds axons will most likely require a systems approach incorporating proteome analyses.

7.4
Proteomics in Studies of Axon Injury Responses

The brief description above of distinct stages in the axon injury response directs our attention to the contribution of posttranscriptional events. Lesion-induced rupture of the membrane is followed by calcium and other ion fluxes that stimulate diverse processes within the axon – including proteolysis, local protein synthesis, and posttranslational modifications for signaling such as phosphorylation. Although proteomics is the approach of choice for characterizing the protein ensembles and mechanisms involved, there are a number of constraints and problems inherent in carrying out proteomics in the nervous system. Tissue lysates or fluids contain many tens of thousands of proteins with differing abundances that can range over seven orders of magnitude [39]. The challenge of addressing such complexity is compounded in the nervous system due to the anatomical complexity at tissue level, the multiplicity of cell types at any given site, and the morphological complexity at the subcellular level [40]. Proteomics in the nervous system must therefore deal with highly complex samples, typically available in very restricted quantity. Proteomic studies carried out on whole nerve or ganglia or brain extract are heavily biased to the identification of abundant cytoskeletal or housekeeping proteins (see, e.g., [41–43]), and it is very difficult to progress beyond this level unless one applies high-resolution sample preparation methods or very efficient targeted enrichment protocols [39]. Techniques such as laser-assisted microdissection [44] or FACS sorting of labeled cells of interest [45] have recently been adapted for transcriptome analyses in neurosciences, and their application to proteome studies may pay dividends. The availability of well-defined protocols to isolate synaptosomes or postsynaptic densities, coupled with affinity chromatography to enrich specific receptor complexes or specifically modified components, have enabled comprehensive characterization of the synaptic proteome on multiple levels [46–48]. The first draft overview of the synapse comprises approximately 1000 proteins, and fewer than 20% of these have been characterized to function in the nervous system [46]. These numbers highlight the potential of proteomic approaches to lead us into terra incognita. Although axon proteomics currently lags behind the synapse in terms of comprehensiveness of available data sets, interesting mechanistic insights have nevertheless been obtained, as detailed below.

7.5
Proteomics of Retrograde Injury Signals – From Local Translation to Signal Identification

Local translation of importin β was shown to be important for the formation of retrograde signaling complexes in injured axons [19]. Perlson *et al.* [12,49] set out to identify signaling molecules retrogradely transported by this complex after injury by a nonbiased differential proteomics approach. They took advantage of the relative anatomical simplicity of molluscan nerve to obtain retrogradely concentrated axoplasm free of glia or serum contamination, and further focused the analyses by dividing the axoplasm into soluble, vesicular, and precipitate fractions by differential centrifugation [12,49]. The fractions underwent differential 2D-PAGE to identify injury-correlated retrogradely transported proteins. Usage of gels at different pI ranges allowed resolution of approximately 4000 spots by silver staining, and 172 of these were found to differ between lesioned versus control nerves. Mass spectrometric sequencing of 134 differential spots allowed their assignment to over 40 different proteins, some belonging to a vesicular ensemble blocked by the lesion, and others comprising an upregulated ensemble highly enriched in calpain cleavage products of an intermediate filament termed RGP51 (retrograde protein of 51 kDa). RPG51 is related in sequence to the mammalian type III intermediate filament vimentin. Inhibition of RGP51 expression by RNA interference inhibits regenerative outgrowth of adult Lymnaea neurons in culture [49]. These results implicated regulated proteolysis in the formation of retrograde injury signaling complexes after nerve lesion and suggested that this signaling modality utilizes a wide range of protein components.

The RGP51 findings in Lymnaea motivated examination of potential roles for the type III intermediate filaments peripherin and vimentin in mammals. Axoplasm from uninjured rat sciatic nerve does not contain appreciable amounts of soluble vimentin or peripherin [20]. Following axonal injury, vimentin is produced by local translation of axonal mRNA, in a similar manner as previously described for importin β. The newly synthesized vimentin undergoes calpain-mediated proteolysis, as was previously observed for RGP51 in Lymnaea model, generating a number of vimentin fragments that lack the capacity to polymerize into filaments. Vimentin immunoprecipitates with dynein from injury axoplasm, suggesting its involvement in retrograde signaling mechanisms. NLS-peptide pull-down experiments using axoplasm from injured sciatic nerve revealed that vimentin associates with importin in rodent DRG neurons. Association experiments with purified proteins *in vitro* demonstrated direct binding of vimentin to importin β, thus potentially creating additional sites for protein–protein interactions with the complex without occupying the NLS binding site on importin α [20]. It was subsequently shown that phosphorylated forms of the MAP kinases Erk1 and Erk2 bind to vimentin in axoplasm after nerve injury, thus linking phospho-Erks to the dynein retrograde motor via vimentin and importin β [20]. Strikingly, the phospho-Erks are protected from dephosphorylation while being bound to vimentin. Pull-down and ELISA experiments revealed robust calcium-dependent binding of phospho-Erks to the second coiled-coil domain of vimentin, with little or no binding of nonphosphorylated Erk to vimentin under these conditions. Geometric and electrostatic complementarity docking showed that vimentin binding to phospho-Erk may cover the region containing the phosphorylated residues in the kinase, and binding competition experiments with Erk peptides supports a structure wherein vimentin interacts with residues above and below the cleft containing the phosphorylated residues in Erk [50]. The same peptides inhibited pErk binding to the dynein complex in sciatic nerve axoplasm and interfered with the protection from phosphatases by vimentin.

In addition to the biochemical evidence for the role of vimentin in the binding of Erk to dynein, retrograde tracing experiments in vimentin knockout mice support a role for vimentin in the retrograde transport of pErk. Injured axons from mice lacking vimentin do not accumulate pErk at the ligature in a lesion-ligation experiment. Furthermore, vimentin-null mice have an attenuated conditioning lesion response in the vimentin-dependent subpopulation of DRG neurons. *In vivo*, vimentin knockout mice suffer from delayed recovery of sensory functions following sciatic nerve lesion. These results support an essential role for newly synthesized and calpain-cleaved axonal vimentin in protecting Erk from dephosphorylation, allowing its retrograde transport and signaling as part of the conditioning lesion response following axonal damage [20,51]. These findings would not have been possible without the initial study using proteomics in axoplasm, taking advantage of reduced glial contamination in the invertebrate model. Conversely, the lack of genome sequence information in molluscs required *de novo* deciphering of the spectra of most of the peptides analyzed in that study, and many of these have still not been assigned to the relevant proteins [49].

7.6
Differential Proteomics in Central versus Peripheral Axon Tracts

Differences in the regenerative response of central versus peripheral neurons are usually attributed to differences in the environment in these two compartments, but might also derive from different intrinsic characteristics of central versus peripheral axonal responses. This possibility has been emphasized in sensory neurons by the work of Woolf and colleagues, who show a difference between central and peripheral branches of the DRG in mounting a regenerative response to conditional lesions [52]. Recently, Katano *et al.* [53] published the first attempt to use proteomics to compare central and peripheral DRG axons. Peripheral and central DRG nerve lysates from the lumbar spinal region of rats aged 5 weeks underwent 2D-PAGE focused to pIs in the pH 5–6 range [53]. The authors detected ~800 protein spots but reported on the characterization of only 1, uniquely found in the peripheral fraction and identified as an isoform of collapsin response mediator protein-2 (CRMP-2).

The new isoform, named periCRMP-2, differs from CRMP-2 at its C-terminus. periCRMP-2 expression was decreased upon sciatic nerve injury, and its true functional significance for central versus peripheral injury responses awaits future work [53]. Although the limited scope of the analysis conducted by Katano *et al.* [53] preclude any broad conclusions, they have demonstrated the potential for proteomics to shed new light on this important question.

7.7
Proteomics in Regenerating or Degenerating Axons

In addition to the work described above, designed to address retrograde signaling and differential characteristics of the axonal response to injury, other studies have used proteomics to analyze regeneration or degeneration processes within axons. Willis *et al.* [54] used metabolic labeling with ^{35}S-methionine/cysteine coupled with 2D-PAGE to estimate protein synthesis in the axonal compartment of DRG neurons. Isolated axons underwent metabolic labeling *in vitro*, and the labeled axonal preparations were resolved on 2D gels. Unlabeled lysates from whole DRG cultures were run in parallel and stained for total protein. Superimposition of radioactive and nonradioactive stained gel images revealed aligned spots that were excised from the preparative gels, trypsin digested, and subjected to MALDI TOF/TOF MS, supplemented by MS/MS sequencing. This approach took advantage of labeling in isolated axons to focus on the proteins of interest, while carrying out the actual identification from a less-defined cellular lysate fractionated in parallel. Careful validation of protein assignments in follow-up experiments at both protein and mRNA level in axons allowed the identification of approximately 40 proteins, almost certainly an underestimate of the true number of locally synthesized proteins since over 100 radioactive spots were resolved in the metabolic labeling gels. A number of the labeled spots could not be aligned with stained spots on the whole DRG lysate gels, suggesting that some of the locally synthesized proteins are of low abundance relative to total cellular protein. The confirmed assignments revealed a diverse ensemble of proteins and their encoding mRNAs – including proteins with important roles in cytoskeleton, stress response, endoplasmic reticulum, and general metabolism, as well as proteins associated with neurodegenerative diseases [54]. As noted above, adult retinal ganglion axons that regenerate poorly are also deficient in local protein synthesis [30], so it is tempting to speculate that the diverse and robust local synthetic profile revealed by the work of Willis *et al.* [54] fulfills an important role in axon regrowth and repair [32].

Jimenez *et al.* [55] used gel-based proteomics to study temporal changes in the protein content of rat sciatic nerve after crush lesion. Extracts of whole nerves were collected at 5, 10, and 35 days after injury and analyzed by 2D-PAGE. Approximately 1500 protein spots were resolved from each sample and 121 of these seemed to be changed at one or more time points [55]. Cluster analyses grouped these proteins mainly by cellular origin, reflecting the difficulty in obtaining insights from analyses conducted on whole-tissue lysates. Nonetheless, in addition to the ubiquitous housekeeping and stress response proteins typically observed in gel-based proteomics of whole tissues, this study highlighted a number of components involved in synthesis and maturation or degradation of proteins. Finally, a very recent study of interest was conducted on the Wlds mouse, taking advantage of established methods for isolating synaptic compartments to compare Wlds versus wild-type synaptic regions from the striatum [56]. Sixteen differential proteins were identified, and 50% of these could be classified as regulators of mitochondrial stability. Subsequent analyses demonstrated that additional mitochondrial proteins are also modified in Wlds synapses, although these were not identified in the initial proteomics screen [56]. Taken together, these studies emphasize the importance of local synthesis, degradation, and energy supply in long-term regeneration.

7.8
Moving Forward – Technical Developments with Potential Application in Neuroproteomics

Most of the proteomics studies described above have either taken advantage of MS for qualitative identification of proteins from partially purified complexes or lysates or used comparative 2D gel-based methods for semi-quantitative analyses. However, the complexity of the tissue and the processes involved in nerve injury suggest that true progress in this field will require more advanced methodologies with higher resolution and the possibility of quantification. Much effort has been invested in recent years in the development of nongel-based approaches for quantitative proteomics, primarily taking advantage of differential stable isotopic labeling of samples. For example, stable isotope labeling with amino acids in culture (SILAC) is a method based on metabolic incorporation of "heavy" (usually ^{13}C or ^{15}N) amino acids by cultured cells [57]. Typically, two identical cell populations are grown in culture, one with a "light" and the other a "heavy" form of a particular amino acid. The cells incorporate the nonradioactive, stable isotope containing amino acids into newly synthesized proteins, with complete incorporation usually achieved after five cell doublings. Cells are then harvested and extracted, and the protein extracts or fractions of interest are then mixed, proteolytically digested, and analyzed by LC–MS/MS. Relative protein abundances can then be determined from "light" versus "heavy" isotope signal intensities in the MS. So far, there have been few applications of SILAC in neuroscience, and those primarily in studies of glia in neurodegeneration [58,59]. The requirement to maintain cells over a long period in culture is a limitation for most neurobiological studies, and the technique is not easily adaptable for *in vivo* experiments or tissue analyses.

Alternative methods of quantification using stable isotopes in mass spectrometry have been developed, based on modification of the sample *after* extraction from the cell or tissue of interest. The first version of this idea was isotope coded affinity tagging (ICAT), wherein proteins are modified by a biotinylated cysteine-targeted affinity tag, containing a linker in either light form with eight hydrogen atoms or heavy form with eight deuterium atoms [60]. Labeled proteins are mixed and digested, and labeled peptides can then be purified by affinity chromatography and analyzed by mass spectrometry. In contrast to SILAC, ICAT can be performed on native samples extracted directly from cells or tissues of interest and is therefore also more easily applicable to samples obtained from neurobiological experiments [61]. A limitation of the original ICAT technique was that the biotin affinity tag linked to the peptides caused shifts in their chromatographic and spectroscopic properties in comparison to unmodified peptides, thus complicating the analysis. Although second- and third-generation ICAT reagents allow for cleavage of the biotin moiety before MS analysis, thus solving this problem, the technique is still limited to cysteine-containing peptides, which typically comprise less than 20% of the total peptide ensemble in a sample. Recently, an improved approach has been developed called iTRAQ (isobaric tags for relative and absolute quantification). iTRAQ is based on a set of amine-targeted reagents that yield derivatized peptides that are indistinguishable in MS, but upon fragmentation in MS/MS exhibit differential low-mass signature ions that allow quantification [62]. The first-generation iTRAQ system comprised four tags allowing cross comparison of up to four different samples in one experiment, and an eightplex reagent system is currently under advanced development. Although there have been few applications of iTRAQ in neuroscience so far [63,64], the technique has major advantages over ICAT in that multiple peptides are labeled per protein, thus increasing reliability of both protein identification and quantification [61].

7.9
Conclusions

A successful axonal response to injury requires retrograde signaling to induce changes in the cell body response and mobilization of outgrowth programs while integrating growth-promoting and growth-inhibiting signals from the environment. Since there is no transcription within axons, by definition all short-term responses to injury within axons are dependent on posttranscriptional processes. A systems-level understanding of this process clearly requires proteomic approaches, but few such studies have been performed to date, and most of these have used gel-based approaches with insufficient attention to issues of sample complexity and enrichment of the compartment of interest. Future work should incorporate selective tissue and sample preparation methods with LC–MS and quantitative approaches such as iTRAQ labeling. Combining these technical improvements with recent progress on delineating the mechanisms involved has the potential to revolutionize our understanding of the responses to injury in lesioned nerve.

Acknowledgments

We gratefully acknowledge research funding from the Dr Miriam and Sheldon Adelson Medical Research Foundation (AMRF), the Christopher Reeve Foundation (CRF), and the International Institute for Research in Paraplegia (IFP).

References

1 Yamashita, T., Fujitani, M., Yamagishi, S., Hata, K. and Mimura, F. (2005) Multiple signals regulate axon regeneration through the nogo receptor complex. *Molecular Neurobiology*, **32**, 105–111.

2 Goldberg, J.L. (2004) Intrinsic neuronal regulation of axon and dendrite growth. *Current Opinion in Neurobiology*, **14**, 551–557.

3 Rossi, F., Gianola, S. and Corvetti, L. (2007) Regulation of intrinsic neuronal properties for axon growth and regeneration. *Progress in Neurobiology*, **81**, 1–28.

4 Ziv, N.E. and Spira, M.E. (1993) Spatiotemporal distribution of Ca2+ following axotomy and throughout the recovery process of cultured *Aplysia* neurons. *The European Journal of Neuroscience*, **5**, 657–668.

5 Ziv, N.E. and Spira, M.E. (1995) Axotomy induces a transient and localized elevation of the free intracellular calcium concentration to the millimolar range. *Journal of Neurophysiology*, **74**, 2625–2637.

6 Mandolesi, G., Madeddu, F., Bozzi, Y., Maffei, L. and Ratto, G.M. (2004) Acute physiological response of mammalian central neurons to axotomy: ionic regulation and electrical activity. *FASEB Journal*, **18**, 1934–1936.

7 Iwata, A., Stys, P.K., Wolf, J.A., Chen, X.H., Taylor, A.G., Meaney, D.F. and Smith, D.H. (2004) Traumatic axonal injury induces proteolytic cleavage of the voltage-gated sodium channels modulated by tetrodotoxin and protease inhibitors. *Journal of Neuroscience*, **24**, 4605–4613.

8 Wolf, J.A., Stys, P.K., Lusardi, T., Meaney, D. and Smith, D.H. (2001) Traumatic axonal injury induces calcium influx modulated by tetrodotoxin-sensitive sodium channels. *Journal of Neuroscience*, **21**, 1923–1930.

9 Howard, M.J., David, G. and Barrett, J.N. (1999) Resealing of transected myelinated mammalian axons *in vivo*: evidence for involvement of calpain. *Neuroscience*, **93**, 807–815.

10 Ambron, R.T. and Walters, E.T. (1996) Priming events and retrograde injury signals. A new perspective on the cellular and molecular biology of nerve regeneration. *Molecular Neurobiology*, **13**, 61–79.

11 Hanz, S. and Fainzilber, M. (2006) Retrograde signaling in injured nerve – the axon reaction revisited. *Journal of Neurochemistry*, **99**, 13–19.

12 Perlson, E., Hanz, S., Medzihradszky, K.F., Burlingame, A.L. and Fainzilber, M. (2004) From snails to sciatic nerve: retrograde injury signaling from axon to soma in lesioned neurons. *Journal of Neurobiology*, **58**, 287–294.

13 Ambron, R.T., Schmied, R., Huang, C.C. and Smedman, M. (1992) A signal sequence mediates the retrograde transport of proteins from the axon periphery to the cell body and then into the nucleus. *Journal of Neuroscience*, **12**, 2813–2818.

14 Ambron, R.T., Zhang, X.P., Gunstream, J.D., Povelones, M. and Walters, E.T. (1996) Intrinsic injury signals enhance growth survival, and excitability of *Aplysia* neurons. *Journal of Neuroscience*, **16**, 7469–7477.

15 Schmied, R. and Ambron, R.T. (1997) A nuclear localization signal targets proteins to the retrograde transport system thereby evading uptake into organelles in *Aplysia* axons. *Journal of Neurobiology*, **33**, 151–160.

16 Sung, Y.J., Povelones, M. and Ambron, R.T. (2001) RISK-1: a novel MAPK homologue in axoplasm that is activated and retrogradely transported after nerve injury. *Journal of Neurobiology*, **47**, 67–79.

17 Sung, Y.J., Walters, E.T. and Ambron, R.T. (2004) A neuronal isoform of protein kinase G couples mitogen-activated protein kinase nuclear import to axotomy-induced long-term hyper-excitability in *Aplysia* sensory neurons. *Journal of Neuroscience*, **24**, 7583–7595.

18 Smith, D.S. and Skene, J.H. (1997) A transcription-dependent switch controls competence of adult neurons for distinct modes of axon growth. *Journal of Neuroscience*, **17**, 646–658.

19 Hanz, S., Perlson, E., Willis, D., Zheng, J.Q., Massarwa, R., Huerta, J.J., Koltzenburg, M., Kohler, M., van Minnen, J., Twiss, J.L. and Fainzilber, M. (2003) Axoplasmic importins enable retrograde injury signaling in lesioned nerve. *Neuron*, **40**, 1095–1104.

20 Perlson, E., Hanz, S., Ben-Yaakov, K., Segal-Ruder, Y., Seger, R. and Fainzilber, M. (2005) Vimentin-dependent spatial translocation of an activated MAP kinase in injured nerve. *Neuron*, **45**, 715–726.

21 Cavalli, V., Kujala, P., Klumperman, J. and Goldstein, L.S. (2005) Sunday Driver links axonal transport to damage signaling. *The Journal of Cell Biology*, **168**, 775–787.

22 Coleman, M. (2005) Axon degeneration mechanisms: commonality amid diversity. *Nature Reviews. Neuroscience*, **6**, 889–898.

23 Zhou, F.Q. and Snider, W.D. (2006) Intracellular control of developmental and regenerative axon growth. *Philosophical transactions of the Royal Society of London. Series B Biological Sciences*, **361**, 1575–1592.

24 Gitler, D. and Spira, M.E. (1998) Real time imaging of calcium-induced localized proteolytic activity after axotomy and its relation to growth cone formation. *Neuron*, **20**, 1123–1135.

25 Erez, H., Malkinson, G., Prager-Khoutorsky, M., De Zeeuw, C.I., Hoogenraad, C.C. and Spira, M.E. (2007) Formation of microtubule-based traps controls the sorting and concentration of vesicles to restricted sites of regenerating neurons after axotomy. *The Journal of Cell Biology*, **176**, 497–507.

26 Spira, M.E., Oren, R., Dormann, A. and Gitler, D. (2003) Critical calpain-dependent ultrastructural alterations underlie the transformation of an axonal segment into a growth cone after axotomy of cultured *Aplysia* neurons. *The Journal of Comparative Neurology*, **457**, 293–312.

27 Dent, E.W., Tang, F. and Kalil, K. (2003) Axon guidance by growth cones and branches: common cytoskeletal and signaling mechanisms. *Neuroscientist*, **9**, 343–353.

28 Robles, E., Huttenlocher, A. and Gomez, T.M. (2003) Filopodial calcium transients regulate growth cone motility and guidance through local activation of calpain. *Neuron*, **38**, 597–609.

29 Buki, A. and Povlishock, J.T. (2006) All roads lead to disconnection? Traumatic axonal injury revisited. *Acta Neuro-chirurgica*, **148**, 181–193; discussion, 193–184.

30 Verma, P., Chierzi, S., Codd, A.M., Campbell, D.S., Meyer, R.L., Holt, C.E. and Fawcett, J.W. (2005) Axonal protein synthesis and degradation are necessary for efficient growth cone regeneration. *Journal of Neuroscience*, **25**, 331–342.

31 Zheng, J.Q., Kelly, T.K., Chang, B., Ryazantsev, S., Rajasekaran, A.K., Martin, K.C. and Twiss, J.L. (2001) A functional role for intra-axonal protein synthesis during axonal regeneration from adult sensory neurons. *Journal of Neuroscience*, **21**, 9291–9303.

32 Willis, D.E. and Twiss, J.L. (2006) The evolving roles of axonally synthesized proteins in regeneration. *Current Opinion in Neurobiology*, **16**, 111–118.

33 Perry, V.H., Lunn, E.R., Brown, M.C., Cahusac, S. and Gordon, S. (1990) Evidence that the rate of Wallerian degeneration is controlled by a single autosomal dominant gene. *The European Journal of Neuroscience*, **2**, 408–413.

34 Fainzilber, M. and Twiss, J.L. (2006) Tracking in the Wlds – the hunting of the SIRT and the luring of the Draper. *Neuron*, **50**, 819–821.

35 Zhai, R.G., Cao, Y., Hiesinger, P.R., Zhou, Y., Mehta, S.Q., Schulze, K.L., Verstreken, P. and Bellen, H.J. (2006) *Drosophila* NMNAT maintains neural integrity independent of its NAD synthesis activity. *PLoS Biology*, **4**, e416.

36 Conforti, L., Fang, G., Beirowski, B., Wang, M.S., Sorci, L., Asress, S., Adalbert, R., Silva, A. and Bridge, K., Huang, X.P., Magni, G., Glass, J.D. and Coleman, M.P. (2006) NAD+ and axon degeneration revisited: Nmnat1 cannot substitute for WldS to delay Wallerian degeneration., *Cell Death and Differentiation.* **14** (1), 116–127.

37 Awasaki, T., Tatsumi, R., Takahashi, K., Arai, K., Nakanishi, Y., Ueda, R. and Ito, K. (2006) Essential role of the apoptotic cell engulfment genes draper and ced-6 in programmed axon pruning during *Drosophila* metamorphosis. *Neuron*, **50**, 855–867.

38 MacDonald, J.M., Beach, M.G., Porpiglia, E., Sheehan, A.E., Watts, R.J. and Freeman, M.R. (2006) The *Drosophila* cell corpse engulfment receptor Draper mediates glial clearance of severed axons. *Neuron*, **50**, 869–881.

39 Hopf, C., Bantscheff, M. and Drewes, G. (2007) Pathway proteomics and chemical proteomics team up in drug discovery. *Neurodegenerative Diseases*, **4**, 270–280.

40 Anderson, C.N. and Grant, S.G. (2006) High throughput protein expression screening in the nervous system-needs and limitations. *The Journal of Physiology*, **575**, 367–372.

41 Ding, Q., Wu, Z., Guo, Y., Zhao, C., Jia, Y., Kong, F., Chen, B., Wang, H., Xiong, S. and Que, H. (2006) Proteome analysis of up-regulated proteins in the rat spinal cord induced by transection injury. *Proteomics*, **6**, 505–518.

42 Kang, S.K., So, H.H., Moon, Y.S. and Kim, C.H. (2006) Proteomic analysis of injured spinal cord tissue proteins using 2-DE and MALDI-TOF MS. *Proteomics*, **6**, 2797–2812.

43 Konishi, H., Namikawa, K. and Kiyama, H. (2006) Annexin III implicated in the microglial response to motor nerve injury. *Glia*, **53**, 723–732.

44 Burnet, P.W., Eastwood, S.L. and Harrison, P.J. (2004) Laser-assisted microdissection: methods for the molecular analysis of psychiatric disorders at a cellular resolution. *Biological Psychiatry*, **55**, 107–111.

45 Lobo, M.K., Karsten, S.L., Gray, M., Geschwind, D.H. and Yang, X.W. (2006) FACS-array profiling of striatal projection neuron subtypes in juvenile and adult mouse brains. *Nature Neuroscience*, **9**, 443–452.

46 Grant, S.G. (2006) The synapse proteome and phosphoproteome: a new paradigm for synapse biology. *Biochemical Society Transactions*, **34**, 59–63.

47 Trinidad, J.C., Specht, C.G., Thalhammer, A., Schoepfer, R. and Burlingame, A.L. (2006) Comprehensive identification of phosphorylation sites in postsynaptic density preparations. *Molecular & Cellular Proteomics*, **5**, 914–922.

48 Vosseller, K., Trinidad, J.C., Chalkley, R.J., Specht, C.G., Thalhammer, A., Lynn, A.J., Snedecor, J.O., Guan, S. and Medzihradszky, K.F., Maltby, D.A., Schoepfer, R. and Burlingame, A.L. (2006) O-linked *N*-acetylglucosamine proteomics of postsynaptic density preparations using lectin weak affinity chromatography and mass spectrometry. *Molecular & Cellular Proteomics*, **5**, 923–934.

49 Perlson, E., Medzihradszky, K.F., Darula, Z., Munno, D.W., Syed, N.I., Burlingame, A.L. and Fainzilber, M. (2004) Differential proteomics reveals multiple components in retrogradely transported axoplasm after nerve injury. *Molecular & Cellular Proteomics*, **3**, 510–520.

50 Perlson, E., Michaelevski, I., Kowalsman, N., Ben-Yaakov, K., Shaked, M., Seger, R., Eisenstein, M. and Fainzilber, M. (2006) Vimentin binding to phosphorylated Erk

sterically hinders enzymatic dephosphorylation of the kinase. *Journal of
Molecular Biology*, **364**, 938–944.

51 Helfand, B.T., Chou, Y.H., Shumaker,
D.K. and Goldman, R.D. (2005)
Intermediate filament proteins partici-
pate in signal transduction. *Trends in Cell
Biology*, **15**, 568–570.

52 Neumann, S. and Woolf, C.J. (1999)
Regeneration of dorsal column fibers into
and beyond the lesion site following adult
spinal cord injury. *Neuron*, **23**, 83–91.

53 Katano, T., Mabuchi, T., Okuda-Ashitaka,
E., Inagaki, N., Kinumi, T. and Ito, S.
(2006) Proteomic identification of a novel
isoform of collapsin response mediator
protein-2 in spinal nerves peripheral
to dorsal root ganglia. *Proteomics*, **6**,
6085–6094.

54 Willis, D., Li, K.W., Zheng, J.Q., Chang,
J.H., Smit, A., Kelly, T., Merianda, T.T.,
Sylvester, J., van Minnen, J. and Twiss,
J.L. (2005) Differential transport and local
translation of cytoskeletal injury-
response, and neurodegeneration protein
mRNAs in axons. *Journal of Neuroscience*,
25, 778–791.

55 Jimenez, C.R., Stam, F.J., Li, K.W.,
Gouwenberg, Y., Hornshaw, M.P., De
Winter, F., Verhaagen, J. and Smit, A.B.
(2005) Proteomics of the injured rat
sciatic nerve reveals protein expression
dynamics during regeneration. *Molecular
& Cellular Proteomics*, **4**, 120–132.

56 Wishart, T.M., Paterson, J.M., Short,
D.M., Meredith, S., Robertson, K.A.,
Sutherland, C., Cousin, M.A., Dutia,
M.B. and Gillingwater, T.H. (2007)
Differential proteomic analysis of
synaptic proteins identifies potential
cellular targets and protein mediators of
synaptic neuroprotection conferred by
the slow Wallerian degeneration (Wlds)
gene. *Molecular & Cellular Proteomics*, **6**,
1318–1330.

57 Ong, S.E. and Mann, M. (2006) A
practical recipe for stable isotope labeling

by amino acids in cell culture (SILAC).
Nature Protocols, **1**, 2650–2660.

58 McLaughlin, P., Zhou, Y., Ma, T., Liu, J.,
Zhang, W., Hong, J.S., Kovacs, M. and
Zhang, J. (2006) Proteomic analysis of
microglial contribution to mouse strain-
dependent dopaminergic neurotoxicity.
Glia, **53**, 567–582.

59 Zhou, Y., Wang, Y., Kovacs, M., Jin, J. and
Zhang, J. (2005) Microglial activation
induced by neurodegeneration: a
proteomic analysis. *Molecular & Cellular
Proteomics*, **4**, 1471–1479.

60 Gygi, S.P., Rist, B., Gerber, S.A., Turecek,
F., Gelb, M.H. and Aebersold, R. (1999)
Quantitative analysis of complex
protein mixtures using isotope-coded
affinity tags. *Nature Biotechnology*, **17**,
994–999.

61 Tannu, N.S. and Hemby, S.E. (2006)
Methods for proteomics in neuroscience.
Progress in Brain Research, **158**, 41–82.

62 Ross, P.L., Huang, Y.N., Marchese, J.N.,
Williamson, B., Parker, K., Hattan, S.,
Khainovski, N., Pillai, S. and Dey, S.,
Daniels, S., Purkayastha, S., Juhasz, P.,
Martin, S., Bartlet-Jones, M., He, F.,
Jacobson, A. and Pappin, D.J. (2004)
Multiplexed protein quantitation in
Saccharomyces cerevisiae using amine-
reactive isobaric tagging reagents.
Molecular & Cellular Proteomics, **3**,
1154–1169.

63 Liu, T., D'Mello, V., Deng, L., Hu, J.,
Ricardo, M., Pan, S., Lu, X., Wadsworth,
S., Siekierka, J., Birge, R. and Li, H.
(2006) A multiplexed proteomics
approach to differentiate neurite
outgrowth patterns. *Journal of Neuroscience Methods*, **158**, 22–29.

64 Salim, K., Kehoe, L., Minkoff, M.S.,
Bilsland, J.G., Munoz-Sanjuan, I. and
Guest, P.C. (2006) Identification of
differentiating neural progenitor cell
markers using shotgun isobaric tagging
mass spectrometry. *Stem Cells and
Development*, **15**, 461–470.

8
Genomics Approaches to the Study of Neurodegeneration

Jeanine Jochems, Peter Buckley, and James Eberwine

8.1
Introduction

Neurodegeneration is not only an unavoidable part of normal brain aging but is also involved in numerous diseases, such as Alzheimer's, Huntington's, and Parkinson's diseases, and amyotrophic lateral sclerosis (ALS), and it occurs as a result of brain injury. There are many processes that are believed to occur to protect young brains that seem to break down in an aged or a diseased brain. The ability to study how these processes work and why they break down is crucial for understanding neurodegeneration. Only once that we have gained complete understanding of the protective processes can we begin to enhance them and stop the destructive ones, thus furthering treatment and hopefully curing these neurodegenerative diseases.

The effects of neurodegeneration in society are significant. It is projected by the organization Alzheimer's Worldwide that by the year 2010 the number of people living with Alzheimer's disease (AD) will be about 7.4 million. Although numbers vary, it seems that the occurrence of Huntington's disease (HD) numbers around 1 in 2000 people, while 4–6 million people are estimated to be affected by Parkinson's disease (PD). The incidence of amyotrophic lateral sclerosis is significant all over the world. A sampling of annual statistics shows 32 000 cases in the United States, 20 000 cases in Brazil, 9000 cases in Germany, and more than 140 000 cases in China.

According to the International Brain Injury Association, brain injury is the leading cause of death and disability as well as of seizure disorders worldwide. Injuries can happen in many ways, including automobile accidents, falls, and while participating in sports. In the United States it is estimated that 5.3 million people are living with disability related to a traumatic brain injury (TBI) and approximately 50 000 people die annually as a result of brain injuries. About 1 million annual hospitalizations in the European Union are attributed to brain injuries. Many kinds of physical, cognitive, behavioral, and emotional impairments, both temporary and permanent, are caused by brain injuries.

Each disease mentioned has trademark pathological, physical, and behavioral distinctions. Different brain areas are affected, but the effects can be widespread,

Neural Degeneration and Repair: Gene Expression Profiling, Proteomics, and Systems Biology
Edited by Hans Werner Müller
Copyright © 2008 WILEY-VCH Verlag GmbH & Co. KGaA, Weinheim
ISBN: 978-3-527-31707-3

causing a variety of changes. Although modulation in the levels and effectiveness of neurotransmitter are usually the direct cause of behavioral changes, ultimately, these variations are induced by genetic alterations. Many studies have been done to explore what these genetic shifts are and exactly how they affect the phenotype.

8.2
Causes of Neurodegeneration

8.2.1
Alzheimer's Disease

AD is a progressive disease resulting in loss of memory, thinking and language skills, as well as behavioral changes. There are two cellular, morphological abnormalities that are associated with AD: extracellular amyloid β plaques, which are protein fragments clumped together that form outside and around neurons, and intraneuronal neurofibrillary tangles (NFT). These insoluble twisted fibers, largely composed of the tau protein, build up inside neurons in the AD brain [1].

The cholinergic system has been most widely studied in AD research. Numerous animal and human studies have shown that enhancing cholinergic transmission improves memory and vice versa. In 1978, Perry *et al.* suggested a correlation between AD dementia and alterations in the cholinergic system. Atri *et al.* [2] showed that encoding of new memories is impaired by using drugs to block muscarinic cholinergic receptors but retrieval of older memories is not affected, while others have shown that drug activation of nicotinic receptors enhances the encoding of new information [3]. Borchelt *et al.* [4] showed that transgenic mice with the presenilin 1 mutation, associated with familial AD, have increased levels of amyloid β, a peptide whose accumulation in the brain contributes to memory problems by interacting with high-affinity choline transporter, thus impairing acetylcholine release. Treatment of AD model mice with an antibody against this amyloid β peptide has been shown to alleviate memory deficits [5]. Even today, drugs that enhance cholinergic function are the most commonly prescribed treatments for AD.

8.2.2
Huntington's Disease

HD is caused by a rare but dominant genetic mutation, a trinucleotide repeat expansion, in the huntingtin gene. There is a CAG repeat, which translates to long stretches of polyglutamine in the resulting protein. This mutant protein forms aggregates, which localize in the nucleus more than normal huntingtin [1]. It is argued as to whether this is what causes cell death or not [6], but along with cell death in HD are physical effects, such as a lack of coordination; cognitive effects, such as some memory and learning difficulties; and psychiatric effects, including reduced emotional display, anxiety, and/or depression.

Wyttenbach *et al.* [7] showed that the mutant polyglutamine huntingtin proteins compromise CRE-mediated transcription in HD neurons. Similar effects have been reported in the Sp1 transcriptional pathway [8]. Inclusion bodies are also a hallmark of HD; however, it does not seem that the presence of these bodies is correlated with death in cultured neurons expressing abnormal huntingtin. Studies have also shown decreased levels of GABA in the caudate nucleus, an area known to be involved in learning and memory, in severely demented HD brains [9]. Interestingly, Pearson *et al.* [10] found that although levels of GABA were decreased in HD compared to healthy brains, those of patients that had exhibited mild chorea had lower levels of GABA than those with more severe chorea. It is obvious that this requires further examination.

8.2.3
Parkinson's Disease

PD is a neurodegenerative disorder affecting muscle control, movement, speech, and posture. It can also cause disturbances in mood, sleep, cognition, and sensation. The pathological distinction of PD is the presence of Lewy bodies, which are hyaline-like protein inclusions in the cytoplasm of dopaminergic neurons. The presence of these bodies leads to the loss of these dopaminergic neurons, and with reduced dopamine levels, excessive muscle contraction occurs, causing the above-mentioned symptoms [1].

Dopamine and its associated markers have been shown in many studies to be significantly decreased in many areas of Parkinson's affected brains. Although it appears to be related to neurodegeneration in PD, no study has been able to show a significant correlation between the level of dopamine integrity and severity of rest tremor [11]. Noradrenergic, serotonergic, cholinergic, and other systems have also been studied and levels of these neurotransmitters may also be associated with changes in the PD brain.

8.2.4
Amyotrophic Lateral Sclerosis

Amyotrophic lateral sclerosis is an almost invariably fatal, fast-progressing neurodegenerative disease in which both upper and lower motor neurons degenerate or die, becoming incapable of sending messages to muscles. Like PD, ALS is characterized by the presence of inclusion bodies, made up of varied accumulations of phosphorylated neurofilaments. It was found that these bodies are sometimes immunoreactive for an antibody against SOD1, which acts as a detoxifier of free radicals. At one time it seemed like this might be a promising finding, but experiments with transgenic mice have shown that this mutation does not always cause loss of affected motor neurons [1].

Many different potential mechanisms have been studied for ALS. Metabolism, specifically alterations in levels and distribution of glutamate, may be a mediator in neurodegeneration in ALS [12]. Decreased levels of cholinergic acetyl transferase, which is a marker of motor neuron activity, have been found in spinal cords of those affected by ALS. Dangond *et al.* [13] used microarray analysis and expression profiling to study other possible genetic links in ALS, finding alterations in many pathways, such as signal transduction, cytoskeletal organization, and mitochondrial function, as well as finding evidence that oxidative stress is a possible factor in neuronal cell death in ALS. It is yet unknown which of these mechanisms have a role in the neurodegeneration in ALS and to what extent.

8.2.5
Common Processes Leading to Pathological Protein Aggregation in Neurodegenerative Diseases

The importance of genomics is evident in all of these diseases. All proteins, for example, the tau protein that composes the NFTs in AD, are encoded in DNA and transcribed to RNA, which is eventually translated into protein. In many cases, there are also modifications made to the RNA before translation and/or to the protein after initial translation. The schematic in Figure 8.1 illustrates this process and how variations in RNA splicing can lead to differing proteins. If we can find out what the changes in these transcription, translation, and modification processes are, we may be able to find out what is causing these NFTs to form. These same processes produce the alpha-synuclein protein that composes Lewy bodies in PD and can be analyzed in a similar manner. Genomics analysis can also be of benefit to learn more about the inclusions in ALS, as well as find further information about the SOD1 gene and its role. As HD is known to be caused by a genetic mutation, it is obvious that genomics analysis is important. Continued research may find additional genes affected by the mutant huntingtin and hopefully yield information that can be used in finding potential cures.

8.2.6
Aging

There are many types of decreased neuronal functions in the aging brain and even more processes believed to have a part in causing them. Mukherjee *et al.* [14] found that the number of dopamine receptors declines with age at varying rates throughout brain regions. Volkow *et al.* [15] have shown that decreases in dopamine activity have negative effects on motor function and may also affect performance on frontal brain region related tasks. Numerous studies have shown the significance of BDNF and serotonin on neuronal plasticity and neurogenesis and the way they work together in the brain, as well as the effects of malfunction in either of their systems [16]. Free radicals, caused by oxidative stress, can make the cell membrane more permeable via peroxidation of the membrane lipids, which ultimately lowers the level of neuronal activity [1]. In a young, healthy brain, there are protections against this, but where production of free radicals is increased or these protective processes are decreased, neurons can die. For example, when illness or injury occurs, the damaged tissues must be replaced, which requires

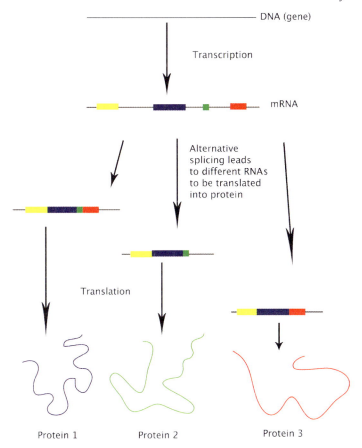

Figure 8.1 Translation of gene into protein. A gene is transcribed into mRNA with different exons, represented by different colored sections, and intronic sequences, which will be spliced out of the RNA before translation. Exons are sometimes also excluded from the RNA to be translated, causing very different proteins to be created.

energy, causing the release of free radicals that then build up to such an abundance that the defense system may no longer be able to keep up with the elimination [17]. Gage *et al.* [18] found a correlation between performance on tests for learning and place navigation and regional glucose utilization, where younger rats had higher levels of glucose activity than older rats. This supports the idea that brain glucose levels have an effect on learning and memory. Studies have also shown the effects of stress, specifically the release of corticosteroids on cognitive function. Wright *et al.* [19] found that stress-induced spatial memory deficits were most effectively reduced by higher doses of the corticosterone synthesis inhibitor, metyrapone.

Levels of neurotransmitters change in aging brains even of healthy individuals, thus it is unknown if the difference in diseased brains is due to a differing mechanism, an altered pattern of change, or a result of threshold phenomena. It is certainly easy to hypothesize that neurodegenerative diseases accelerate the aging process, and there are many similarities between a diseased brain tissue and healthy aged tissue to support this. There is evidence in AD, PD, ALS, and HD, as well as in aged brains, of the role of free radicals in neuronal cell death. Prolonged Ca^{2+} influx into neurons can also cause cell death by excitotoxicity. This can be caused by an increase in available extracellular glutamate. This increase can be a result of glutamate transporter loss (as in ALS spinal cord), a reduction in GluR2 (a subunit of the glutamate receptor that controls conductance of AMPA receptors to Ca^{2+}) RNA expression, and/or editing, leading to continuous Ca^{2+} influx. There is also evidence that a reduction in protein synthesis, such as the reduced amount of tyrosine hydroxylase (a dopamine synthesizing enzyme) in the neurons of a PD brain, can cause neuronal death [1].

All of these causes of neurodegeneration have been studied for years, and although some treatments to make life easier for those affected have come out of these studies, cures are still not available. There are many systems involved in the normal functioning of neurons, and the way that these interact is complex. In experimenting with neurodegeneration, it has so far not been completely clear which systems and interactions are most important but progress is being made every day.

8.3
Gene Expression Studies in Traumatic Brain and Spinal Cord Injury

8.3.1
Methodological Considerations

The majority of methods for studying the genomics of neurodegeneration have been on a large scale. Whole brains are used for imaging studies or large amounts of tissue have been used for *in situ* hybridization, immunohistochemistry, or reverse transcription (RT) PCR. There are unfortunately some fundamental problems with these methods. One problem is that when using a number of cells, a heterogeneous mixture is obtained that will not yield results indicating what is actually occurring at the cellular and genetic level in individual cells [20], but the amount of RNA necessary for experimentation is much greater than what is available in a single cell. Van Gelder *et al.* [21] developed a method, which could be used for amplifying the RNA from a single cell, allowing for improved genomics investigation. The procedure begins with the reverse transcription of the cell's RNA to the first strand of cDNA, on which the second strand of cDNA is made. After purification, this double-stranded cDNA is then transcribed into RNA, which due to the continuous nature of RNA polymerase yields a large number of antisense RNA strands. A schematic of this procedure is presented in Figure 8.2.

Begin with RNA from single cell

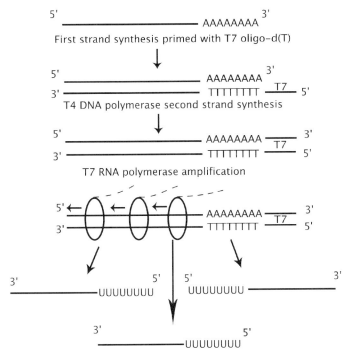

Figure 8.2 aRNA schematic. Primed with a T7 oligo-d(T) primer, a first strand of cDNA is synthesized on the RNA from a single cell. After denaturing the cDNA from the RNA, a second strand cDNA is then synthesized complementary to the first. T7 RNA polymerase is used to transcribe (and linearly amplify about 1000 times) the cDNA into RNA. The procedure can be repeated to further amplify and obtain necessary amounts of RNA.

Another issue with the above-mentioned methods is that it is possible to consider only a limited number of RNAs at a time. The development of microarray technology by Schena *et al.* [22] meant that a system became available for studying the expression of many RNAs from the same sample at the same time. A number of target cDNAs can be amplified using PCR and then printed onto glass microscope slides from a 96-well plate using a special arraying machine. After denaturing the cDNAs, fluorescently labeled mRNA can then be hybridized to this array. Scanning with a laser will then reveal to which of the hundreds of cDNA targets the fluorescent RNA has bound. On the basis of the intensity of the spots, the level of expression of specific RNAs in the sample in question can be determined (Figure 8.3).

Researchers have accepted these methods as ways to enhance their experiments and discover even more of the genetic responses associated with neurodegeneration. Here, traumatic brain injury will be used as an example of a few of the studies that

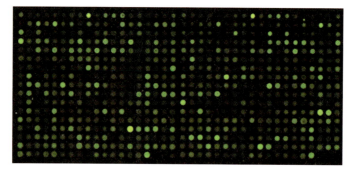

Figure 8.3 Microarray Image. Cy3-labeled cDNA from rat hippocampal total poly-A$^+$ mRNA is hybridized to a National Institute of Aging (NIA) mouse 15 000 cDNA microarray slide. Fluorescent spot intensity allows for qualitative and quantitative assessment of the expression profile for represented genes in rat hippocampal cells. These studies were done in collaboration with Dr Kevin Becker, NIA.

use microarrays and/or single cell aRNA amplification to determine genetic changes occurring before or during the cell death process. Many of these studies used similar methods on different areas of the brain and spinal cord and have found different results, indicating the possibility of varied responses to injury in individual neuron types.

8.3.2
Spinal Cord

Hu *et al.* [23] used microarray analysis to identify changes in gene expression in spinal cord samples following proximal spinal root avulsion. The L4–L6 ventral spinal roots were torn as described in the spinal root avulsion technique in Hammarberg *et al.* [24]. Three days post injury, rats were sacrificed and spinal cords were sectioned. RNA was extracted and amplified using RT-PCR, and the resulting cDNA probes were labeled with ^{32}P and hybridized to commercial nylon membrane microarrays. The expression of most genes involved in normal neuronal activity was decreased, including metabolic, ion channel, transporter, and exocytosis protein coding genes. Significant increases were found in preapoptotic genes (caspase-1 and -3, Fas antigen, and Bax), cell cycle related genes, transcription and translation related genes, oncogenes, and tumor suppressor related genes. It seems like cells may be trying to rebuild via transcription and translation, but this action would be in competition with preapoptotic processes indicated by the increase in related genes. These results may seem somewhat contradictory, but considering that the sample used was a heterogeneous mixture of many cells, it probably implies that different cells were at different stages in their postinjury reaction. This is a place where using single cell aRNA amplification could have been of benefit to the study.

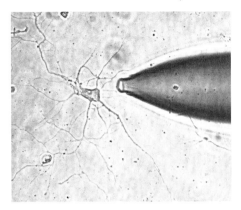

Figure 8.4 Cell collection. Single cells are visualized under a microscope and the cytoplasm collected by aspiration using a glass micropipette that is controlled by micromanipulators.

8.3.3
Traumatic Brain Injury

O'Dell *et al.* [20] studied the alterations of gene expression in the injured cerebral cortex of rats. They used the lateral fluid percussion method of traumatic brain injury, where a bolus of saline is rapidly injected causing mechanical deformation of brain tissue in the closed cranial cavity. Brains were collected and sliced 12 and 24 hours post injury. Terminal transferase dUTP nick end labeling (TUNEL), a common method for detecting cells in the final stages of apoptosis by incorporating labeled dUTPs at nicks in the DNA with the help of terminal transferase enzyme, was then used to identify cells undergoing apoptosis. Reverse transcription was done *in situ* directly on the brain section. The aRNA amplification procedure described above was then used on single cells after they were mechanically separated from the tissue section using micromanipulators, in a manner similar to what is seen in Figure 8.4. Reverse Northern blot, using target cDNAs that were both general cell function and apoptosis associated, was the method employed to identify the mRNAs present in the cells at the time of collection. Genes known to be responsible for cell survival and repair were shown to generally decrease in expression in TUNEL positive cells compared to those from sham-injured brains, at the 12 hours post-injury time point, and then return to sham levels at 24 hours post injury. Levels of mRNA coding for the GluR2 subunit, which usually prevents calcium from entering the cell via AMPA receptors and thus guarding against excitotoxicity, were found to be decreased 12 hours post injury. Increases were found in caspase-2 coding mRNA at 24 hours. Caspase-2 has been shown to be an initiator of apoptosis. These results lead to a possible conclusion that cells at first are attempting to rebuild, but for some reason are not able and progress into an apoptotic state.

In Marciano *et al.* [25] the hippocampus, specifically the CA3 and dentate gyrus, was the focus area for gaining the understanding of the genomic responses after experimental brain injury. A controlled cortical impact at 5.0 m/s to a depth of 1 mm was used as an injury method. Mice were euthanized at 24 hours post injury, brains were sectioned, and TUNEL labeling as well as caspase-3 antibody immunolabeling was carried out. First, strand cDNA synthesis was done *in situ*, and then, using microdissection, single cells were collected in each of the three categories: caspase-3+/TUNEL+, caspase-3+/TUNEL−, and nonlabeled (caspase-3−/TUNEL−). The aRNA amplification was performed, and then labeled cDNA probes were made and hybridized to microarrays with 8734 randomly selected mouse target genes. In general observation, the numbers of genes with altered expression post injury vary in the two different areas of the hippocampus on the basis of staining. No cells from sham-injured animals stained TUNEL+ and only a few were found to stain for caspase-3, showing that the genetic changes are in some way a result of a TBI-induced apoptotic cascade. It is hypothesized that the cells that stained caspase-3+/TUNEL− have not yet broken down their nuclear membrane but have already started an apoptotic cascade. Across both regions, the uninjured cells expressed about two thirds of the mRNAs. In the caspase-3+/TUNEL− cells, an overall expression increase up to 88% of the mRNAs was evident, while in the caspase-3+/TUNEL+ cells expression was greatly declined. In the latter, the percentage of genes expressed was region specific, showing that the cascades must be different in different cell types. Highly conserved cellular isoform of the prion protein, which is shown to have neuroprotective properties, was observed as highly upregulated. It was also found that cells that stain the same in immunohistochemical analysis do not show the same gene expression. This study shows that the apoptotic process is diverse and dependent on the mRNA expression of individual neurons.

Similar to the O'Dell study, von Gertten *et al.* [26] studied the genomics response to TBI of the rat cerebral cortex, but in addition to the collection of samples 1 day post injury they also collected samples 4 days post injury, hoping to find the differences in the primary and secondary responses. Weight drop, of 24 g from a height of 9.3 cm that compressed the tissue to a maximum of 3 mm, was the injury method used in this study. Brain tissue was homogenized, RNA was isolated, and fluorescent cDNA probes were made using a reverse transcription reaction. Microarrays with 6200 clones from the TIGR (The Institute for Genomic Research) rat gene index were used. The number of genes with increased expression compared to baseline was found to be significantly higher at 1 day than at 4 days post injury in the following categories: cell communication, cell death, cell proliferation, metabolism, and transcription. This shows that there is a difference in the genetic response between the two time points. At 4 days post injury, a significant immune response was present in immunohistochemical analysis that was not present at 1 day post injury. This could be part of the secondary response to injury and could help in understanding secondary responses and find treatments to avoid the delayed effects of injury.

8.4
Concluding Remarks

These types of studies of neurodegenerative diseases as well as TBI are crucial in advancing the medical field, leading to better diagnoses and treatment of neurodegeneration and each of its causes. We see a great example of this in the recommendation of the O'Dell study that early intervention after TBI is important so that the downregulation in neuroprotective factor mRNAs can be prevented or compensated for, before too many cells can no longer protect themselves from neurodegeneration. The findings of von Gertten indicate that it may be useful to monitor immune responses of TBI patients and possibly treat them to minimize harmful responses and/or increase helpful ones. The other two studies described show that researchers must forge ahead in order to optimize results and further increase the understanding of the impact of gene expression in neurodegeneration. It is important that studies of this nature using the methods presented here are continued, as they are likely to lead to cures for diseases that are at present a terrible experience for all affected. The next experiments done could be the ones to lead to a cure.

References

1 Kanazawa, I.2001 How do neurons die in neurodegenerative diseases? *Trends in Molecular Medicine*, **7**, 339.

2 Atri, A., Sherman, S., Norman, K.A., Kirchhoff, B.A., Nicolas, M.M, Greicius, M.D., Cramer, S.C., Breiter, H.C., Hasselmo, M.E. and Stern, C.E. (2004) Blockade of central cholinergic receptors impairs new learning and increases proactive interference in a word paired-associate memory task. *Behavioral Neuroscience*, **118**, 223.

3 Buccafusco, J.J., Letchworth, S.R., Bencherif, M. and Lippiello, P.M. 2005 Long-lasting cognitive improvement with nicotinic receptor agonists: mechanisms of pharmacokinetic–pharmacodynamic discordance. *Trends in Pharmacological Sciences*, **26**, 352.

4 Borchelt, D.R., Thinakaran, G., Eckman, C.B., Lee, M.K., Davenport, F., Ratovitsky, T., Prada, C.M., Kim, G., Seekins, S., Yager, D., Slunt, H.H., Wang, R., Seeger, M., Levey, A.I., Gandy, S.E., Copeland, N.G., Jenkins, N.A., Price, D.L., Younkin, S.G. and Sisodia, S.S. (1996) Familial Alzheimer's disease-linked presenilin 1 variants elevate Abeta1-42/1-40ratio *in vitro* and *in vivo*. *Neuron*, **17**, 1005.

5 Bales, K.R., Tzavara, E.T., Wu, S., Wade, M.R., Bymaster, F.P., Paul, S.M. and Nomikos, G.G. (2006) Cholinergic dysfunction in a mouse model of Alzheimer disease is reversed by an anti-A beta antibody. *Journal of Clinical Investigation*, **116**, 825.

6 Sugars, K.L. and Rubinsztein, D.C. 2003 Transcriptional abnormalities in Huntington disease. *Trends in Genetics*, **19**, 233.

7 Wyttenbach, A., Swartz, J., Kita, H., Thykjaer, T., Carmichael, J., Bradley, J., Brown, R., Maxwell, M., Schapira, A., Orntoft, T.F., Kato, K. and Rubinsztein, D.C. (2001) Polyglutamine expansions cause decreased CRE-mediated transcription and early gene expression changes prior to cell death in an inducible cell model of Huntington's disease. *Human Molecular Genetics*, **10**, 1829.

8 Dunah, A.W., Jeong, H., Griffin, A., Kim, Y.M., Standaert, D.G., Hersch, S.M., Mouradian, M.M., Young, A.B., Tanese, N. and Krainc, D. (2002) Sp1 and TAFII130 transcriptional activity disrupted in early Huntington's disease. *Science*, **296**, 2238.

9 Reynolds, G.P., Pearson, S.J. and Heathfield, K.W. 1990 Dementia in Huntington's disease is associated with neurochemical deficits in the caudate nucleus not the cerebral cortex. *Neuroscience Letters*, **113**, 95.

10 Pearson, S.J., Heathfield, K.W. and Reynolds, G.P. 1990 Pallidal GABA and chorea in Huntington's disease. *Journal of Neural Transmission. General Section*, **81**, 241.

11 Brooks, D.J. and Piccini, P. 2006 Imaging in Parkinson's disease: the role of monoamines in behavior. *Biological Psychiatry*, **59**, 908.

12 Plaitakis, A., Constantakakis, E. and Smith, J. 1988 The neuroexcitotoxic amino acids glutamate and aspartate are altered in the spinal cord and brain in amyotrophic lateral sclerosis. *Annals of Neurology*, **24**, 446.

13 Dangond, F., Hwang, D., Camelo, S., Pasinelli, P., Frosch, M.P., Stephanopoulos, G., Stephanopoulos, G., Brown, R.H. Jr and Gullans, S.R. (2004) Molecular signature of late-stage human ALS revealed by expression profiling of postmortem spinal cord gray matter. *Physiological Genomics*, **16**, 229.

14 Mukherjee, J., Christian, B.T., Dunigan, K.A., Shi, B., Narayanan, T.K., Satter, M. and Mantil, J. (2004) Brain imaging of 18F-fallypride in normal volunteers: blood analysis distribution, test–retest studies, and preliminary assessment of sensitivity to aging effects on dopamine D-2/D-3 receptors. *Synapse*, **46**, 170.

15 Volkow, N.D., Gur, R.C., Wang, G.J., Fowler, J.S., Moberg, P.J., Ding, Y.S., Hitzemann, R., Smith, G. and Logan, J. (1998) Association between decline in brain dopamine activity with age and cognitive and motor impairment in healthy individuals. *The American Journal of Psychiatry*, **155**, 344.

16 Mattson, M.P., Maudsley, S. and Martin, B. 2004 BDNF and 5-HT: a dynamic duo in age-related neuronal plasticity and neurodegenerative disorders. *Trends in Neurosciences*, **27**, 589.

17 Semsei, I. 2000 On the nature of aging. *Mechanisms of Ageing and Development*, **117**, 93.

18 Gage, F.H., Kelly, P.A. and Bjorklund, A. 1984 Regional changes in brain glucose metabolism reflect cognitive impairments in aged rats. *Journal of Neuroscience*, **4**, 2856.

19 Wright, R.L., Lightner, E.N., Harman, J.S., Meijer, O.C. and Conrad, C.D. 2006 Attenuating corticosterone levels on the day of memory assessment prevents chronic stress-induced impairments in spatial memory. *The European Journal of Neuroscience*, **24**, 595.

20 O'Dell, D.M., Raghupathi, R., Crino, P.B., Eberwine, J.H. and McIntosh, T.K. 2000 Traumatic brain injury alters the molecular fingerprint of TUNEL-positive cortical neurons *in vivo*: a single-cell analysis. *Journal of Neuroscience*, **20**, 4821.

21 van Gelder, R.N., von Zastrow, M.E., Yool, A., Dement, W.C., Barchas, J.D. and Eberwine, J.H. (1990) Amplified RNA synthesized from limited quantities of heterogeneous cDNA. *Proceedings of the National Academy of Sciences of the United States of America*, **87**, 1663.

22 Schena, M., Shalon, D., Davis, R.W. and Brown, P.O. 1995 Quantitative monitoring of gene expression patterns with a complementary DNA microarray. *Science*, **270**, 467.

23 Hu, J., Fink, D. and Mata, M. 2002 Microarray analysis suggests the involvement of proteasomes lysosomes, and matrix metalloproteinases in the response of motor neurons to root avulsion. *The European Journal of Neuroscience*, **16**, 1409.

24 Hammarberg, H., Piehl, F., Risling, M. and Cullheim, S. 2000 Differential regulation of trophic factor receptor mRNAs in spinal motoneurons after sciatic nerve transection and ventral root avulsion in the rat. *The Journal of Comparative Neurology*, **426**, 587.

25 Marciano, P.G., Brettschneider, J., Manduchi, E., Davis, J.E., Eastman, S., Raghupathi, R., Saatman, K.E., Speed, T.P., Stoeckert, C.J. Jr, Eberwine, J.H. and McIntosh, T.K. (2004) Neuron-specific mRNA complexity responses during hippocampal apoptosis after traumatic brain injury. *Journal of Neuroscience*, **24**, 2866.

26 von Gertten, C., Flores Morales, A., Holmin, S., Mathiesen, T. and Nordqvist, A.C. 2005 Genomic responses in rat cerebral cortex after traumatic brain injury. *BMC Neuroscience*, **6**, 69.

9

Redox Proteomics and Metabolic Proteins in Brain of Subjects with Alzheimer's Disease, Mild Cognitive Impairment, and Models Thereof

Rukhsana Sultana, Tanea Reed, and D. Allan Butterfield

9.1
Oxidative Stress

Under normal physiological conditions, generation of reactive oxygen species (ROS) and reactive nitrogen species (RNS) is counterbalanced with an abundance of antioxidant defense mechanisms [1]. ROS/RNS are important mediators in biological signaling processes, widely used as second messengers to propagate proinflammatory or growth stimulatory signals [2,3]. When the generation of ROS/RNS exceeds the endogenous limit of antioxidant defense systems, oxidative or nitrosative stress result [4]. Oxidative stress may be caused by an imbalance in the prooxidant and antioxidant systems. ROS/RNS can react with macromolecules that may cause reversible and/or irreversible modifications leading to structural, functional, and stability modulations [5–12].

Oxidative damage of proteins is one of the modifications that lead to a severe failure of biological functions and cell death [13]. Protein oxidation is normally assessed in a cell by the formation of protein carbonyls and 3-nitrotyrosine (3-NT). Protein carbonyls are formed by free radical-mediated oxidation of amino acid residue side chains (histidine, arginine, lysine residues, among others) [14–16] and also lead to damage of proteins by advanced lipid peroxidation end products (ALEs) and glycation/glycoxidation of Lys amino groups, forming advanced glycation end products (AGE). 3-NTs are formed by nitration of tyrosine residues, which in a protein play an important role in regulating protein function, usually by phosphorylation, a prominent protein regulation mechanism. Addition of nitrite to the protein at the tyrosine residue sterically hinders or prevents tyrosine phosphorylation and may also change the structure of proteins, thereby rendering a protein dysfunctional that may lead to cell death [17]. Regulation of cellular homeostasis through posttranslational modification of proteins is one of the major responses to oxidative and nitrosative stress that may alter the structure of proteins and cause reversible and/or irreversible modifications of proteins [18–21]. Reversible modification usually occurs at Cys and Met amino acid residues by various enzymatic systems [21–23].

Neural Degeneration and Repair: Gene Expression Profiling, Proteomics, and Systems Biology
Edited by Hans Werner Müller
Copyright © 2008 WILEY-VCH Verlag GmbH & Co. KGaA, Weinheim
ISBN: 978-3-527-31707-3

Protein modifications such as carbonylation, nitration, and protein–protein cross-linking are generally associated with the loss of function and may lead to either unfolding and degradation of damaged proteins or aggregation that leads to accumulation as cytoplasmic inclusions, as observed in age-related neurodegenerative disorders [24,25]. Oxidized proteins are typically dysfunctional or nonfunctional and are highly sensitive to proteolytic degradation by the proteasome [26,27], so this issue has both physiological and pathological significance [28,29]. The increase in the level of oxidized protein in Alzheimer's disease (AD) is associated with the loss of the activity of the 20S proteasome, a major enzyme for the degradation of oxidized proteins [30–33]. Recent studies have shown that prolonged oxidized proteins are more resistant to degradation by 20S proteasome [34,35]. Therefore, accumulation of oxidatively modified proteins disrupts cellular functions either by the loss of catalytic ability or by the interruption of regulatory pathways [36].

A number of sensitive assays are available for detection of oxidatively modified proteins. Previously, immunoprecipitation techniques were used to identify selective oxidatively modified proteins. But this technique requires a thorough knowledge of the protein of interest and the availability of a specific antibody. Earlier, immunoprecipitation techniques were used in our laboratory to identify HNE modification of creatine kinase (CK), the glutamate transporter (GLT-1), glutathione-S-transfersase (GST) and the multidrug resistant protein-1 (MRP-1) in AD brain [37,38] and elevated protein carbonyls in CK [39]. However, such methods are both time consuming and laborious; in addition, posttranslational modification can sometime change the structure of proteins, which could then prevent the formation of the appropriate antigen–antibody complex.

Proteomics represents a much more convenient way to identify a large number of proteins in a sample at one time. However, a disadvantage of using proteomic analysis to identify oxidatively modified proteins is that carbonylated abundant proteins with a low "specific carbonyl content" appear prominent on immunoblots, while proteins present at low levels but with a high specific carbonyl content may be missed. In our laboratory, we used redox proteomics to identify oxidatively modified proteins in various diseases, including neurodegenerative diseases such as AD (Figure 9.1). In this chapter, we discuss the application of redox proteomics in the identification of oxidatively modified proteins involved in energy metabolism in AD, mild cognitive impairment (MCI) and models thereof.

9.2
Redox Proteomics

Proteomics is the large-scale study of proteins, particularly their structures and functions. Proteome analysis is "the analysis of the entire PROTEin complement expressed by a genOME." It involves the systematic separation, identification, and quantification of many proteins simultaneously from a single sample. The term "proteomics" was termed to be analogous with "genomics," and while it is often viewed as the "next step," proteomics is much more complicated than genomics [40]. Most important,

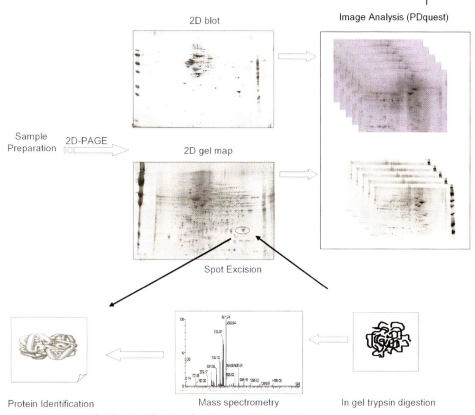

Figure 9.1 Protocol for the identification of oxidized proteins by redox proteomics.

while the genome is relatively invariable, the proteome differs and is constantly changing through its biochemical interactions with the genome and the environment. Proteomic analysis encompasses the qualitative, quantitative, and functional characterization of the entire protein profile of a given cell, tissue, and/or organism. The large increase in protein diversity is thought to be due to posttranslational modification and alternative splicing of proteins. This diversity implies that proteins cannot be fully characterized by gene expression analysis alone, making proteomics a useful tool for characterizing cells and tissues of interest. Accordingly, proteomics seeks to determine protein structure, modifications, localizations, and protein–protein interactions, as well as protein expression levels.

In addition to a variety of new approaches, proteomics still relies heavily on two-dimensional electrophoresis as a means of protein separation. This procedure incorporates both isoelectric focusing and sodium dodecyl sulfate–polyacrylamide gel electrophoresis (SDS-PAGE) to separate proteins first by their isoelectric point and then by their relative mobility [41]. Two-dimensional-polyacrylamide gel electrophoresis (2D-PAGE) represents undoubtedly one of the most commonly used techniques for protein separation, but non-SDS-PAGE methods are also employed.

2D-high performance liquid chromatography (2D-HPLC) achieves separation of a protein mixture by eluting the sample through a series of columns coupled with mass spectroscopy (MS) analysis [42,43]. Alternatively, expression profiling can also be obtained by labeling a mixture of two samples with different isotopes that bind to specific amino acid side chains. The resulting isotopic labeling is further analyzed by a mass spectrometer. This technique is referred as isotopically coded affinity tags (ICAT) [44].

The other key tool of proteomics is MS [45]. It is by combining two-dimensional electrophoresis and mass spectroscopy that proteomics achieves great power. First, the gel-separated proteins are digested into peptides by specific proteases, and an eluted peptide mixture is acquired. Matrix-assisted laser desorption/ionization (MALDI) is performed to produce a mass spectrum or "peptide mass fingerprint." The second step in protein identification often relies on the fragmentation of individual peptides in the mixture to gain sequence information. Electrospray ionization (ESI) is performed in conjunction with tandem mass spectrometry. Both mass spectrum and sequence information can be searched against databases to identify proteins.

9.2.1
Two-Dimensional Electrophoresis (2-DE)

2D-PAGE [46], in which proteins are separated according to their isoelectric point (pI) by isoelectric focusing in the first dimension and according to size (relative migration) by SDS-PAGE in the second dimension, has a unique capacity for the resolution of complex mixtures of proteins, permitting the simultaneous analysis of hundreds or even thousands of gene products. Thousands of different proteins can thus be separated and information such as the protein pI, the molecular migration rate (M_r), and the amount of each protein obtained [47]. Because the first dimension separates on the basis of charge, isoelectric focusing uses pH gradients that can be established by adding ampholytes to an acrylamide gel. The use of narrow range IEF strips enables the investigator to separate proteins over a wide range of pH with a unit pH difference of 1. However, the normally employed IEF strip pH range, that is 3–10, limits the identification of highly basic proteins. To characterize specific proteins in a complex protein mixture, the proteins of interest must be completely soluble under electrophoresis conditions. Different treatments and conditions are required to solubilize different types of protein samples; some proteins are naturally found in complexes with membranes, nucleic acids, or other proteins; some proteins form various nonspecific aggregates; and some proteins precipitate when they are removed from their normal environment. Solubilization of membrane proteins often requires ionic detergent not compatible with isoelectric focusing [48]. Chaotropic agents, such as urea and thiourea, coupled with nonionic or zwitterionic detergents can be used to solubilize proteins and avoid protein precipitation during the IEF and the SDS gel. The use of immobilized pH IEF strips improves the reproducibility among the samples and also eliminates the typical cathodic drift associated with previously used tube gels. This, together with detection of low-abundance proteins and proteins of high isoelectric point, is the main limitation of two-dimensional electrophoresis [49]. The third limitation of 2D-PAGE is the insensitivity to proteins of high trypsin content. Plasma samples are thought to be a better sample for investigating protein expression in neurological diseases because of its ease of collection. However, removal of high-abundance proteins such as albumin and IgG (approximately 70% of the protein mass of plasma) is necessary to identify lower-abundant proteins that these two proteins may be masking.

9.2.2
Mass Spectrometry and Database Searching

In proteome analysis, mass spectrometry can identify electrophoretically separated proteins with two different approaches. The simplest approach is peptide mass fingerprinting (PMF) technique, in which the protein spot of interest is digested in-gel with a specific enzyme, the resulting peptides are extracted from the gel, and the molecular weights of these peptides are measured with MS. Database search programs can create theoretical PMFs for all proteins in the database and compare them to those obtained experimentally. ESI yields partial amino acid sequences from the peptides (sequence tags). Database searches are then performed using both molecular weight and sequence information. PMF is usually obtained with MALDI-TOF and sequence tags by nano-ESI tandem mass spectrometry (MS/MS). The sensitivity of protein identification by MS is in the femtomole range. The development of proteomics databases has facilitate the identification of a protein from its peptide sequence derived from the mass spectrum (Table 9.1). For instance, Swiss-Prot, the first major protein database, allows protein identification by using computer algorithms [50] freely accessible online. These search engines provide a theoretical protease digestion of the proteins contained in the database. Comparison of the resulting theoretical peptide masses with the experimental masses obtained from the in-gel digested proteins leads to protein identification. Several factors have to be considered to obtain correct protein identification, such as the protein size and the probability of a single peptide to occur in the whole database. Search engines produce a probability score for each entry, which is calculated by a mathematical

Table 9.1 Mass spectrometry search engines for peptide mass fingerprinting.

Search engine	URL
Mascot	http://www.matrixscience.com
MOWSE	http://www.hgmp.mrc.ac.uk/Bioinformatics/Webapp/mowse
Profound	http://prowl.rockefeller.edu/profound_bin/WebProFound.exe
MS-fit	http://prospector.ucsf.edu/ucsfhtml4.0/msfit.htm
Peptident	http://ca.expasy.org/tools/peptident.html
Mass Search	http://cbrg.inf.ethz.ch
Peptide Search	http://www.mann.emblheidelberg.de
ExPASy	http://www.expasy.ch/tools

algorithm that is specific for each search engine. Any hit with a score higher than that for statistical significance from the search engine is considered statistically significant and has an excellent chance to be the protein cut from a given spot. In addition, the molecular weight and the isoelectric point of the protein are calculated based on the position in the 2D map to avoid any false identification. Immuno-chemical methods also are performed to validate protein identity.

9.3
Oxidative Damage in AD

AD is the most common form of dementia involving a number of cellular and biochemical lesions [8,9,51–53]. It is characterized by synaptic loss, nerve cell loss, and the deposition of extracellular plaques that consists of 40–42 amino acid long amyloid β (Aβ) peptides and intracellular neurofibrilary tangles [54]. Familial or inherited AD, which manifests at an early age, is often associated with mutations in amyloid precursor protein (APP), presenilin-1 (PS-1), and presenilin-2 (PS-2), whereas the sporadic form, which manifests at later stages of life, is reported to be multifactorial, including induced expression of APP [55–57]. The exact biochemical mechanism of the pathogenesis of AD is still unknown, but several hypotheses have been proposed to explain AD pathogenesis including amyloid cascade, excitoxicity, oxidative stress, and inflammation [8,9,58–63]. However, it is difficult to know a priori if the oxidative modifications observed are the primary contributors or the secondary effects of the disease [64].

Evidences indicates that ROS and RNS levels are increased in AD brain, which can cause oxidative damage, which may play a role in the subsequent pathogenesis of AD [53,65–68]. There are postmortem studies on the brains of AD patients and in animal models of AD that showed indirect markers of oxidative damage and changes in antioxidant enzymes [69–74], protein carbonyl, protein nitration, lipid peroxidation, advanced glycation end products, and DNA and RNA oxidation products [5,11,53,65,75–77]. Further, the presence of ferritin, hemoxygenase, and iron suggests the prevalence of oxidative stress in AD [78]. β-Amyloid has been shown by our laboratory and others as central to oxidative stress and neurodegeneration in AD. The ability of β-amyloid to produce free radicals mediates the oxidation of unsaturated membrane lipids, disruption of the neuronal membrane, and, ultimately, cell death [58]. Some researchers have recently proposed that oxidative stress precedes Aβ deposition [79,80] and that deposition of Aβ could be a compensatory mechanism to protect the cells from the small oligomeric toxic form of Aβ [81]. In fact, others have proposed that Aβ has many physiological roles, which include free-radical scavenging ability as supported by superoxide dismutase-like activity *in vitro* [82] and as a redox-active metal sequestration [83–85]. Further, Aβ can also indirectly produce free radicals via the induction of a local immune response leading to inflammation [59,86–89]. This notion is consistent with the reported increase in cellular and soluble mediators of inflammation in postmortem AD tissue or mouse models thereof [59,86–89].

In AD brain and plasma, several proteins have been identified as targets of oxidative stress [9,25,90–94]. Immunohistochemical studies have revealed an increase in carbonyl formation in AD brain [76]. However, no oxidatively modified proteins were actually identified. A band of oxidized protein at 78 kDa on one-dimensional oxyblots in AD plasma was observed [95]. A recent study revealed that several isoforms of fibrinogen α-chain precursor protein and α-1-antitrypsin exhibited a greater specific oxidation in AD plasma [96].

Several targets of protein nitration in AD have been identified [92,94]. In AD brain and CSF increased levels of nitrated proteins have been found [68,92,94], implying a role for RNS in AD pathology. Increased levels of 3-NT immunoreactivity were observed in the brain of AD subjects when compared to aged matched controls [68], and DiTyr and 3-NT levels were reported to be elevated consistently in the hippocampus, IPL, and neocortical regions of the AD brain and in ventricular cerebrospinal fluid (VF) [68,97]. The increased 3-NT residues and free adducts in CSF of AD subjects probably reflect increased leakage of mitochondrial electron equivalents and protein nitrating agents with resultant and increased protein nitration in brain tissue [75].

Our redox proteomics studies identified the oxidatively modified proteins, indexed either by increased carbonyl levels or by increased 3-nitrotyrosine levels, in AD inferior parietal lobule and hippocampus [9,53,90–94]. Previous studies from our laboratory demonstrated a pattern of protein modification in AD brain suggesting a correspondence among amyloid deposition, neurofibrillary tangle formation, microglial accumulation, and tissue oxidation [76]. The amyloid-rich inferior parietal lobule and hippocampal regions showed increased levels of oxidative damage compared with absence of oxidative modification in cerebellum of AD brain. We first identified cytosolic creatine kinase BB isoform, β-actin, glutamine synthase, ubiquitin carboxy-terminal hydrolase L-1, dihydropyrimidinase-related protein 2, α-enolase, phosphoglycerate mutase 1 (PGM1), gamma-soluble *N*-ethylmaleimide-sensitive factor attachment protein (SNAP), peptidyl-prolyl *cis/trans* isomerase 1 (Pin1), glyceraldehyde 3-phosphate dehydrogenase (GAPDH), voltage-dependent anion channel protein-1 (VDAC-1), triosephosphate isomerase, ATP synthase alpha chain, and carbonic anhydrase 2 as targets of protein oxidation in AD brain; and further studies showed that the oxidatively modified proteins are generally functionally inactive [7,38,98–100]. The oxidatively modified proteins in AD brain are involved in diverse functions including energy-related enzymes, neurotrasmitter-related proteins, proteasome-related proteins, cholinergic system, pH regulation protein, structural proteins, and are related to pathological observations in AD, including neurofibrillary tangles, senile plaques, and entrance of AD neurons into the cell cycle [9,53].

Creatine kinase BB isoform, α-enolase, γ-enolase, lactate dehydrogenase (LDH), phosphoglycerate mutase 1 (PGM1), glyceraldehyde 3-phosphate dehydrogenase (GAPDH), VDAC-1, triosephosphate isomerase, and ATP synthase alpha chain are energy-related proteins that are more affected by protein oxidation in AD brain. Consequently, these oxidatively modified proteins are more prone to inactivation in AD brain. In this chapter, we discuss the consequence of protein modification on cell energy.

9.4
Role of Identified Energy-Related Proteins in AD Brain

Energy metabolism is crucial for the normal function of cells, such as neurotransmission, muscular contractions, and signaling pathways. Impairment of cerebral energy metabolism can induce dementia by altering cellular functions [101,102]. The brain uses approximately 20% of the body's glucose consumption, although it is only 2% of the entire body mass. Glucose metabolism is the main source of energy in the brain, and, hence, impairment of cerebral energy metabolism might be an important cause of dementia in AD [103]. Glucose enters cells by specific transporters, called glucose transporters, from the exterior to the cytosol. Several glucose transporters were found to be oxidatively modified in AD, which can be attributed to the decreased energy metabolism seen in AD [104]. The AD brain was reported to have altered glucose utilization and consequently impaired energy metabolism [105–107]. This effect was demonstrated as early as the 1950s by different methods and has been reproduced extensively by modern methods, including positron emission tomography (PET), single photon emission computed tomography (SPECT), and functional magnetic resonance imaging [105,108,109]. Hence, glucose utilization can be used as a sensitive neurophysiological test or evidence of brain atrophy on MRI [110].

Impairment of oxidative energy metabolism leads to increased expression of the Alzheimer's APP [102] and to cytoskeletal disorganization, including the appearance of epitopes associated with paired helical filaments/tangles [111]. Further, a decrease in ATP levels could cause disturbances in cholesterol homeostasis, cholinergic defects, disruption of ion homeostasis, altered protein synthesis, sorting, transport and degradation of proteins, and maintenance of synaptic transmission, all detrimental to cell viability. Such changes can also lead to exposure of phosphatidylserine to the outer membrane leaflet, a signal for apoptosis [112,113]. Moreover, an ATP shortage can also induce hypothermia, causing abnormal tau phosphorylation through differential inhibition of kinase and phosphatase [114].

Our group identified CK, ENO1, TPI, GAPDH, LDH, PGM1, and α-ATPase as oxidized proteins using redox proteomics, which suggests that these proteins are involved directly or indirectly in altered ATP production in AD brain [39,90–94]. The identification of these proteins as oxidized correlated with the altered energy metabolism in AD brain [105,107,108]. Further, previous studies from our laboratory and others have shown altered function of the enzymes involved in glucose metabolism in AD brain [39,76,93,94,115,116].

The creatine/phosphocreatine system functions as a spatial energy buffer between the cytosol and mitochondria, using a unique mitochondrial CK isoform. The mitochondrial CK isoform exists in the intermembrane space of the mitochondria and the octameric form of CK keeps the membrane permeability transition pore closed. However, the presence of free radicals promotes opening of the pore and subsequent apoptosis. In the AD brain, CK is oxidized and shows diminished activity [76]. ATP synthase α-chain is a part of the complex V of oxidative phosphorylation that promotes ATP synthesis and release [117]. A previous study showed cytosolic accumulation of ATP synthase α-chain with neurofibrillary tangles in

AD [118], and our laboratory identified this protein as an oxidized protein [53]. Oxidation of ATP synthase alpha suggests impaired function and also interactions between the subunits leading to reduced activity of F_1F_0-ATPase (ATP synthase, complex V) that could compromise brain ATP synthesis and induce damaging ROS production and, if severe, could lead to neuronal death. Further, mitochondria have recently been described to play an important role in APP metabolism [119].

Among the oxidized proteins identified, α-enolase, γ-enolase, triose phosphate isomerase, GAPDH, PGM1, and LDH are part of glycolysis, and the reactions catalyzed by these enzymes are shown in Figure 9.2. Abnormal oxidation of enolase, triosephosphate isomerase, GAPDH, PGM1, and LDH might account for decreased

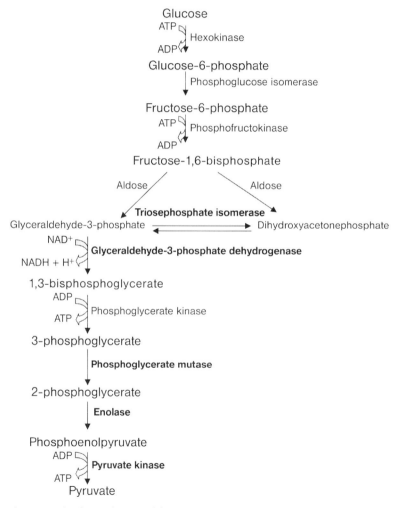

Figure 9.2 Glycolytic pathways and the enzymes involved in these pathways. Proteins that are identified as oxidized in AD brain are highlighted.

enzyme activity, which, in turn, could lead to decreased glycolysis and hypometabolism [116]. Most of the identified oxidized proteins were found to be formed by glycolysis, suggesting the sensitivity of these proteins to oxidative stress. Moreover, since glycolysis is the first step in the energy production pathway, impartment of glycolysis would compromise the total cellular ATP production [7,39,53,90–92]. Consequently, our redox proteomics observations suggest a possible relationship between glycolytic enzymatic impairment and reduced glucose metabolism in AD.

9.5
Oxidative Stress in MCI

MCI is a syndrome defined as cognitive decline greater than that expected for an individual's age and education level, but that does not interfere notably with activities of daily life [120]. Considered a transition stage between the normal condition and AD [121], MCI shows a number of features similar to AD including cholinergic dysfunction, white-matter lesions and cerebral infarctions, extracellular amyloid deposition, and intracellular neurofibrillary tangle formation. Further, several gene mutations associated with AD have been observed in subjects with MCI including mutations in APP and PS-1 and the presence of APOE4, which clearly raises the risk of progression from amnestic MCI to Alzheimer's disease [122–124]. Therefore, the MCI stage may provide an opportunity to clarify whether increased oxidative damage is an important factor in the pathogenesis of neuronal death in AD or a secondary consequence of AD.

Similar to AD, MCI shows an increasing trend in oxidative stress as indicated by decreased levels of antioxidant system such as Vitamin A, Vitamin C, Vitamin E, Uric acid, and so on, and activity of antioxidant enzymes like GPx and SOD in MCI plasma [125–128]. In addition, an increase in oxidative damage to proteins and lipids was reported in MCI brain [129,130]. An increase in isoprostane $8,12$-iso-$PF_{2\alpha}$-VI – a specific marker of *in vivo* lipid peroxidation – was also reported in CSF, plasma, and urine of MCI subjects compared to controls. Further, elevated levels of DNA and RNA oxidation were reported in MCI brain [131,132]. The data so far available on MCI suggest that oxidative stress may be an early event in the pathogenesis of the disease and may be of importance in MCI progression to AD [133].

Our group recently reported oxidation of enolase, glutamine synthase, and Pin1 in subjects with MCI using redox proteomics, and all three proteins were previously identified as targets of oxidation in AD brain [53,90–94,98]. This finding provides a link between oxidative modification of enolase and impaired energy metabolism, which is a characteristic feature of AD.

9.6
Models of Alzheimer's Disease

Animal models of AD are useful in providing insight into the neurochemical and cellular changes associated with this disorder and also to develop a therapy. Several

Table 9.2 Energetically related proteins found to be oxidatively modified in AD, MCI, and various AD models.

Proteins	SAMP8	Aβ synaptosomes	C. elegans	ICV	MCI	AD
α-Enolase	×				×	×
Adenosine kinase			×			
Aldolase 3	×					
Arginine kinase			×			
ATP synthase α1	×		×			×
Creatine kinase	×					×
Glutamate ammonia ligase				×		
Glutamate dehydrogenase		×				
Glyceraldehyde 3-phosphate dehydrogenase				×		×
H⁺ transporting ATP synthase		×				
Lactate dehydrogenase	×					×
Malate dehydrogenase			×			
Medium chain acyl CoA dehydrogenase			×			
Phosphoglycereate mutase 1				×		×
Pyruvate dehydrogenase				×		
Pyruvate kinase M2					×	
Short-chain acyl CoA dehydrogenase			×			
Transketolase			×			
Triosephosphate isomerase	×					×

knock-in and knock-out models were constructed to study the role of the genetic mutations of AD, such as APP, PS-1, PS-1/APP, tau, and Tau/APP/PS-1 animal models, which show some pathological markers of AD [134–136]. Further, these animal models also enable us to study the consequences of oxidation of proteins on cellular functions, as exemplified by the gracile axonal dystrophy (GAD) mouse model that has a defective UCHL-1 protein, an oxidized protein in AD brain [90,93,137]. A comparative analysis of the oxidized proteins in AD and models of AD is shown in Table 9.2.

9.6.1
Cell Culture Model

An *in vitro* study using Aβ (1–42) examined neuronal cells as a model relevant to AD [138,139]. Neuronal cell cultures treated with 10 μM Aβ (1–42) showed an increased oxidation in the metabolic protein, GAPDH. This enzyme converts glyceraldehyde 3-phosphate to 1,3-bisphosphoglycerate through glycolysis and produces energy, so any loss of function can greatly influence the energy used for the remaining events in glycolysis [140–142]. Moreover, oxidative modification of GAPDH can lead to neurotoxicity [143]. Further, GAPDH serves as a NO sensor [144]. Consequently, oxidative modification of GAPDH conceivably could be involved in the elevated RNS associated with AD.

9.6.2
SAMP 8

The senescence-accelerated mouse (SAM) is a model of accelerated aging through phenotypic selection from a common genetic pool of the AKR/J strain of mice [145,146]. In particular, the SAMP8 (senescence – accelerated – prone) substrain mouse demonstrates normal physical aging but develops learning and memory deficits as well as Aβ (Abeta) deposition as early as 6–8 months [147–149]. Along with these characteristics, the aged SAMP8 mouse showed increased oxidative stress [150] that is associated with mitochondrial dysfunction [151,152].

The age-dependent deposition of Aβ peptide can be significantly reduced by antisense oligonucleotide to APP or by Aβ antibody to diminish oxidative stress, a process that improves memory defects [148,153–155]. Since the antisense oligonucleotide can cross the blood–brain barrier, the neurons can internalize it to effectively lower APP levels [156]. Current research has shown that at 12 months SAMP8 mice have higher levels of protein oxidation and lipid peroxidation compared to that of 4-month-old SAMP8 mice [157]. Compared to AD, the SAMP8 mouse model through reverse transcription–polymerase chain reaction showed that levels of the proapoptotic factor, bcl-2α, and presenillin-2 mRNA were significantly increased [158,159]. In terms of energetically related genes, Δ-9-desaturase mRNA levels decrease in the SAMP8 mouse model, which can alter the membrane fluidity and signal transduction in the synapse [160]. The mRNA of glycogen debranching enzyme isoform-like gene in SAMP8 mice may result in dysfunction of the central nervous system [158,159]. In aged SAMP8, glutamine synthase activity and gluathione peroxidase are decreased [150,161,162].

Glucose metabolism decreased along with decreased hexokinase activity in the female SAMP8 mouse [163,164]. Hexokinase activity is crucial in energy metabolism, as this enzyme catalyzes the first step of glycolysis. GLUT-1 transporter, located in the BBB, decreased in the SAMP8 mouse, which can correspond to reduced energy metabolism in this model of aging. There were several energetically related proteins that were found to be oxidatively modified in the SAMP8 mouse model including α-enolase, lactate dehydrogenase, triosephosphate isomerase, aldolase 3, creatine kinase, and ATP synthase α1 [157]. α-Enolase, lactate dehydrogenase, triosephosphate isomerase, creatine kinase, and ATP synthase α1 are found as commonly oxidized proteins between AD brain and SAMP8 mice brain [90–94,157]. It is interesting to speculate that since Aβ accumulates in both AD and SAMP8 brain, the oxidative stress induced by this peptide may be a link between the two systems.

9.6.3
Synaptosomal Model

Synaptosomes are resealed presynaptic nerve terminals that take up glucose and oxygen, intake K^+, excrete Na^+, and maintain membrane potential. Therefore, synaptosomes are an excellent model for investigating changes at the synapse. In AD, synapse loss has been thought to be an early event [165–167]. Synapse loss can lead to neuronal miscommunication developing into memory deficiencies, one of the first symptoms of AD [168,169]. Synaptosomes treated with $10 \mu M$ Aβ (1–42) partially duplicate the effects of Aβ (1–42) in the AD brain [170,171]. These results also showed an increase in overall protein oxidation and the oxidation of the energy-related enzymes H$^+$ transporting ATP synthase and glutamate dehydrogenase [7].

H$^+$ transporting ATP synthase is a multisubunit enzyme involved in the transport of ions by an H$^+$ gradient [172]. Through a rotational mechanism, all the subunits must align together in the proper conformation to produce ATP [173,174]. Improper function of this enzyme leads to a lag in the H$^+$ potential and the ability of the subunits to properly align to form ATP. Misalignment of these subunits consequently affects production of ATP, thereby decreasing ATP available in the cell to drive biological processes [175–177]. Glutamate dehydrogenase, which uses NAD$^+$ as a cofactor, is essential to the reversible conversion of α-ketoglutarate to glutamate. NAD$^+$ is used in electron transfer to produce NADH and create energy. NAD$^+$ regulates this enzyme and the ratio of NAD$^+$ and NADH is crucial to the directionality of the enzyme [178]. The malfunction of this enzyme can lead to increased levels of the amino acid, glutamate, and therefore excitotoxicity. In this direction of the reaction, ATP consumption is high; therefore, energy metabolism is inefficient. The reverse reaction produces α-ketoglutarate, which can flow into the TCA cycle to produce ATP.

9.6.4
Intracerebral Ventricular Model

Casamenti *et al.* [179] looked at the lingering effects of intracerebral injection of Aβ (1–42) *in vivo* into the nucleus basalis magnocellularis (NBM) to imitate the cholinergic dysfunction found in AD [180–183]. NBM is found in the basal forebrain, in which most of the brain's cholinergic neurons are located. Injection into the nucleus magnocellularis has profound effects on neighboring brain regions such as the cortex and hippocampus [184,185]. The cortex is responsible for reasoning, judgment, learning, and visuospatial activities. By a redox proteomics approach, several enzymes involved in energy metabolism, including glutamine synthetase, glyceraldehyde 3-phosphate dehydrogenase, pyruvate dehydrogenase, and phosphoglycerate mutase 1, were found to be oxidized in these regions. Glutamine synthetase (i.e., glutamate ammonia ligase) was the only energy-related enzyme found to be oxidized in the cortex. This protein was also shown to be oxidized in old mice [186] and in AD [90].

The hippocampus is the principal area in which long-term and short-term memory are processed. In normal aging, shrinkage in hippocampal volume as well as deterioration of the gyri and sulcus [187–189] are observed. The three energy-related enzymes oxidized in the hippocampus by Aβ (1–42) injection in NBM are glyceraldehyde 3-phosphate dehydrogenase (mentioned above), pyruvate dehydrogenase, and phosphoglyceromutase 1. Pyruvate dehydrogenase is the E$_1$ component of a multienzyme complex that decarboxylates pyruvate to form acetyl CoA and carbon dioxide [190]. There are roughly 30 copies of pyruvate dehydrogenase in this enzyme complex that use thiamin pyrophosphate (TPP) as a prosthetic group. The disruption of this component inhibits the function of the entire complex, thus significantly halting acetyl CoA production; this molecule is the linker step of glycolysis to the TCA cycle for more ATP production. Phosphoglyceromutase 1 simply rearranges the phosphate group on 3-phosphoglycerate to 2-phosphoglycerate in glycolysis. This isomerization is crucial for the following steps of glycolysis to form phosphoenolpyruvate through a dehydration step catalyzed by enolase. Any malfunction of phosphoglyceromutase 1 can lead to an increase in 3-phosphoglycerate and lower levels of 2-phosphoglycerate, thus preventing proper ATP production [191,192].

9.6.5
Caenorhabditis elegans Model

The transgenic worm *Caenorhabditis elegans* (*C. elegans*) expresses human Aβ (1–42) making it a valuable model of study. In the *C. elegans* model, protein oxidation occurs before fibril deposition of Aβ (1–42) peptide [81]. This observation further supports the notion that Aβ (1–42) toxicity is caused by oligomers of Aβ rather than fibrils. Several models of the transgenic *C. elegans* worm have been used for proteomic analysis. This section will focus only on the CL4176 and CL2337 models, since these models are the only ones that contain oxidatively modified energy-related proteins. The CL4176 model expresses human Aβ (1–42) in its body wall muscle, while the CL2337 model expresses a green fluorescent protein fusion protein (GFP) that quickly aggregates GFP. In the model of transgenic *C. elegans* that expresses human Aβ, several proteins including medium- and short-chain acyl-CoA dehydrogenases, transketolase, arginine kinase, adenosine kinase, and malate dehydrogenase were found to be oxidatively modified [49].

The CL2337 *C. elegans* model yielded oxidatively modified glutamate dehydrogenase and ATP synthase α chain. These two proteins were the same as found to undergo excess carbonylation in the Aβ synaptosome model. This is interesting because these proteins are seen in the transgenic *C. elegans* model that rapidly aggregates GFP instead of expressing human Aβ (1–42) and may reflect the effects of protein aggregation rather than Aβ or GFP *per se*.

9.7
Conclusions

Protein oxidation occurs during neurodegeneration and has been demonstrated to induce tertiary structural changes in proteins causing alteration in bioenergetics. These changes have been implicated in impairment of cellular functions that could eventually lead to cell death. The appearance of a common set of proteins in AD, MCI, and various models of AD suggests that Aβ plays an important role in oxidation of proteins. We hypothesize that the oxidation of glycolytic proteins such as enolase,

GADPH, LDH, and PGM1 function to downregulate intracellular energy metabolism with consequent generation of ROS through respiratory control mechanisms. Therefore, the identification of molecular mechanisms that function to minimize protein oxidation under conditions of oxidative stress is crucial to the understanding of the underlying mechanisms associated with AD. Therapeutic interventions that decrease the formation of ROS and restore homeostatic balances may be a promising therapeutic strategy for MCI and AD, studies for which are underway in our laboratory.

Acknowledgments

This work was supported in part by NIH grants (AG-05119 and AG-10836).

References

1 Stadtman, E.R. and Levine, R.L. (2003) Free radical-mediated oxidation of free amino acids and amino acid residues in proteins. *Amino Acids*, **25** (3–4), 207–218.

2 Mikkelsen, R.B. and Wardman, P. (2003) Biological chemistry of reactive oxygen and nitrogen and radiation-induced signal transduction mechanisms. *Oncogene*, **22** (37), 5734–5754.

3 Thannickal, V.J., Day, R.M., Klinz, S.G., Bastien, M.C., Larios, J.M. and Fanburg, B.L. (2000) Ras-dependent and -independent regulation of reactive oxygen species by mitogenic growth factors and TGF-beta1. *FASEB Journal*, **14** (12), 1741–1748.

4 Sies, H. and Cadenas, E. (1985) Oxidative stress: damage to intact cells and organs. *Philosophical Transactions of the Royal Society of London. Series B Biological Sciences*, **311** (1152), 617–631.

5 Aksenov, M.Y., Aksenova, M.V., Butterfield, D.A., Geddes, J.W. and Markesbery, W.R. (2001) Protein oxidation in the brain in Alzheimer's disease. *Neuroscience*, **103** (2), 373–383.

6 Baynes, J.W. and Thorpe, S.R. (2000) Glycoxidation and lipoxidation in atherogenesis. *Free Radical Biology and Medicine*, **28** (12), 1708–1716.

7 Boyd-Kimball, D., Castegna, A., Sultana, R., Poon, H.F., Petroze, R., Lynn, B.C., Klein, J.B. and Butterfield, D.A. (2005) Proteomic identification of proteins oxidized by Abeta(1–42) in synaptosomes: implications for Alzheimer's disease. *Brain Research*, **1044** (2), 206–215.

8 Butterfield, D.A. (2002) Amyloid beta-peptide (1–42)-induced oxidative stress and neurotoxicity: implications for neurodegeneration in Alzheimer's disease brain. A review. *Free Radical Research*, **36** (12), 1307–1313.

9 Butterfield, D.A., Perluigi, M. and Sultana, R. (2006) Oxidative stress in Alzheimer's disease brain: new insights from redox proteomics. *European Journal of Pharmacology*, **545** (1), 39–50.

10 Nakamura, K., Hori, T., Sato, N., Sugie, K., Kawakami, T. and Yodoi, J. (1993) Redox regulation of a src family protein tyrosine kinase p56lck in T cells. *Oncogene*, **8** (11), 3133–3139.

11 Smith, M.A. and Perry, G. (1996) Alzheimer disease: protein–protein interaction and oxidative stress. *Boletin de Estudios Medicos Y Biologicos*, **44** (1–4), 5–10.

12 Staal, F.J., Anderson, M.T., Staal, G.E., Herzenberg, L.A. and Gitler, C. (1994) Redox regulation of signal transduction: tyrosine phosphorylation and calcium influx. *Proceedings of the National Academy of Sciences of the United States of America*, **91** (9), 3619–3622.

13 Shen, J., Yang, X., Dong, A., Petters, R.M., Peng, Y.W., Wong, F. and Campochiaro, P.A. (2005) Oxidative damage is a potential cause of cone cell death in retinitis pigmentosa. *Journal of Cellular Physiology*, **203** (3), 457–464.

14 Butterfield, D.A. and Stadtman, E.R. (1997) Protein oxidation processes in aging brain. *Advances in Cell Aging and Gerontology*, **2**, 161–191.

15 Davies, K.J. (2001) Degradation of oxidized proteins by the 20S proteasome. *Biochimie*, **83** (3–4), 301–310.

16 Shacter, E. (2000) Quantification and significance of protein oxidation in biological samples. *Drug Metabolism Reviews*, **32** (3–4), 307–326.

17 Lafon-Cazal, M., Culcasi, M., Gaven, F., Pietri, S. and Bockaert, J. (1993) Nitric oxide superoxide and peroxynitrite: putative mediators of NMDA-induced cell death in cerebellar granule cells. *Neuropharmacology*, **32** (11), 1259–1266.

18 Calabrese, V., Scapagnini, G., Colombrita, C., Ravagna, A., Pennisi, G., Giuffrida Stella, A.M., Galli, F. and Butterfield, D.A. (2003) Redox regulation of heat shock protein expression in aging and neurodegenerative disorders associated with oxidative stress: a nutritional approach. *Amino Acids*, **25** (3–4), 437–444.

19 Calabrese, V., Scapagnini, G., Ravagna, A., Bella, R., Butterfield, D.A., Calvani, M., Pennisi, G. and Giuffrida Stella, A.M. (2003) Disruption of thiol homeostasis and nitrosative stress in the cerebrospinal fluid of patients with active multiple sclerosis: evidence for a protective role of acetylcarnitine. *Neurochemical Research*, **28** (9), 1321–1328.

20 Poon, H.F., Calabrese, V., Scapagnini, G. and Butterfield, D.A. (2004) Free radicals: key to brain aging and heme oxygenase as a cellular response to oxidative stress. *Journals of Gerontology. Series A Biological Sciences and Medical Sciences*, **59** (5), 478–493.

21 Stadtman, E.R. and Berlett, B.S. (1997) Reactive oxygen-mediated protein oxidation in aging and disease. *Chemical Research in Toxicology*, **10** (5), 485–494.

22 Budanov, A.V., Sablina, A.A., Feinstein, E., Koonin, E.V. and Chumakov, P.M. (2004) Regeneration of peroxiredoxins by p53-regulated sestrins homologs of bacterial AhpD. *Science*, **304** (5670), 596–600.

23 Levine, R.L., Wehr, N., Williams, J.A., Stadtman, E.R. and Shacter, E. (2000) Determination of carbonyl groups in oxidized proteins. *Methods in Molecular Biology*, **99**, 15–24.

24 Dalle-Donne, I., Scaloni, A. and Butterfield, D.A. (2006) *Redox Proteomics: From Protein Modifications to Cellular Dysfunction and Diseases*, John Wiley & Sons, Ltd, Hoboken, NJ.

25 Dalle-Donne, I., Scaloni, A., Giustarini, D., Cavarra, E., Tell, G., Lungarella, G., Colombo, R., Rossi, R. and Milzani, A. (2005) Proteins as biomarkers of oxidative/nitrosative stress in diseases: the contribution of redox proteomics. *Mass Spectrometry Reviews*, **24** (1), 55–99.

26 Grune, T., Reinheckel, T. and Davies, K.J. (1997) Degradation of oxidized proteins in mammalian cells. *FASEB Journal*, **11** (7), 526–534.

27 Stadtman, E.R., Oliver, C.N., Levine, R.L., Fucci, L. and Rivett, A.J. (1988) Implication of protein oxidation in protein turnover aging, and oxygen toxicity. *Basic Life Science*, **49**, 331–339.

28 Fucci, L., Oliver, C.N., Coon, M.J. and Stadtman, E.R. (1983) Inactivation of key metabolic enzymes by mixed-function oxidation reactions: possible implication in protein turnover and ageing. *Proceedings of the National Academy of Sciences of the United States of America*, **80** (6), 1521–1525.

29 Shacter, E., Williams, J.A., Lim, M. and Levine, R.L. (1994) Differential susceptibility of plasma proteins to oxidative modification: examination by Western blot immunoassay. *Free Radical Biology and Medicine*, **17** (5), 429–437.

30 Keller, J.N., Hanni, K.B. and Markesbery, W.R. (2000) Impaired proteasome function in Alzheimer's disease. *Journal of Neurochemistry*, **75** (1), 436–439.

31 Petropoulos, I., Conconi, M., Wang, X., Hoenel, B., Bregegere, F., Milner, Y. and Friguet, B. (2000) Increase of oxidatively modified protein is associated with a decrease of proteasome activity and content in aging epidermal cells. *Journals of Gerontology. Series A Biological Sciences and Medical Sciences*, **55** (5), B220–B227.

32 Starke-Reed, P.E. and Oliver, C.N. (1989) Protein oxidation and proteolysis during aging and oxidative stress. *Archives of Biochemistry and Biophysics*, **275** (2), 559–567.

33 Szweda, P.A., Friguet, B. and Szweda, L.I. (2002) Proteolysis free radicals, and aging. *Free Radical Biology and Medicine*, **33** (1), 29–36.

34 Rivett, A.J. (1986) Regulation of intracellular protein turnover: covalent modification as a mechanism of marking proteins for degradation. *Current Topics in Cellular Regulation*, **28**, 291–337.

35 Sitte, N., Huber, M., Grune, T., Ladhoff, A., Doecke, W.D., Von Zglinicki, T. and Davies, K.J. (2000) Proteasome inhibition by lipofuscin/ceroid during postmitotic aging of fibroblasts. *FASEB Journal*, **14** (11), 1490–1498.

36 Stadtman, E.R. and Levine, R.L. (2000) Protein oxidation. *Annals of the New York Academy of Sciences*, **899**, 191–208.

37 Lauderback, C.M., Hackett, J.M., Huang, F.F., Keller, J.N., Szweda, L.I., Markesbery, W.R. and Butterfield, D.A. (2001) The glial glutamate transporter GLT-1, is oxidatively modified by 4-hydroxy-2-nonenal in the Alzheimer's disease brain: the role of Abeta 1–42. *Journal of Neurochemistry*, **78** (2), 413–416.

38 Sultana, R. and Butterfield, D.A. (2004) Oxidatively modified GST and MRP1 in Alzheimer's disease brain: implications for accumulation of reactive lipid peroxidation products. *Neurochemical Research*, **29**, 2215–2220.

39 Aksenova, M., Butterfield, D.A., Zhang, S.X., Underwood, M. and Geddes, J.W. (2002) Increased protein oxidation and decreased creatine kinase BB expression and activity after spinal cord contusion injury. *Journal of Neurotrauma*, **19** (4), 491–502.

40 Roix, J. and Misteli, T. (2002) Genomes proteomes, and dynamic networks in the cell nucleus. *Histochemistry and Cell Biology*, **118** (2), 105–116.

41 Rabilloud, T. (2002) Two-dimensional gel electrophoresis in proteomics: old, old fashioned, but it still climbs up the mountains. *Proteomics*, **2**, 3–10.

42 Stevens, S.M., Jr, Kem, W.R. and Prokai, L. (2002) Investigation of cytolysin variants by peptide mapping: enhanced protein characterization using complementary ionization and mass spectrometric techniques. *Rapid Communications in Mass Spectrometry*, **16** (22), 2094–2101.

43 Wagner, Y., Sickmann, A., Meyer, H.E. and Daum, G. (2003) Multidimensional nano-HPLC for analysis of protein complexes. *Journal of the American Society for Mass Spectrometry*, **14** (9), 1003–1011.

44 Smolka, M.B., Zhou, H., Purkayastha, S. and Aebersold, R. (2001) Optimization of the isotope-coded affinity tag-labeling procedure for quantitative proteome analysis. *Analytical Biochemistry*, **297** (1), 25–31.

45 Anderson, N.L., Matheson, A.D. and Steiner, S. (2000) Proteomics: applications in basic and applied biology. *Current Opinion in Biotechnology*, **11** (4), 408–412.

46 O'Farrell, P.H. (1975) High resolution two-dimensional electrophoresis of proteins. *The Journal of Biological Chemistry*, **250** (10), 4007–4021.

47 Tilleman, K., Stevens, I., Spittaels, K., Haute, C.V., Clerens, S., Van Den Bergh, G., Geerts, H., Van Leuven, F., Vandesande, F. and Moens, L. (2002) Differential expression of brain proteins in glycogen synthase kinase-3 transgenic mice: a proteomics point of view. *Proteomics*, **2** (1), 94–104.

48 Santoni, V., Molloy, M. and Rabilloud, T. (2000) Membrane proteins and proteomics: un amour impossible? *Electrophoresis*, **21** (6), 1054–1070.

49 Boyd-Kimball, D., Poon, H.F., Lynn, B.C., Cai, J., Pierce, W.M., Jr, Klein, J.B., Ferguson, J., Link, C.D. and Butterfield, D.A. (2006) Proteomic identification of proteins specifically oxidized in *Caenorhabditis elegans* expressing human Abeta(1–42): implications for Alzheimer's disease. *Neurobiology of Aging*, **27** (9), 1239–1249.

50 Hoogland, C., Sanchez, J.C., Tonella, L., Binz, P.A., Bairoch, A., Hochstrasser, D.F. and Appel, R.D. (2000) The 1999 SWISS-2DPAGE database update. *Nucleic Acids Research*, **28** (1), 286–288.

51 Beal, M.F. (1998) Mitochondrial dysfunction in neurodegenerative diseases. *Biochimica et Biophysica Acta*, **1366** (1–2), 211–223.

52 Mecocci, P., Beal, M.F., Cecchetti, R., Polidori, M.C., Cherubini, A., Chionne, F., Avellini, L., Romano, G. and Senin, U. (1997) Mitochondrial membrane fluidity and oxidative damage to mitochondrial DNA in aged and AD human brain. *Molecular and Chemical Neuropathology*, **31** (1), 53–64.

53 Sultana, R., Perluigi, M. and Butterfield, D.A. (2006) Redox proteomics identification of oxidatively modified proteins in Alzheimer's disease brain and *in vivo* and *in vitro* models of AD centered around Abeta (1–42). *Journal of Chromatography. B, Analytical Technologies in the Biomedical and Life Sciences*, **833** (1), 3–11.

54 Katzman, R. and Saitoh, T. (1991) Advances in Alzheimer's disease. *FASEB Journal*, **5** (3), 278–286.

55 Cohen, M.L., Golde, T.E., Usiak, M.F., Younkin, L.H. and Younkin, S.G. (1988) *in situ* hybridization of nucleus basalis neurons shows increased beta-amyloid mRNA in Alzheimer disease. *Proceedings of the National Academy of Sciences of the United States of America*, **85** (4), 1227–1231.

56 Palmert, M.R., Golde, T.E., Cohen, M.L., Kovacs, D.M., Tanzi, R.E., Gusella, J.F., Usiak, M.F., Younkin, L.H. and Younkin, S.G. (1988) Amyloid protein precursor messenger RNAs: differential expression in Alzheimer's disease. *Science*, **241** (4869), 1080–1084.

57 Trojanowski, J.Q. and Lee, V.M. (2002) The role of tau in Alzheimer's disease. *The Medical Clinics of North America*, **86** (3), 615–627.

58 Butterfield, D.A., Drake, J., Pocernich, C. and Castegna, A. (2001) Evidence of oxidative damage in Alzheimer's disease brain: central role for amyloid beta-peptide. *Trends in Molecular Medicine*, **7** (12), 548–554.

59 Ho, G.J., Drego, R., Hakimian, E. and Masliah, E. (2005) Mechanisms of cell signaling and inflammation in Alzheimer's disease. *Current Drug Targets – Inflammation and Allergy*, **4** (2), 247–256.

60 Hynd, M.R., Scott, H.L. and Dodd, P.R. (2004) Glutamate-mediated excitotoxicity and neurodegeneration in Alzheimer's disease. *Neurochemistry International*, **45** (5), 583–595.

61 Markesbery, W.R. (1997) Oxidative stress hypothesis in Alzheimer's disease. *Free Radical Biology and Medicine*, **23** (1), 134–147.

62 Rego, A.C. and Oliveira, C.R. (2003) Mitochondrial dysfunction and reactive oxygen species in excitotoxicity and apoptosis: implications for the pathogenesis of neurodegenerative diseases. *Neurochemical Research*, **28** (10), 1563–1574.

63 Tuppo, E.E. and Arias, H.R. (2005) The role of inflammation in Alzheimer's disease. *The International Journal of*

Biochemistry and Cell Biology, **37** (2), 289–305.

64 Ischiropoulos, H. and Beckman, J.S. (2003) Oxidative stress and nitration in neurodegeneration: cause effect, or association? *Journal of Clinical Investigation*, **111** (2), 163–169.

65 Butterfield, D.A. and Lauderback, C.M. (2002) Lipid peroxidation and protein oxidation in Alzheimer's disease brain: potential causes and consequences involving amyloid beta-peptide-associated free radical oxidative stress. *Free Radical Biology and Medicine*, **32** (11), 1050–1060.

66 Markesbery, W.R. and Carney, J.M. (1999) Oxidative alterations in Alzheimer's disease. *Brain Pathology*, **9** (1), 133–146.

67 Smith, M.A., Nunomura, A., Zhu, X., Takeda, A. and Perry, G. (2000) Metabolic metallic, and mitotic sources of oxidative stress in Alzheimer disease. *Antioxidants and Redox Signalling*, **2** (3), 413–420.

68 Smith, M.A., Richey Harris, P.L., Sayre, L.M., Beckman, J.S. and Perry, G. (1997) Widespread peroxynitrite-mediated damage in Alzheimer's disease. *Journal of Neuroscience*, **17** (8), 2653–2657.

69 Calabrese, V., Butterfield, D.A. and Stella, A.M. (2003) Nutritional antioxidants and the heme oxygenase pathway of stress tolerance: novel targets for neuroprotection in Alzheimer's disease. *Italian Journal of Biochemistry*, **52** (4), 177–181.

70 Choi, J., Rees, H.D., Weintraub, S.T., Levey, A.I., Chin, L.S. and Li, L. (2005) Oxidative modifications and aggregation of Cu Zn-superoxide dismutase associated with Alzheimer and Parkinson diseases. *The Journal of Biological Chemistry*, **280** (12), 11648–11655.

71 Dore, S. (2002) Decreased activity of the antioxidant heme oxygenase enzyme: implications in ischemia and in Alzheimer's disease. *Free Radical Biology and Medicine*, **32** (12), 1276–1282.

72 Lovell, M.A., Ehmann, W.D., Butler, S.M. and Markesbery, W.R. (1995) Elevated thiobarbituric acid-reactive substances and antioxidant enzyme activity in the brain in Alzheimer's disease. *Neurology*, **45** (8), 1594–1601.

73 Lovell, M.A., Xie, C., Gabbita, S.P. and Markesbery, W.R. (2000) Decreased thioredoxin and increased thioredoxin reductase levels in Alzheimer's disease brain. *Free Radical Biology and Medicine*, **28** (3), 418–427.

74 Ramassamy, C., Averill, D., Beffert, U., Bastianetto, S., Theroux, L., Lussier-Cacan, S., Cohn, J.S., Christen, Y., Davignon, J., Quirion, R. and Poirier, J. (1999) Oxidative damage and protection by antioxidants in the frontal cortex of Alzheimer's disease is related to the apolipoprotein E genotype. *Free Radical Biology and Medicine*, **27** (5–6), 544–553.

75 Good, P.F., Werner, P., Hsu, A., Olanow, C.W. and Perl, D.P. (1996) Evidence of neuronal oxidative damage in Alzheimer's disease. *American Journal of Pathology*, **149** (1), 21–28.

76 Hensley, K., Hall, N., Subramaniam, R., Cole, P., Harris, M., Aksenov, M., Aksenova, M., Gabbita, S.P., Wu, J.F., Carney, J.M., Lovell, M., Markesbery, W.R. and Butterfield, D.A. (1995) Brain regional correspondence between Alzheimer's disease histopathology and biomarkers of protein oxidation. *Journal of Neurochemistry*, **65** (5), 2146–2156.

77 Sayre, L.M., Zelasko, D.A., Harris, P.L., Perry, G., Salomon, R.G. and Smith, M.A. (1997) 4-Hydroxynonenal-derived advanced lipid peroxidation end products are increased in Alzheimer's disease. *Journal of Neurochemistry*, **68** (5), 2092–2097.

78 Rottkamp, C.A., Raina, A.K., Zhu, X., Gaier, E., Bush, A.I., Atwood, C.S., Chevion, M., Perry, G. and Smith, M.A. (2001) Redox-active iron mediates amyloid-beta toxicity. *Free Radical Biology and Medicine*, **30** (4), 447–450.

79 Pratico, D., Uryu, K., Leight, S., Trojanoswki, J.Q. and Lee, V.M. (2001) Increased lipid peroxidation precedes amyloid plaque formation in an animal model of Alzheimer amyloidosis. *Journal of Neuroscience*, **21** (12), 4183–4187.

80 Yan, S.D., Yan, S.F., Chen, X., Fu, J., Chen, M., Kuppusamy, P., Smith, M.A., Perry, G., Godman, G.C., Nawroth, P., Zweier, J.L. and Stern, D. (1995) Non-enzymatically glycated tau in Alzheimer's disease induces neuronal oxidant stress resulting in cytokine gene expression and release of amyloid beta-peptide. *Nature Medicine*, **1** (7), 693–699.

81 Drake, J., Link, C.D. and Butterfield, D.A. (2003) Oxidative stress precedes fibrillar deposition of Alzheimer's disease amyloid beta-peptide (1–42) in a transgenic *Caenorhabditis elegans* model. *Neurobiology of Aging*, **24** (3), 415–420.

82 Curtain, C.C., Ali, F., Volitakis, I., Cherny, R.A., Norton, R.S., Beyreuther, K., Barrow, C.J., Masters, C.L., Bush, A.I. and Barnham, K.J. (2001) Alzheimer's disease amyloid-beta binds copper and zinc to generate an allosterically ordered membrane-penetrating structure containing superoxide dismutase-like subunits. *Journal of Biological Chemistry*, **276** (23), 20466–20473.

83 Obrenovich, M.E., Joseph, J.A., Atwood, C.S., Perry, G. and Smith, M.A. (2002) Amyloid-beta: a (life) preserver for the brain. *Neurobiology of Aging*, **23** (6), 1097–1099.

84 Opazo, C., Huang, X., Cherny, R.A., Moir, R.D., Roher, A.E., White, A.R., Cappai, R., Masters, C.L., Tanzi, R.E., Inestrosa, N.C. and Bush, A.I. (2002) Metalloenzyme-like activity of Alzheimer's disease beta-amyloid. Cu-dependent catalytic conversion of dopamine cholesterol, and biological reducing agents to neurotoxic H(2)O(2). *The Journal of Biological Chemistry*, **277** (43), 40302–40308.

85 Zou, K., Gong, J.S., Yanagisawa, K. and Michikawa, M. (2002) A novel function of monomeric amyloid beta-protein serving as an antioxidant molecule against metal-induced oxidative damage. *Journal of Neuroscience*, **22** (12), 4833–4841.

86 Casserly, I. and Topol, E. (2004) Convergence of atherosclerosis and Alzheimer's disease: inflammation cholesterol, and misfolded proteins. *Lancet*, **363** (9415), 1139–1146.

87 Colton, C.A. (1994) Microglial oxyradical production: causes and consequences. *Neuropathology and Applied Neurobiology*, **20** (2), 208–209.

88 Mohmmad Abdul, H., Sultana, R., Keller, J.N., St Clair, D.K., Markesbery, W.R. and Butterfield, D.A. (2006) Mutations in amyloid precursor protein and presenilin-1 genes increase the basal oxidative stress in murine neuronal cells and lead to increased sensitivity to oxidative stress mediated by amyloid beta-peptide (1–42) HO and kainic acid: implications for Alzheimer's disease. *Journal of Neurochemistry*, **96** (5), 1322–1335.

89 Summers, W.K. (2004) Alzheimer's disease, oxidative injury, and cytokines. *Journal of Alzheimer's Disease*, **6** (6), 651–657, discussion 673–681.

90 Castegna, A., Aksenov, M., Aksenova, M., Thongboonkerd, V., Klein, J.B., Pierce, W.M., Booze, R., Markesbery, W.R. and Butterfield, D.A. (2002) Proteomic identification of oxidatively modified proteins in Alzheimer's disease brain. Part I: creatine kinase BB glutamine synthase, and ubiquitin carboxy-terminal hydrolase L-1. *Free Radical Biology and Medicine*, **33** (4), 562–571.

91 Castegna, A., Aksenov, M., Thongboonkerd, V., Klein, J.B., Pierce, W.M., Booze, R., Markesbery, W.R. and Butterfield, D.A. (2002) Proteomic identification of oxidatively modified proteins in Alzheimer's disease brain. Part II: dihydropyrimidinase-related protein 2 alpha-enolase and heat shock cognate 71. *Journal of Neurochemistry*, **82** (6), 1524–1532.

92 Castegna, A., Thongboonkerd, V., Klein, J.B., Lynn, B., Markesbery, W.R. and Butterfield, D.A. (2003) Proteomic identification of nitrated proteins in Alzheimer's disease brain. *Journal of Neurochemistry*, **85** (6), 1394–1401.

93 Sultana, R., Boyd-Kimball, D., Poon, H.F., Cai, J., Pierce, W.M., Klein, J.B., Merchant, M., Markesbery, W.R. and Butterfield, D.A. (2006) Redox proteomics identification of oxidized proteins in Alzheimer's disease hippocampus and cerebellum: an approach to understand pathological and biochemical alterations in AD. *Neurobiology of Aging*, **27** (11), 1564–1576.

94 Sultana, R., Poon, H.F., Cai, J., Pierce, W.M., Merchant, M., Klein, J.B., Markesbery, W.R. and Butterfield, D.A. (2006) Identification of nitrated proteins in Alzheimer's disease brain using a redox proteomics approach. *Neurobiology of Disease*, **22** (1), 76–87.

95 Yu, H.L., Chertkow, H.M., Bergman, H. and Schipper, H.M. (2003) Aberrant profiles of native and oxidized glycoproteins in Alzheimer plasma. *Proteomics*, **3** (11), 2240–2248.

96 Choi, J., Malakowsky, C.A., Talent, J.M., Conrad, C.C. and Gracy, R.W. (2002) Identification of oxidized plasma proteins in Alzheimer's disease. *Biochemical and Biophysical Research Communications*, **293** (5), 1566–1570.

97 Hensley, K., Maidt, M.L., Yu, Z., Sang, H., Markesbery, W.R. and Floyd, R.A. (1998) Electrochemical analysis of protein nitrotyrosine and dityrosine in the Alzheimer brain indicates region-specific accumulation. *Journal of Neuroscience*, **18** (20), 8126–8132.

98 Butterfield, D.A., Poon, H.F., St Clair, D., Keller, J.N., Pierce, W.M., Klein, J.B. and Markesbery, W.R. (2006) Redox proteomics identification of oxidatively modified hippocampal proteins in mild cognitive impairment: insights into the development of Alzheimer's disease. *Neurobiology of Disease*, **22** (2), 223–232.

99 Choi, J., Levey, A.I., Weintraub, S.T., Rees, H.D., Gearing, M., Chin, L.S. and Li, L. (2004) Oxidative modifications and down-regulation of ubiquitin carboxyl-terminal hydrolase L1 associated with idiopathic Parkinson's and Alzheimer's diseases. *Journal of Biological Chemistry*, **279** (13), 13256–13264.

100 Gong, B., Cao, Z., Zheng, P., Vitolo, O.V., Liu, S., Staniszewski, A., Moolman, D., Zhang, H., Shelanski, M. and Arancio, O. (2006) Ubiquitin hydrolase Uch-L1 rescues beta-amyloid-induced decreases in synaptic function and contextual memory. *Cell*, **126** (4), 775–788.

101 Blass, J.P., Sheu, R.K. and Cedarbaum, J.M. (1988) Energy metabolism in disorders of the nervous system. *Revue Neurologique (Paris)*, **144** (10), 543–563.

102 Blass, J.P., Sheu, R.K. and Gibson, G.E. (2000) Inherent abnormalities in energy metabolism in Alzheimer disease. Interaction with cerebrovascular compromise. *Annals of the New York Academy of Sciences*, **903**, 204–221.

103 Vannucci, R.C. and Vannucci, S.J. (2000) Glucose metabolism in the developing brain. *Seminars in Perinatology*, **24** (2), 107–115.

104 Harr, S.D., Simonian, N.A. and Hyman, B.T. (1995) Functional alterations in Alzheimer's disease: decreased glucose transporter 3 immunoreactivity in the perforant pathway terminal zone. *Journal of Neuropathology and Experimental Neurology*, **54** (1), 38–41.

105 Messier, C. and Gagnon, M. (1996) Glucose regulation and cognitive functions: relation to Alzheimer's disease and diabetes. *Behavioural Brain Research*, **75** (1–2), 1–11.

106 Rapoport, S.I. (1999) *in vivo* PET imaging and postmortem studies suggest potentially reversible and irreversible stages of brain metabolic failure in Alzheimer's disease. *European Archives of*

Psychiatry and Clinical Neuroscience, **249** (Suppl. 3), 46–55.

107 Vanhanen, M. and Soininen, H. (1998) Glucose intolerance cognitive impairment and Alzheimer's disease. *Current Opinion in Neurology*, **11** (6), 673–677.

108 Geddes, J.W., Pang, Z. and Wiley, D.H. (1996) Hippocampal damage and cytoskeletal disruption resulting from impaired energy metabolism. Implications for Alzheimer disease. *Molecular and Chemical Neuropathology*, **28** (1–3), 65–74.

109 Ibanez, V., Pietrini, P., Alexander, G.E., Furey, M.L., Teichberg, D., Rajapakse, J.C., Rapoport, S.I., Schapiro, M.B. and Horwitz, B. (1998) Regional glucose metabolic abnormalities are not the result of atrophy in Alzheimer's disease. *Neurology*, **50** (6), 1585–1593.

110 Reiman, E.M., Caselli, R.J., Yun, L.S., Chen, K., Bandy, D., Minoshima, S., Thibodeau, S.N. and Osborne, D. (1996) Preclinical evidence of Alzheimer's disease in persons homozygous for the epsilon 4 allele for apolipoprotein E. *New England Journal of Medicine*, **334** (12), 752–758.

111 Cheng, B. and Mattson, M.P. (1992) Glucose deprivation elicits neuro-fibrillary tangle-like antigenic changes in hippocampal neurons: prevention by NGF and bFGF. *Experimental Neurology*, **117** (2), 114–123.

112 Castegna, A., Lauderback, C.M., Mohmmad-Abdul, H. and Butterfield, D.A. (2004) Modulation of phospho-lipid asymmetry in synaptosomal membranes by the lipid peroxidation products 4-hydroxynonenal and acrolein: implications for Alzheimer's disease. *Brain Research*, **1004** (1–2), 193–197.

113 Mohmmad Abdul, H. and Butterfield, D.A. (2005) Protection against amyloid beta-peptide (1–42)-induced loss of phospholipid asymmetry in synapto-somal membranes by tricyclodecan-9-xanthogenate (D609) and ferulic acid ethyl ester: implications for Alzheimer's disease. *Biochimica et Biophysica Acta*, **1741** (1–2), 140–148.

114 Planel, E., Miyasaka, T., Launey, T., Chui, D.H., Tanemura, K., Sato, S., Murayama, O., Ishiguro, K., Tatebayashi, Y. and Takashima, A. (2004) Alterations in glucose metabolism induce hypothermia leading to tau hyperphosphorylation through differential inhibition of kinase and phosphatase activities: implications for Alzheimer's disease. *Journal of Neuroscience*, **24** (10), 2401–2411.

115 Iwangoff, P., Armbruster, R., Enz, A. and Meier-Ruge, W. (1980) Glycolytic enzymes from human autoptic brain cortex: normal aged and demented cases. *Mechanisms of Ageing and Development*, **14** (1–2), 203–209.

116 Meier-Ruge, W., Iwangoff, P. and Reichlmeier, K. (1984) Neurochemical enzyme changes in Alzheimer's and Pick's disease. *Archives of Gerontology and Geriatrics*, **3** (2), 161–165.

117 Junge, W., Lill, H. and Engelbrecht, S. (1997) ATP synthase: an electrochemical transducer with rotatory mechanics. *Trends in Biochemical Sciences*, **22** (11), 420–423.

118 Sergeant, N., Wattez, A., Galvan-valencia, M., Ghestem, A., David, J.P., Lemoine, J., Sautiere, P.E., Dachary, J., Mazat, J.P., Michalski, J.C., Velours, J., Mena-Lopez, R. and Delacourte, A. (2003) Association of ATP synthase alpha-chain with neurofibrillary degeneration in Alzheimer's disease. *Neuroscience*, **117** (2), 293–303.

119 Busciglio, J., Pelsman, A., Wong, C., Pigino, G., Yuan, M., Mori, H. and Yankner, B.A. (2002) Altered metabolism of the amyloid beta precursor protein is associated with mitochondrial dysfunction in Down's syndrome. *Neuron*, **33** (5), 677–688.

120 Petersen, R.C. (2004) Mild cognitive impairment as a diagnostic entity. *Journal of Internal Medicine*, **256** (3), 183–194.

121 Visser, P.J., Verhey, F.R., Ponds, R.W. and Jolles, J. (2001) Diagnosis of preclinical Alzheimer's disease in a clinical setting. *International Psychogeriatrics*, **13** (4), 411–423.

122 Almkvist, O., Axelman, K., Basun, H., Jensen, M., Viitanen, M., Wahlund, L.O. and Lannfelt, L. (2003) Clinical findings in nondemented mutation carriers predisposed to Alzheimer's disease: a model of mild cognitive impairment. *Acta Neurologica Scandinavica Supplementum*, **179**, 77–82.

123 Nacmias, B., Piccini, C., Bagnoli, S., Tedde, A., Cellini, E., Bracco, L. and Sorbi, S. (2004) Brain-derived neurotrophic factor apolipoprotein E genetic variants and cognitive performance in Alzheimer's disease. *Neuroscience Letters*, **367** (3), 379–383.

124 Traykov, L., Rigaud, A.S., Baudic, S., Smagghe, A., Boller, F. and Forette, F. (2002) Apolipoprotein E epsilon 4 allele frequency in demented and cognitively impaired patients with and without cerebrovascular disease. *Journal of the Neurological Sciences*, **203–204**, 177–181.

125 Barnes, D.E. and Yaffe, K. (2005) Vitamin E and donepezil for the treatment of mild cognitive impairment. *New England Journal of Medicine*, **353** (9), 951–952, author reply 951–952.

126 Guidi, I., Galimberti, D., Lonati, S., Novembrino, C., Bamonti, F., Tiriticco, M., Fenoglio, C., Venturelli, E., Baron, P., Bresolin, N. and Scarpini, E. (2006) Oxidative imbalance in patients with mild cognitive impairment and Alzheimer's disease. *Neurobiology of Aging*, **27** (2), 262–269.

127 Mecocci, P., Mariani, E., Cornacchiola, V. and Polidori, M.C. (2004) Antioxidants for the treatment of mild cognitive impairment. *Neurological Research*, **26** (5), 598–602.

128 Rinaldi, P., Polidori, M.C., Metastasio, A., Mariani, E., Mattioli, P., Cherubini, A., Catani, M., Cecchetti, R., Senin, U. and Mecocci, P. (2003) Plasma antioxidants are similarly depleted in mild cognitive impairment and in Alzheimer's disease. *Neurobiology of Aging*, **24** (7), 915–919.

129 Butterfield, D.A., Reed, T., Perluigi, M., De Marco, C., Coccia, R., Cini, C. and Sultana, R. (2006) Elevated protein-bound levels of the lipid peroxidation product 4-hydroxy-2-nonenal, in brain from persons with mild cognitive impairment. *Neuroscience Letters*, **397** (3), 170–173.

130 Keller, J.N., Schmitt, F.A., Scheff, S.W., Ding, Q., Chen, Q., Butterfield, D.A. and Markesbery, W.R. (2005) Evidence of increased oxidative damage in subjects with mild cognitive impairment. *Neurology*, **64** (7), 1152–1156.

131 Ding, Q., Markesbery, W.R., Cecarini, V. and Keller, J.N. (2006) Decreased RNA and increased RNA oxidation, in Ribosomes from early Alzheimer's disease. *Neurochemical Research*. **31** (5), 705–710.

132 Wang, J., Markesbery, W.R. and Lovell, M.A. (2006) Increased oxidative damage in nuclear and mitochondrial DNA in mild cognitive impairment. *Journal of Neurochemistry*, **96** (3), 825–832.

133 Markesbery, W.R., Kryscio, R.J., Lovell, M.A. and Morrow, J.D. (2005) Lipid peroxidation is an early event in the brain in amnestic mild cognitive impairment. *Annals of Neurology*, **58** (5), 730–735.

134 German, D.C. and Eisch, A.J. (2004) Mouse models of Alzheimer's disease: insight into treatment. *Reviews in the Neurosciences*, **15** (5), 353–369.

135 Siman, R., Reaume, A.G., Savage, M.J., Trusko, S., Lin, Y.G., Scott, R.W. and Flood, D.G. (2000) Presenilin-1 P264L knock-in mutation: differential effects on abeta production amyloid deposition, and neuronal vulnerability. *Journal of Neuroscience*, **20** (23), 8717–8726.

136 Terwel, D., Lasrado, R., Snauwaert, J., Vandeweert, E., Van Haesendonck, C., Borghgraef, P. and Van Leuven, F. (2005) Changed conformation of mutant

Tau-P301L underlies the moribund tauopathy absent in progressive, nonlethal axonopathy of Tau-4R/2N transgenic mice. *The Journal of Biological Chemistry*, **280** (5), 3963–3973.

137 Castegna, A., Thongboonkerd, V., Klein, J., Lynn, B.C., Wang, Y.L., Osaka, H., Wada, K. and Butterfield, D.A. (2004) Proteomic analysis of brain proteins in the gracile axonal dystrophy (gad) mouse a syndrome that emanates from dysfunctional ubiquitin carboxyl-terminal hydrolase L-1, reveals oxidation of key proteins. *Journal of Neurochemistry*, **88** (6), 1540–1546.

138 Boyd-Kimball, D., Sultana, R., Poon, H.F., Mohmmad-Abdul, H., Lynn, B.C., Klein, J.B. and Butterfield, D.A. (2005) Gamma-glutamylcysteine ethyl ester protection of proteins from Abeta(1–42)-mediated oxidative stress in neuronal cell culture: a proteomics approach. *Journal of Neuroscience Research*, **79** (5), 707–713.

139 Sultana, R., Newman, S.F., Abdul, H.M., Cai, J., Pierce, W.M., Klein, J.B., Merchant, M. and Butterfield, D.A. (2006) Protective effect of D609 against amyloid-beta1–42-induced oxidative modification of neuronal proteins: redox proteomics study. *Journal of Neuroscience Research*, **84** (2), 409–417.

140 Dhar-Chowdhury, P., Harrell, M.D., Han, S.Y., Jankowska, D., Parachuru, L., Morrissey, A., Srivastava, S., Liu, W., Malester, B., Yoshida, H. and Coetzee, W.A. (2005) The glycolytic enzymes glyceraldehyde-3-phosphate dehydrogenase, triose-phosphate isomerase, and pyruvate kinase are components of the K(ATP) channel macromolecular complex and regulate its function. *Journal of Biological Chemistry*, **280** (46), 38464–38470.

141 Sirover, M.A. (1997) Role of the glycolytic protein, glyceraldehyde-3-phosphate dehydrogenase, in normal cell function and in cell pathology. *Journal of Cellular Biochemistry*, **66** (2), 133–140.

142 Tatton, W.G., Chalmers-Redman, R.M., Elstner, M., Leesch, W., Jagodzinski, F.B., Stupak, D.P., Sugrue, M.M. and Tatton, N.A. (2000) Glyceraldehyde-3-phosphate dehydrogenase in neuro-degeneration and apoptosis signaling. *Journal of Neural Transmission*, (Suppl. 60), 77–100.

143 Chuang, D.M., Hough, C. and Senatorov, V.V. (2005) Glyceraldehyde-3-phosphate dehydrogenase apoptosis, and neurodegenerative diseases. *Annual Review of Pharmacology and Toxicology*, **45**, 269–290.

144 Hara, M.R., Cascio, M.B. and Sawa, A. (2006) GAPDH as a sensor of NO stress. *Biochimica et Biophysica Acta*, **1762** (5), 502–509.

145 Miyamoto, M. (1997) Characteristics of age-related behavioral changes in senescence-accelerated mouse SAMP8 and SAMP10. *Experimental Gerontology*, **32** (1–2), 139–148.

146 Takeda, T., Hosokawa, M. and Higuchi, K. (1997) Senescence-accelerated mouse (SAM): a novel murine model of senescence. *Experimental Gerontology*, **32** (1–2), 105–109.

147 Flood, J.F. and Morley, J.E. (1998) Learning and memory in the SAMP8 mouse. *Neuroscience and Biobehavioral Reviews*, **22** (1), 1–20.

148 Kumar, V.B., Farr, S.A., Flood, J.F., Kamlesh, V., Franko, M., Banks, W.A. and Morley, J.E. (2000) Site-directed antisense oligonucleotide decreases the expression of amyloid precursor protein and reverses deficits in learning and memory in aged SAMP8 mice. *Peptides*, **21** (12), 1769–1775.

149 Morley, J.E., Kumar, V.B., Bernardo, A.E., Farr, S.A., Uezu, K., Tumosa, N. and Flood, J.F. (2000) Beta-amyloid precursor polypeptide in SAMP8 mice affects learning and memory. *Peptides*, **21** (12), 1761–1767.

150 Butterfield, D.A., Howard, B.J., Yatin, S., Allen, K.L. and Carney, J.M. (1997) Free radical oxidation of brain proteins in accelerated senescence and its

modulation by *N-tert*-butyl-alpha-phenylnitrone. *Proceedings of the National Academy of Sciences of the United States of America*, **94** (2), 674–678.

151 Fujibayashi, Y., Yamamoto, S., Waki, A., Konishi, J. and Yonekura, Y. (1998) Increased mitochondrial DNA deletion in the brain of SAMP8 a mouse model for spontaneous oxidative stress brain. *Neuroscience Letters*, **254** (2), 109–112.

152 Nishikawa, T., Takahashi, J.A., Fujibayashi, Y., Fujisawa, H., Zhu, B., Nishimura, Y., Ohnishi, K., Higuchi, K., Hashimoto, N. and Hosokawa, M. (1998) An early stage mechanism of the age-associated mitochondrial dysfunction in the brain of SAMP8 mice: an age-associated neurodegeneration animal model. *Neuroscience Letters*, **254** (2), 69–72.

153 Banks, W.A., Farr, S.A., Butt, W., Kumar, V.B., Franko, M.W. and Morley, J.E. (2001) Delivery across the blood–brain barrier of antisense directed against amyloid beta: reversal of learning and memory deficits in mice overexpressing amyloid precursor protein. *Journal of Pharmacology and Experimental Therapeutics*, **297** (3), 1113–1121.

154 Banks, W.A., Robinson, S.M., Verma, S. and Morley, J.E. (2003) Efflux of human and mouse amyloid beta proteins 1–40 and 1–42 from brain: impairment in a mouse model of Alzheimer's disease. *Neuroscience*, **121** (2), 487–492.

155 Poon, H.F., Joshi, G., Sultana, R., Farr, S.A., Banks, W.A., Morley, J.E., Calabrese, V. and Butterfield, D.A. (2004) Antisense directed at the Abeta region of APP decreases brain oxidative markers in aged senescence accelerated mice. *Brain Research*, **1018** (1), 86–96.

156 Kumar, V.B., Franko, M.W., Farr, S.A., Armbrecht, H.J. and Morley, J.E. (2000) Identification of age-dependent changes in expression of senescence-accelerated mouse (SAMP8) hippocampal proteins by expression array analysis. *Biochemical and Biophysical Research Communications*, **272** (3), 657–661.

157 Poon, H.F., Castegna, A., Farr, S.A., Thongboonkerd, V., Lynn, B.C., Banks, W.A., Morley, J.E., Klein, J.B. and Butterfield, D.A. (2004) Quantitative proteomics analysis of specific protein expression and oxidative modification in aged senescence-accelerated-prone 8 mice brain. *Neuroscience*, **126** (4), 915–926.

158 Wei, X., Zhang, Y. and Zhou, J. (1999) Alzheimer's disease-related gene expression in the brain of senescence accelerated mouse. *Neuroscience Letters*, **268** (3), 139–142.

159 Wei, X., Zhang, Y. and Zhou, J. (1999) Differential display and cloning of the hippocampal gene mRNas in senescence accelerated mouse. *Neuroscience Letters*, **275** (1), 17–20.

160 Kumar, V.B., Vyas, K., Buddhiraju, M., Alshaher, M., Flood, J.F. and Morley, J.E. (1999) Changes in membrane fatty acids and delta-9 desaturase in senescence accelerated (SAMP8) mouse hippocampus with aging. *Life Sciences*, **65** (16), 1657–1662.

161 Okatani, Y., Wakatsuki, A., Reiter, R.J. and Miyahara, Y. (2002) Melatonin reduces oxidative damage of neural lipids and proteins in senescence-accelerated mouse. *Neurobiology of Aging*, **23** (4), 639–644.

162 Sato, E., Oda, N., Ozaki, N., Hashimoto, S., Kurokawa, T. and Ishibashi, S. (1996) Early and transient increase in oxidative stress in the cerebral cortex of senescence-accelerated mouse. *Mechanisms of Ageing and Development*, **86** (2), 105–114.

163 Kurokawa, T., Sato, E., Inoue, A. and Ishibashi, S. (1996) Evidence that glucose metabolism is decreased in the cerebrum of aged female senescence-accelerated mouse: possible involvement of a low hexokinase activity. *Neuroscience Letters*, **214** (1), 45–48.

164 Shimano, Y. (1998) Studies on aging through analysis of the glucose

metabolism related to the ATP–production of the senescence accelerated mouse (SAM). *Hokkaido Igaku Zasshi*, **73** (6), 557–569.

165 Bendiske, J., Caba, E., Brown, Q.B. and Bahr, B.A. (2002) Intracellular deposition microtubule destabilization, and transport failure: an ''early'' pathogenic cascade leading to synaptic decline. *Journal of Neuropathology and Experimental Neurology*, **61** (7), 640–650.

166 Masliah, E., Mallory, M., Alford, M., DeTeresa, R., Hansen, L.A., McKeel, D.W., Jr and Morris, J.C. (2001) Altered expression of synaptic proteins occurs early during progression of Alzheimer's disease. *Neurology*, **56** (1), 127–129.

167 Scheff, S.W., Price, D.A., Schmitt, F.A. and Mufson, E.J. (2005) Hippocampal synaptic loss in early Alzheimer's disease and mild cognitive impairment. *Neurobiology of Aging*, **27** (10), 1372–1384.

168 Lassmann, H. (1996) Patterns of synaptic and nerve cell pathology in Alzheimer's disease. *Behavioural Brain Research*, **78** (1), 9–14.

169 Reddy, P.H., Mani, G., Park, B.S., Jacques, J., Murdoch, G., Whetsell, W., Jr, Kaye, J. and Manczak, M. (2005) Differential loss of synaptic proteins in Alzheimer's disease: implications for synaptic dysfunction. *Journal of Alzheimer's Disease*, **7** (2), 103–117, discussion 173–180.

170 Eckert, G.P., Wood, W.G. and Muller, W.E. (2005) Membrane disordering effects of beta-amyloid peptides. *Subcellular Biochemistry*, **38**, 319–337.

171 Gylys, K.H., Fein, J.A., Yang, F., Wiley, D.J., Miller, C.A. and Cole, G.M. (2004) Synaptic changes in Alzheimer's disease: increased amyloid-beta and gliosis in surviving terminals is accompanied by decreased PSD-95 fluorescence. *American Journal of Pathology*, **165** (5), 1809–1817.

172 Weber, J. and Senior, A.E. (2003) ATP synthesis driven by proton transport in F1F0-ATP synthase. *FEBS Letters*, **545** (1), 61–70.

173 Cross, R.L. (2000) The rotary binding change mechanism of ATP synthases. *Biochimica et Biophysica Acta*, **1458** (2–3), 270–275.

174 Fillingame, R.H. (1992) H+ transport and coupling by the F0 sector of the ATP synthase: insights into the molecular mechanism of function. *Journal of Bioenergetics and Biomembranes*, **24** (5), 485–491.

175 McCabe, M.G., Bourgain, R. and Maguire, D.J. (2003) How proton translocation across mitochondrial inner membranes drives the Fo rotor of ATP synthase. *Advances in Experimental Medicine and Biology*, **540**, 133–138.

176 Nath, S. (2003) Molecular mechanisms of energy transduction in cells: engineering applications and biological implications. *Advances in Biochemical Engineering/Biotechnology*, **85**, 125–180.

177 Strajbl, M., Shurki, A. and Warshel, A. (2003) Converting conformational changes to electrostatic energy in molecular motors: the energetics of ATP synthase. *Proceedings of the National Academy of Sciences of the United States of America*, **100** (25), 14834–14839.

178 Opie, L.H. and Owen, P. (1975) Effects of increased mechanical work by isolated perfused rat heart during production or uptake of ketone bodies. Assessment of mitochondrial oxidized to reduced free nicotinamide–adenine dinucleotide ratios and oxaloacetate concentrations. *The Biochemical Journal*, **148** (3), 403–415.

179 Casamenti, F., Prosperi, C., Scali, C., Giovannelli, L. and Pepeu, G. (1998) Morphological biochemical and behavioural changes induced by neurotoxic and inflammatory insults to the nucleus basalis. *International Journal of Developmental Neuroscience*, **16** (7–8), 705–714.

180 Bales, K.R., Tzavara, E.T., Wu, S., Wade, M.R., Bymaster, F.P., Paul, S.M. and

Nomikos, G.G. (2006) Cholinergic dysfunction in a mouse model of Alzheimer disease is reversed by an anti-A beta antibody. *Journal of Clinical Investigation*, **116** (3), 825–832.

181 Goekoop, R., Scheltens, P., Barkhof, F. and Rombouts, S.A. (2006) Cholinergic challenge in Alzheimer patients and mild cognitive impairment differentially affects hippocampal activation – a pharmacological fMRI study. *Brain*, **129** (Pt 1), 141–157.

182 Muir, J.L., Page, K.J., Sirinathsinghji, D.J., Robbins, T.W. and Everitt, B.J. (1993) Excitotoxic lesions of basal forebrain cholinergic neurons: effects on learning memory and attention. *Behavioural Brain Research*, **57** (2), 123–131.

183 Schliebs, R. (2005) Basal forebrain cholinergic dysfunction in Alzheimer's disease – interrelationship with beta-amyloid, inflammation and neuro-trophin signaling. *Neurochemical Research*, **30** (6–7), 895–908.

184 Boyd-Kimball, D., Sultana, R., Poon, H.F., Lynn, B.C., Casamenti, F., Pepeu, G., Klein, J.B. and Butterfield, D.A. (2005) Proteomic identification of proteins specifically oxidized by intracerebral injection of amyloid beta-peptide (1–42) into rat brain: implications for Alzheimer's disease. *Neuroscience*, **132** (2), 313–324.

185 Giovannini, M.G., Scali, C., Prosperi, C., Bellucci, A., Vannucchi, M.G., Rosi, S., Pepeu, G. and Casamenti, F. (2002) Beta-amyloid-induced inflammation and cholinergic hypofunction in the rat brain *in vivo*: involvement of the p38MAPK pathway. *Neurobiology of Disease*, **11** (2), 257–274.

186 Poon, H.F., Vaishnav, R.A., Getchell, T.V., Getchell, M.L. and Butterfield, D.A. (2006) Quantitative proteomics analysis of differential protein expression and oxidative modification of specific proteins in the brains of old mice. *Neurobiology of Aging*, **27** (7), 1010–1019.

187 Barber, R., McKeith, I.G., Ballard, C., Gholkar, A. and O'Brien, J.T. (2001) A comparison of medial and lateral temporal lobe atrophy in dementia with Lewy bodies and Alzheimer's disease: magnetic resonance imaging volumetric study. *Dementia and Geriatric Cognitive Disorders*, **12** (3), 198–205.

188 Convit, A., de Leon, M.J., Golomb, J., George, A.E., Tarshish, C.Y., Bobinski, M., Tsui, W., De Santi, S., Wegiel, J. and Wisniewski, H. (1993) Hippocampal atrophy in early Alzheimer's disease: anatomic specificity and validation. *The Psychiatric Quarterly*, **64** (4), 371–387.

189 Ishii, K., Sasaki, H., Kono, A.K., Miyamoto, N., Fukuda, T. and Mori, E. (2005) Comparison of gray matter and metabolic reduction in mild Alzheimer's disease using FDG-PET and voxel-based morphometric MR studies. *European Journal of Nuclear Medicine and Molecular Imaging*, **32** (8), 959–963.

190 Patel, M.S. and Korotchkina, L.G. (2001) Regulation of mammalian pyruvate dehydrogenase complex by phospho-rylation: complexity of multiple phosphorylation sites and kinases. *Experimental and Molecular Medicine*, **33** (4), 191–197.

191 Jedrzejas, M.J. (2000) Structure, function, and evolution of phosphoglycerate mutases: comparison with fructose-2,6-bisphosphatase, acid phosphatase, and alkaline phosphatase. *Progress in Biophysics and Molecular Biology*, **73** (2–4), 263–287.

192 van der Oost, J., Huynen, M.A. and Verhees, C.H. (2002) Molecular characterization of phosphoglycerate mutase in archaea. *FEMS Microbiology Letters*, **212** (1), 111–120.

10

Gene Expression Profiling of Gliomas – Improving the Understanding of Glioma Biology and Paving the Way for Molecular Classification

Markus J. Riemenschneider and Guido Reifenberger

10.1
Introduction

Primary tumors of the central nervous system (CNS) account for approximately 2–3% of all cancers. In Western countries, the annual incidence is approximately 15 patients per 100 000 population and the prevalence has been estimated to be approximately 69 patients per 100 000 population [1]. In children, CNS tumors are the second most common form of cancer after leukemias. Primary CNS tumors comprise a heterogeneous group of benign and malignant neoplasms, the most common of which are tumors of glial cells, collectively referred to as gliomas [1]. Gliomas are histologically classified according to the World Health Organization (WHO) classification of tumors of the nervous system [2], which combines tumor typing with the assignment of a defined malignancy grade. These grades range from WHO grade I (benign tumors) to WHO grade IV (highly malignant tumors). The prototypic tumor for a WHO grade I glioma is the pilocytic astrocytoma, which is the most common form of glioma in the pediatric age group, while glioblastoma represents the most common type of WHO grade IV neoplasms and preferentially occurs in adults with a peak incidence between 50 and 60 years of age. At present, the histological classification and grading of gliomas still represents the most important indicator for the biological and clinical behavior of gliomas as well as patient outcome. While patients with WHO grade I tumors can usually be cured by surgical resection, WHO grade II tumors – though still exhibiting a rather slow growth – nearly invariably recur after resection and in the long run tend to progress to anaplastic gliomas of WHO grade III or secondary glioblastomas of WHO grade IV. Therefore, median survival of patients with WHO grade II gliomas is in the range of only 5–8 years after diagnosis. Anaplastic gliomas (WHO grade III) are rapidly growing malignant tumors that, in addition to surgery, require aggressive adjuvant treatment with radio- and/or chemotherapy. However, median survival time comes down to just 2–3 years after diagnosis, except for the subgroup of patients with anaplastic oligodendroglial tumors, who often show significantly longer survival, in particular when the tumors carry combined deletions of chromosomal arms 1p and

Neural Degeneration and Repair: Gene Expression Profiling, Proteomics, and Systems Biology
Edited by Hans Werner Müller
Copyright © 2008 WILEY-VCH Verlag GmbH & Co. KGaA, Weinheim
ISBN: 978-3-527-31707-3

19q [3,4]. As stated above, glioblastoma, the most frequent and most malignant primary brain tumor corresponds to WHO grade IV. Glioblastoma patients exhibit a rapid disease progression despite multimodal aggressive treatment and median survival time – barring a few exceptions – is less than 1 year after initial diagnosis.

The cytogenetic and molecular genetic alterations associated with glioma formation and progression have been intensely studied over the past 20 years. Common aberrations identified in well-differentiated gliomas of WHO grade II include mutations of the *TP53* gene on 17p13 in about 30–50% of diffusely infiltrating astrocytomas [5–7], as well as loss of genetic information on chromosome arms 1p and 19q in up to 80% of oligodendrogliomas [8,9]. The malignant progression to anaplastic gliomas (WHO grade III) and glioblastomas (WHO grade IV) is associated with the accumulation of multiple additional genetic changes that include mutation and/or homozygous deletion of the tumor suppressor genes *CDKN2A*, *RB1*, and *PTEN*; as well as amplification and concomitant overexpression of various proto-oncogenes, such as *EGFR*, *CDK4*, *MDM2*, *MDM4*, and *PDGFRA* [10–16].

The genome-wide search for new tumor suppressor genes and oncogenes, as well as more sophisticated tumor-specific genomic or transcriptional signatures, has been enormously facilitated by the development of novel array-based profiling techniques. Historically, the first arrays date back to the mid- to late 1980s, when robotic devices (so-called gridding robots) made it possible to spot DNA probes on a membrane-type material in a regular pattern [17]. However, spot sizes of these "macroarrays" were rather huge and thus their density was limited to a maximum of about 2000–10 000 spots. This first array generation could be spotted with DNA/cDNA clones, PCR products, or oligonucleotides and was typically labeled with radioactive agents. A common application was the screening of public cDNA libraries for pulling a clone containing the gene of interest when sequencing information was still more restricted than it is today [18]. But macroarrays are still widely used, for example, for gene profiling experiments of moderate scope as it requires only small sample volumes in a standard laboratory setting. In the mid-1990s, miniaturization became a major issue in the development of DNA arrays with the aim of increasing the number of genes assayed in a single experiment. This new generation of "microarrays" now made use of the superior resolution of fluorescence instead of radioactive detection methods. Also, DNA spots were deposited on glass slides to allow intensity measurements with confocal optics for achieving higher detection sensitivity [19]. In addition, the Affymetrix company (Santa Clara, CA, USA) developed and commercialized high-density oligonucleotide microarrays, generated using a unique photolithographic technique [20]. Such oligonucleotide chips are nowadays widely available and may carry hundreds of thousands of probes (each containing several million copies of a given oligonucleotide) that are representative for all known genes or more than 500 000 single-nucleotide polymorphisms (SNPs). It has to be mentioned that similar to the advancements made in expression profiling at the transcriptional level, array-based comparative genomic hybridization (array-CGH) has revolutionized the high-resolution detection of genomic imbalances at the genome-wide level [21,22]. The method is based on the different hybridization efficiency of tumor and reference DNA to a number of predefined hybridization targets (either bacterial artificial chromosomes, BACs, or oligonucleotides) on glass slides. Similar amounts of tumor and reference DNA are labeled with fluorescent dyes and are cohybridized on the microarray. Numerical genomic aberrations, that is, gene amplifications, gains, or deletions, result in color shifts of the fluorescent hybridization signal, which then facilitate automatic detection and statistical interpretation. An advantage the array-CGH has over conventional chromosomal CGH is the much higher resolution that leads to the detection of not only imbalances of defined chromosomal bands or regions but also of single genes.

Finally, significant progress has also been achieved in the field of proteomics. Traditional technologies such as two-dimensional gel electrophoresis (2DE) have been supplemented by new approaches like liquid phase separations combined with mass spectrometry or protein microarrays [23]. However, compared to the degree of automatization reached with microarray analyses at the genomic and transcriptional levels, protein array approaches are still in their infancy and data obtained with these techniques applied to brain tumors are still sparse.

Of the different approaches described above, most advances in the field of brain tumor research have been provided by the use of expression profiling techniques so far. This may be due to the fact that gene expression arrays nowadays are generally available, while array-CGH methodology is less abundantly available. Thus, this chapter will focus on delineating the impact of mRNA expression profiling on some of the most intriguing aspects of brain tumor research. It will be described how expression profiling may contribute to the refinement of glioma classification and how it identified progression-associated molecular changes that may help distinguish between different glioma types and malignancy grades. Moreover, it will report on the identification of pathway-associated expression signatures leading the way to more individualized targeted glioma therapies. Finally, the chapter will point to the emerging issue of molecular heterogeneity within tumors and will discuss how expression profiling of defined tumor cell subpopulations, such as the so-called tumor stem cells, pseudopalisading cells around areas of necrosis, or invading tumor cells may deepen our insight into basic questions of glioma biology.

10.2
Expression Profiling and Glioma Classification

In clinical neurooncology, the histopathological diagnosis still is the most important basis for therapeutic decision-making, as well as one of the most reliable prognostic parameters (Figure 10.1). Classification is carried out according to the WHO classification of tumors of the nervous system, taking into account classical histological as well as defined immunohistochemical parameters [2]. However, histological classification of brain tumors is a challenging task, as the classification criteria is sometimes rather vaguely defined thereby leaving room for a considerable degree of subjectivity and hence interobserver variability. Furthermore, tumors may present with atypical histologies or histological features intermediate between certain tumor types or malignancy grades, thus prohibiting a precise histological diagnosis and

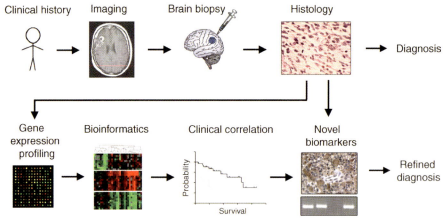

Figure 10.1 Flow chart illustrating the diagnostic assessment of brain tumors in the routine setting (upper panel) and its possible improvement by using microarray-based expression profiling to identify novel diagnostic and prognostic biomarkers (lower panel). The indication for taking a brain biopsy is based on the patient's clinical history, neurological symptoms, and neuroradiological imaging features. Biopsy then is followed by routine histopathological evaluation, which leads to a definite diagnosis constituting the basis for further therapy and prognostic assessments. However, extraction of small amounts of high-quality RNA from tumor tissue and hybridization to DNA microarrays nowadays enables us to analyze the expression of thousands of genes simultaneously. As outlined in this chapter, gene expression analysis followed by adequate bioinformatic analyses is capable of improving tumor classification and predicting the clinical course in tumors with inconclusive histological features. Nevertheless, the routine implication of gene expression profiling in the diagnostic regimen is restricted by the lack of both cost effectiveness and availability of the necessary equipment. However, microarray studies on clinically well-documented patients may reveal novel diagnostic, prognostic, and/or predictive markers, which then can be tested directly and cost effectively in a clinical setting by using, for example, immunohistochemistry or PCR. Such biomarkers will eventually lead to the refinement of brain tumor diagnostics.

making it difficult to predict the individual clinical course. In such cases, the employment of additional molecular information for a refined classification and grading would be highly desirable.

The potential of mRNA expression profiling in glioma classification has been nicely illustrated by the study of Nutt and colleagues, who for the first time showed that gene expression profiling can indeed not only contribute to the classification of histologically challenging cases but may even be superior to the standard histopathological classification [24]. They employed microarray analysis to determine the expression of roughly 12 000 genes in a set of 50 gliomas: 28 glioblastomas and 22 anaplastic oligodendrogliomas. Supervised learning approaches were then used to build a two-class prediction model based on a subset of 14 glioblastomas and 7 anaplastic oligodendrogliomas with classic histology. A 20-feature k-nearest neighbor model correctly classified 18 of the 21 classic cases in leave-one-out cross-validation, compared to pathological diagnoses. This model was then used to predict the classification of histologically nonclassic cases of malignant gliomas. When tumors were classified according to pathology, the survival of patients with non-classic glioblastoma and nonclassic anaplastic oligodendroglioma was not significantly different ($P = 0.19$). Class distinctions according to the model, however, were significantly associated with the survival outcome ($P = 0.05$). Thus, the class prediction model was capable of classifying high-grade, nonclassic glial tumors objectively and reproducibly. Moreover, the model provided a more accurate predictor of prognosis in these nonclassic lesions than did pathological classification. The authors concluded that class prediction models, based on defined molecular profiles, classify diagnostically challenging malignant gliomas in a manner that better correlates with clinical outcome than does standard pathology.

Another study pointing in the same direction is by Freije and colleagues, which underlines the power of expression profiling in predicting patient survival [25]. The authors performed large-scale gene expression analyses on 85 diffusely infiltrating glioma samples of all histological types and grades by employing Affymetrix HG U133 oligonucleotide chips. Remarkably, gene expression profiling turned out to be a more powerful survival predictor than histological grade or patient age. Poor prognosis samples could be further subclassified into three prognostic groups, each with distinct molecular signatures. Moreover, the authors broke down the expression signatures to a list of 44 candidate genes, the expression patterns of which reliably classified gliomas into histologically unrecognized biological and prognostic groups. These findings are trendsetting in two ways: first, they demonstrate that microarray analysis has the potential to identify previously unrecognized, clinically relevant patient subsets even within defined histological glioma grades. Second, as the standard implementation of whole-genome expression chips in the routine diagnostics will not be realistic due to its lack of cost effectiveness, this study points in the right direction of generating diagnostic and prognostic signatures comprising a restricted number of highly distinctive transcripts that can be tested for not only in an experimental but also in a diagnostic setting (Figure 10.1).

An interesting example of how defined molecular alterations directly influence the clinical course of glioma is the distinction between primary and secondary glioblastomas [26]. Though sharing the same histological features of cellular atypia, mitotic figures, necrotic foci with peripheral cellular pseudopalisading, and microvascular hyperplasia, the clinical history of both lesions is strikingly different. Secondary glioblastomas develop slowly through progression from low-grade (WHO grade II) or anaplastic (WHO grade III) glial tumors. In contrast, primary glioblastomas develop rapidly *de novo* and manifest as WHO grade IV tumors from the beginning. At the molecular level, we know that secondary glioblastomas are characterized by frequent mutations in the *TP53* gene (>60%), overexpression of the platelet-derived growth factor receptor (*PDGFRA*), and loss of heterozygosity (LOH) on 17p, 19q, and 10q [26,27]. Primary glioblastomas have frequent amplification/ overexpression of the epidermal growth factor receptor (*EGFR*; amplification in about 40% and overexpression in more than 60% of cases, respectively) and the mouse double minute 2 gene (*MDM2*), *PTEN* mutations, and loss of all or a portion of chromosome 10 [26,27]. In recent studies, there has been emerging evidence that gene expression profiling is capable of corroborating and further dissecting this distinctive molecular phenotype of primary and secondary glioblastomas [28–30]. Tso and colleagues employed large-scale expression analyses to reliably differentiate between primary and secondary lesions [29]. Interestingly, genes expressed in primary glioblastomas were frequently related to stromal response, suggesting the importance of extracellular signaling and host–tumor interaction in these phenotypically highly invasive lesions. Secondary glioblastomas, in contrast, were more adequately described by expression of genes functioning in mitotic cell cycle regulation processes. Nevertheless, also common transcripts between primary and secondary glioblastomas could be detected, which mainly reflected characteristics of hyperprofileration, hypervascularity, and apoptotic resistance shared by both glioblastoma subgroups.

Another study pointing in the same direction is by Godard and colleagues [30]. The authors performed cDNA-array analysis of 53 patient biopsies, comprising the histological groups of low-grade astrocytomas, secondary glioblastomas (respective recurrent high-grade tumors), and newly diagnosed primary glioblastomas. Low-grade astrocytomas had the most specific and consistent expression profiles, while primary glioblastomas exhibited much larger variation between tumors. Secondary glioblastomas displayed features of both other groups. Several sets of genes with highly correlated expression within groups were identified that (a) were associated with specific biological functions and (b) effectively differentiated tumor classes. A prominent gene cluster discriminating primary versus secondary glioblastoma comprised mostly genes known to be involved in angiogenesis, like *VEGF* or *IGFBP2*.

Taken together, these studies demonstrate that gene expression profiling is not only helping the classification of diagnostically challenging tumors, but might also enable the detection of molecular subsets within "classic" histopathological entities. Spoken in terms of therapeutics, this would imply that in addition to the common grade-adapted therapies we employ today, expression profiling could add to tailoring more specific gene pathway-targeted, individualized therapeutic strategies, thereby maximizing therapeutic efficiency and minimizing negative side effects.

One recent study aiming at identifying new molecular subsets of morphologically identical tumors is the work by Mischel and colleagues [28]. The authors employed global gene expression analyses to compare EGFR-expressing and EGFR-nonexpressing primary glioblastomas. Strikingly, EGFR-expressing glioblastomas had a globally distinctive pattern of gene expression compared to EGFR-nonexpressing primary glioblastomas, indicating that they are a biologically relevant subset. Furthermore, a relatively small number of genes could be used to distinguish between EGFR-expressing and EGFR-negative primary glioblastomas, and this list of genes was highly enriched for signaling molecules, many of which could potentially provide therapeutic targets. Not surprisingly, the EGFR-negative primary glioblastomas were not a uniform subclass: at least two further subsets were detected, including one in which a set of contiguous genes in the chromosomal region 12q13–15 were overexpressed, which is consistent with a chromosomal amplification in this area. These data add further proof to the hypothesis that patterns of gene expression can uncover biologically relevant molecular subsets of morphologically identical tumors.

10.3
Progression-Associated Gene Expression Changes in Gliomas

Gliomas usually recur after neurosurgical resection due to their infiltrative behavior, which makes complete surgical resection technically impossible. On recurrence, tumors that had previously manifested as low-grade gliomas (WHO grade II) commonly progress to high-grade lesions, that is, anaplastic glioma (WHO grade III) or glioblastoma (WHO grade IV). Thus, malignant progression represents the main cause of tumor-related death in astrocytoma patients [31,32]. We have mentioned that the malignant transformation is a multiple-step process, which results in the accumulation of genetic alterations. Diffuse astrocytomas of WHO grade II, for example, are characterized by frequent *TP53* mutations, LOH on 17p, and gains of chromosome 7 or 7q. Anaplastic astrocytomas additionally demonstrate frequent allelic losses on 9p, 13q, and 19q, with important target genes being *CDKN2A*, *CDKN2B*, and *p14ARF* at 9p21 as well as the retinoblastoma gene (*RB1*) at 13q14. Glioblastomas carry the most complex genetic aberrations, resulting in the inactivation of various tumor suppressor genes, such as *PTEN*, *TP53*, *RB1*, *CDKN2A*, *CDKN2B*, and *p14ARF*, as well as the amplification of different proto-oncogenes, most commonly the *EGFR*, *CDK4*, *MDM2*, and *PDGFRA* genes [33–35].

While the progression-associated changes on the genomic level have been well characterized, little is known about progression-associated gene expression changes at the transcript level. One of the first studies dealing with this issue was contributed by Sallinen and colleagues who performed cDNA microarray analyses on matched pairs of primary tumors and tumor recurrences in the same glioma patients [36]. They found the upregulation of the insulin-like growth factor binding protein 2 (*IGFBP2*) gene as the most distinct progression-related expression change. Results were confirmed with a high-density tissue microarray of 418 brain tumors. Immunohistochemical analyses proved that strong expression of *IGFBP2* was associated with the progression of gliomas and when expressed in diffuse astrocytomas, it correlated with poor patient survival ($P < 0.0001$).

The study by van den Boom *et al.* compared the transcriptional profile of approximately 6800 genes in primary WHO grade II gliomas and corresponding recurrent high-grade (WHO grade III or IV) gliomas from eight patients by means of oligonucleotide-based microarray analysis and real-time reverse transcription–polymerase chain reaction [37]. Sixty-six genes were identified with mRNA levels differing significantly ($P < 0.01$, >twofold) between primary and recurrent tumors (Figure 10.2). The microarray data were corroborated by real-time reverse transcription polymerase chain reaction analysis of 12 selected genes, including 7 genes with increased expression and 5 genes with reduced expression on progression. In addition, the expression of these 12 genes was determined in an independent series of 43 astrocytic gliomas (9 diffuse astrocytomas, 10 anaplastic astrocytomas, 17 primary and 7 secondary glioblastomas). Transcript levels of nine of the selected genes (*COL4A2*, *FOXM1*, *MGP*, *TOP2A*, *CENPF*, *IGFBP4*, *VEGFA*, *ADD3*, and *CAMK2G*) could be confirmed to differ significantly in WHO grade II astrocytomas as compared to anaplastic astrocytomas and/or glioblastomas.

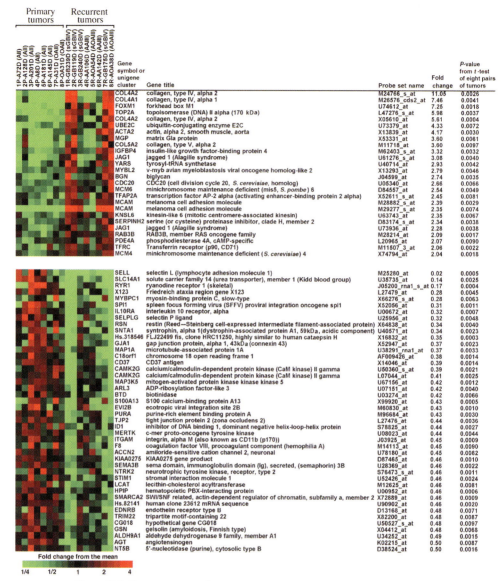

Figure 10.2 Characterization of gene expression profiles associated with glioma progression using oligonucleotide-based microarray analysis (image reprinted with permission from Ref. [37]). The figure shows the 70 probe sets (corresponding to 66 genes) whose mRNA levels differed significantly (*P* < 0.01, >twofold change) when comparing eight pairs of primary and recurrent tumors. Microarray data were corroborated by real-time reverse transcription–polymerase chain reaction analysis. Expression levels of nine of the selected genes (COL4A2, FOXM1, MGP, TOP2A, CENPF, IGFBP4, VEGFA, ADD3, and CAMK2G) differed significantly in WHO grade II astrocytomas as compared to anaplastic astrocytomas and/or glioblastomas in an independent series of 43 astrocytic gliomas. The individual case numbers and diagnoses are given on top of the heat map. AII: diffuse astrocytoma WHO grade II; AAIII: anaplastic astrocytoma WHO grade III; sGBIV: secondary glioblastoma WHO grade IV; OAII: oligoastrocytoma WHO grade II; AOAIII: anaplastic oligoastrocytoma WHO grade III.

In a second study, the authors followed up on their initial study by employing suppression subtractive hybridization and subsequent macroarray hybridization, which also allowed for the enrichment of transcripts highly differentially expressed between glioma grades [38]. Four patients with primary low-grade gliomas of WHO grade II that recurred as secondary glioblastomas (WHO grade IV) were investigated. Eight genes exhibiting differential expression between primary and recurrent tumors in three of the four patients were selected for further analysis using real-time reverse transcription–PCR on a series of 10 pairs of primary low-grade and recurrent high-grade gliomas as well as 42 astrocytic gliomas of different WHO grades. The analyses revealed that five genes, namely, *AMOG* (*ATP1B2*, 17p13.1), *APOD* (3q26.2-qter), *DMXL1* (5q23.1), *DRR1* (*TU3A*, 3p14.2), and *PSD3* (*KIAA09428/ HCA67/EFA6R*, 8p22), were expressed at significantly lower levels in secondary glioblastomas as compared to diffuse astrocytomas of WHO grade II. In addition, *AMOG*, *DRR1*, and *PSD3* transcript levels turned out to be significantly lower in primary glioblastomas than in diffuse astrocytomas. Subsequent promoter methylation studies demonstrated *AMOG* hypermethylation in glioma cell lines and a primary anaplastic astrocytoma with low *AMOG* expression, thus arguing for a role of epigenetic silencing of *AMOG* in malignant glioma cells.

In summary, array-based studies on progression-associated gene expression changes in gliomas are still limited and there seems to be room for additional experimental discoveries. However, from the studies performed on human glioma tissues, a number of interesting novel candidate genes have been derived that now await their further functional characterization in appropriate model systems.

10.4
Expression Signatures Relating to Tumor Location

It has been indicated by previous studies that the distribution of defined genetic alterations may correlate with glioma location [39]. In a recent study, Sharma and colleagues performed gene expression profiling on 41 primary pilocytic astrocytomas to molecularly discriminate tumors with clinically aggressive or indolent phenotypes [40]. While the authors did not succeed in finding an expression signature discriminating the two prognostic subgroups of pilocytic astrocytomas, they identified a gene expression signature that stratified pilocytic astrocytomas by location (supratentorial versus infratentorial). They also identified a gene expression pattern common to pilocytic astrocytomas, normal mouse astrocytes, and neural stem cells from these distinct brain regions, as well as a gene expression pattern shared between pilocytic astrocytoma and ependymoma – another human glial tumor showing ependymal differentiation – that arose supratentorially compared with those originating in the posterior fossa. These results might indicate that glial tumors share intrinsic, lineage-specific molecular signatures that reflect the brain regions in which their nonmalignant cells of origin resided.

Two other studies performed on ependymal gliomas point in the same direction [41,42]. To analyze whether subgroups of ependymoma patients are characterized by specific gene expression patterns that might explain pathophysiological processes on the gene expression level, Korshunov *et al.* used the nearest shrunken centroid classification that identifies minimal combinations of genes that provide best discrimination between two known groups [42,43]. The identified gene expression patterns allowed an accurate classification of 39 ependymoma patients according to tumor location (spinal versus intracranial) and patient age (<16 years versus >16 years) in 87 and 77% of cases, respectively. Of note, the investigated tumor series did not include any spinal ependymomas of WHO grade III histology, suggesting that the differences seen for tumor location were also in part related to tumor grade. Specifically, all WHO grade I ependymomas of spinal location ($n = 4$) displayed a common signature with high-expression levels of *HOXB5*, *PLA2G5*, and *ITIH2*, clearly separating these cases from all intracranial tumors, whereas WHO grade II spinal ependymomas clustered either to the myxopapillary cases or to the group of intracranial tumors, suggesting a molecular heterogeneity of this histologically homogeneous subset. In line with this study, Modena *et al.* identified 98 probe sets differentially expressed between ependymomas located in supra- and infratentorial brain regions, thus corroborating the fact that ependymomas arising in different intracranial locations are molecularly distinct [41]. Several genes involved in CNS development were differentially expressed, including *PAX3*, *NET1*, and *MSX1* upregulated in infratentorial and *MSI2* upregulated in supratentorial tumors. Hence, subgroups of the same histologic tumor type are likely generated by different populations of progenitor cells in their tissues of origin which would argue for the requirement of more diversified therapies.

10.5
Pathway-Associated Expression Signatures and Targeted Therapies

In the preceding paragraphs we have delineated the striking contributions that gene expression profiling has made to the introduction of new molecularly defined tumor subsets. Thus, array-based gene expression analysis adds a considerable level of diversity to our current concept of glioma classification. But how to deal with this diversity? How to exploit it in a way that it provides benefits to glioma patients? The most promising approach in this context can be derived from the fact that all the genes differently regulated on array analyses do not act as individual units but do collaborate in overlapping pathways. With the signatures of these activated pathways known and with powerful biostatisticial tools now in hand, we should be able to extract patterns of pathway activation from the tumor profiles, which then could be directly translated into targeted therapies.

The most groundbreaking step in this direction has been undertaken by Nevins and colleagues in breast, ovarian, and lung cancer patients [44,45]. The authors employed human primary mammary epithelial cell cultures to develop a series of pathway signatures. This was accomplished by adenoviral-mediated introduction of various oncogenic alterations in an otherwise quiescent cell, thereby specifically isolating the subsequent events as defined by the activation/deregulation of the single pathway concerned. Gene expression signatures that reflected the activity of a given pathway were identified using supervised classification methods. Since genes involved in pathways often overlap, several additional statistical approaches were employed to generate refined sets of predictors most exclusive to the respective pathways. In the next step, the pathway signatures were used to identify patterns of pathway dysregulation in expression profiles of human tumors. Indeed, stratification for activation or inactivation of defined signaling pathways showed clinically relevant association with disease outcome and effectively differentiated between specific cancers and tumor subtypes. Moreover, pathway signatures in tumor cell lines could also predict sensitivity to therapeutic agents specifically targeting the respective pathways. Thus, this approach may provide the opportunity to directly extract therapeutically relevant information from given tumor gene expression profiles and to match individual patients with the most appropriate therapeutic strategy.

Despite the fascinating potential of transcriptional profiling in the search of new pathway-related targeted therapies, it has to be noted, however, that gene expression patterns provide only indirect information about signaling pathways. The direct analysis of signal transcription cascades within human tumors requires the investigation of posttranslational modifications of proteins, such as phosphorylation events. In this respect, recent studies aimed at deciphering signaling pathways directly in human glioma tissues using phosphorylation specific antibodies [46–48]. The significance of these approaches becomes evident in the work of Choe *et al.*, in which 45 primary glioblastoma specimens were studied for aberrations in the phosphatidylinositol 3′-kinase (PI3K) pathway on a tissue microarray [46]. Multidimensional scaling, hierarchical clustering, and univariate and multivariate analyses were employed for statistical evaluation of array results. The authors found a pattern of interrelationships between the signaling molecules that reflected the current knowledge of the signaling pathway as derived from *in vitro* experimental studies. Moreover, hierarchical clustering identified potentially meaningful molecular subsets on the basis of PTEN and EGFR expression. These results suggest that phospho-specific antibodies can be used to detect the activation state of key signaling molecules *in vivo* and that analytic tools, such as multidimensional scaling and hierarchical clustering, can help identify biologically meaningful patterns of pathway activation that, in addition to the transcriptional signatures, can be used to stratify patients for therapy with pathway inhibitors.

10.6
Expression Profiling of Selected Tumor Cell Subpopulations – Deciphering Tumor Heterogeneity

State-of-the-art tumor diagnosis and grading are based on the microscopic detection and interpretation of particular microscopic features like count of mitoses, pathological vessel formation, or presence/absence of necroses [2]. This makes perfect sense keeping in mind that all those microscopic appearances are equivalents of defined biologic processes. So the detection of mitotic figures, for example, indicates cell division resulting in more rapid tumor growth. As outlined above, technological progress in gene expression profiling has taken us to a point where mere histological classification can be supplemented and refined by molecular diagnostic approaches. Even within histological tumor types and grades new molecularly defined tumor subsets can be delineated. So the next logical question is whether also the dissection of defined histological features within tumors and the assessment of their expression signatures can deepen our understanding of the basic processes underlying glioma biology or may even generate new prognostic and diagnostic markers in glioma classification. In an interesting study, Dong and colleagues used laser capture microdissection and oligonucleotide arrays to detect molecules differentially expressed in perinecrotic palisades in comparison to nonpalisading tumor cells distant from necrosis [49]. Palisading around necroses is a common phenomenon in glioblastomas with tumor cells more densely packed at the edge of the necrotic zone. Recent extensive studies, investigating this histologic phenomenon, had demonstrated that these palisades represent a dynamic response to local hypoxic stresses [50,51]. So, it is no surprise that Dong *et al.* found exactly those genes that convey response to hypoxic environmental conditions were most commonly altered in pseudopalisading tumor cells. However, in the second step, the authors identified a set of five RNAs (*POFUT2, PTDSR, PLOD2, ATF5,* and *HK2*) that were not only differentially expressed in three initially studied, microdissected glioblastomas but could also provide prognostic information in an independent set of 28 glioblastomas that did not all have perinecrotic palisades. Thus, it appears feasible to derive tissue biomarkers that provide ancillary prognostic and predictive information from the study of defined subpopulations of tumor cells.

A key issue in glioma research to which a similar approach could easily be applied is the better understanding of the molecular mechanisms that convey the migratory and invasive phenotype of glioma cells. Despite the best current surgical, radiation, and chemotherapeutic approaches, nearly all glioma patients experience tumor recurrences that lead to death, primarily because these tumors invade surrounding tissues, thus making local therapeutic approaches ineffective. Interestingly, employing *in situ* analyses has given further evidence that many of the molecules and pathways regulating tumor cell migration and invasion are heterogenic within tumors, meaning that they are altered in defined intratumoral regions, like, for example, the tumor infiltration zone [48,52–54]. Thus, the analysis of the molecular signatures of invading and migrating tumor cells appears particularly promising.

The most interesting work from an array analysis perspective has been contributed by the group of Michael Berens. In an early study employing cDNA microarrays of up to 7000 gene sequences, the authors compared cDNA populations of a glioma cell line (G112) exposed, or not, to a motility-inducing substrate of cell-derived extracellular matrix (ECM) proteins [55]. Validation of differentially regulated genes was performed on additional cell lines and human glioblastoma tissues. The data were analyzed for whether genes involved in pathways of motility, apoptosis, and proliferation were differentially expressed when motility behavior was engaged. Genes known to be involved in cell motility, like tenascin C, neuropilin 2, *GAP43, PARG1* (an inhibitor of Rho), *PLCγ,* and *CD44,* were overexpressed; others, like adducin 3γ and integrins, were downregulated in migrating cells. Interestingly, many key cell cycle components, like cyclin A and B, and proliferation markers,

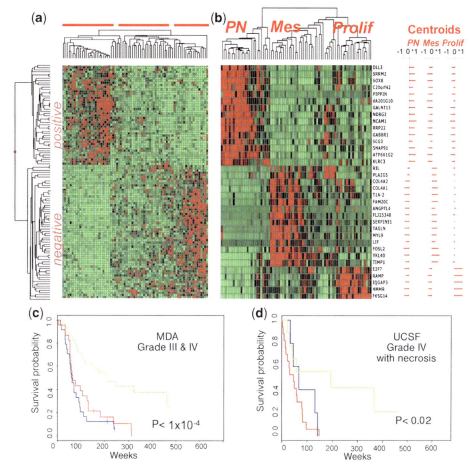

Figure 10.3 Expression profiling identified three major, previously undescribed prognostic subclasses of high-grade astrocytoma that resemble stages in neurogenesis (image reprinted with permission from Ref. [63]). (a) Unsupervised clustering of 76 primary astrocytomas by expression of 108 genes positively or negatively correlated with survival (gene clusters labeled positive or negative) identified three sample clusters. From these clusters, 35 signature genes could be derived to assign tumors to subclasses by means of hierarchical clustering. (b) Subclasses were designated proneural (*PN*), proliferative (*Prolif*), and mesenchymal (*Mes*) to recognize the dominant feature of the gene list that

characterized each subclass. Centroids from *k*-means clustering were depicted using *Z* score-normalized gene expression values (scale from −1 to +1). (c) and (d) Kaplan–Meier plots showing survival of high-grade astrocytoma patients with respect to subclasses. Green, blue, and red lines correspond to *PN*, *Prolif*, and *Mes* subclasses, respectively. *PN* subclass tumors displaying neuronal lineage markers showed longer survival, while *Prolif* and *Mes* cases that are enriched for neural stem cell markers displayed equally short survival *P*-values from log-rank tests shown. Vertical ticks indicate censored survival observations.

like *PCNA*, were strongly downregulated on ECM. Also, genes involved in apoptotic cascades, like *BCL2* and effector caspases, were differentially expressed, suggesting the global downregulation of proapoptotic components in cells exposed to cell-derived ECM. Taken together, these findings are essential as they further prove the hypothesis that cells that migrate do not proliferate and are also protected from apoptotic stimuli [56]. Thus, inhibition of migration would not only be of utmost importance to fight the recurrent nature of gliomas but also to make these tumors more susceptible to radiation or chemotherapy.

In a subsequent study aiming at the identification of new potential therapeutic targets, Hoelzinger *et al.* turned to the investigation of human glioblastoma tissues and collected laser capture-microdissected tumor cells from paired patient tumor cores and white matter invading cell populations [57]. Expression analyses again were performed on 7000 cDNA microarrays and results validated by RT-PCR and immunohistochemistry. Autotaxin (*ATX*), ephrin B3, B-cell lymphoma-w (*BCLW*), and protein tyrosine kinase 2 beta were strongly overexpressed in invasive glioma cells and the known glioblastoma markers insulin-like growth factor binding protein 2 and vimentin were robustly expressed in the tumor core. While the number of interesting candidate genes generated in this study was still limited, the findings nonetheless prove that this approach is highly effective in depicting transcriptional differences between cells of the tumor core and the invasive rim. Additional studies that employ the new generation of high-density whole-genome chips, integrate findings at the genomic, transcriptional and epigenetic levels, and follow up on the functional properties of the differentially expressed genes, are now needed.

The concept of intratumoral heterogeneity has gained additional recent support with the discovery of a potential tumor stem cell fraction in malignant gliomas. These so-called glioma stem cells are characterized by the expression of the CD133 antigen [58–61]. When isolated from human gliomas, CD133-positive cells exhibit stem cell properties, including self-renewal and differentiation capacities in different neural lineages *in vitro*. Moreover, when xenotransplanted into nonobese diabetic, severe combined immunodeficient (NOD-SCID) mice, only a few CD133-positive tumor cells were sufficient to induce gliomas, while the injection of much higher numbers of CD133-negative cells did not result in glioma formation [60]. Although the presence and significance of CD133-positive tumor cells at least in a subset of gliomas are out of question, the exceptional tumor-initiating capabilities of these cells look controversial. In a recent study, Beier *et al.* cultured tumor cells from 22 primary and secondary glioblastomas under medium conditions favoring the growth of neural and cancer stem cells [62]. Remarkably, only a subset of primary glioblastomas contained a significant CD133-positive subpopulation, and also CD133-negative tumor cells with stem cell properties could be identified. While both CD133-positive and CD133-negative tumor cells were similarly tumorigenic in nude mice, CD133-positive cells were characterized by higher proliferation indices, thus suggesting a possible prognostic significance. The authors also employed expression array analysis to compare both tumor cell subpopulations. A total of 117 genes turned out to be differentially regulated. The most striking difference was the upregulation of seven MHC class II proteins in CD133-negative cells, which had not been described in glioblastomas yet and might be exploited for tumor immuno therapy.

Another highly relevant glioma stem cell study employing array analyses is by Phillips *et al.* [63], in which they pinpointed three previously undescribed prognostic subclasses of high-grade astrocytomas to resemble stages in neurogenesis. Sub-classes were designated proneural (*PN*), proliferative (*Prolif*) and mesenchymal (*Mes*) to recognize the dominant feature of the gene list that characterized each subclass. The proneural tumor subclass displayed neuronal lineage markers and showed longer survival, while the proliferative and mesenchymal tumor classes were enriched for neural stem cell markers and displayed equally short survival (Figure 10.3). Upon recurrence, the tumors frequently shifted toward the mesen-chymal subclass. Interestingly, tumor subtypes could predict neurosphere growth of the respective tumor cell lines pointing to a potential functional relevance of the newly identified expression signatures. Finally, the authors derived a robust two-gene (*PTEN* and *DLL3*) prognostic expression model suggesting that Akt and Notch signaling can be considered hallmarks of poor prognosis versus better prognosis in gliomas, respectively. Taken together, these data suggest that a deepened under-standing of neurogenesis may yield novel therapeutic insights into glial malignan-cies and may also add to molecular glioma classification.

10.7
Summary and Outlook

This chapter has provided a brief overview of the tremendous advances that gene expression profiling approaches have provided to the field of glioma research. The most direct way in which this new technique impacts clinical and diagnostic deci-sion processes is the definition of novel gene expression-based and clinically relevant tumor subclasses. The essential next step now will be to validate these expression signatures and break them down to a number of surrogate molecular markers that can be easily and cost-effectively tested for routine diagnosis (Figure 10.1). The search for such new prognostic and predictive biomarkers will be additionally facilitated by the combination of expression array analyses with other global screen-ing techniques, such as array-CGH for genomic and CpG-island microarray analy-ses for epigenetic profiling. The identification of genes synergistically altered in these approaches will most likely be a potent approach to identify new, highly relevant tumor suppressor genes and proto-oncogenes. Powerful bioinformatic tools to integrate such high-dimensional data sets from different platforms are currently being developed.

In addition to its promises in glioma classification, the application of expression array analyses in hypothesis-driven experimental assays may provide significant advances in understanding the complex pathomechanisms underlying glioma growth and resistance to therapy. As not yet mentioned, gene expression arrays, for example, have also been used to indirectly detect gene methylation by comparing glioma cells before and after treatment with demethylating agents, such 5-aza-2′-

desoxycytidin [64]. Other promising ongoing studies include the expression profiling of defined tumor cell subpopulations, like pseudopalisading cells, infiltrating tumor cells, or tumor stem cells, as outlined above. The results of such studies will certainly have a significant impact on our understanding of glioma biology and hopefully will enable us to more effectively target this complex and devastating disease.

References

1 Ohgaki, H. and Kleihues, P. (2005) Epidemiology and etiology of gliomas. *Acta Neuropathologica (Berlin)*, **109**, 93–108.

2 Louis, D.N., Ohgaki, H., Wiestler, O.D. and Cavenee, W.K. (2007) *WHO Classification of Tumours of the Central Nervous System*, IARC Press, Lyon.

3 van den Bent, M.J., Carpentier, A.F., Brandes, A.A., Sanson, M., Taphoorn, M.J., Bernsen, H.J., Frenay, M., Tijssen, C.C., Grisold, W., Sipos, L., Haaxma-Reiche, H., Kros, J.M., van Kouwenhoven, M.C., Vecht, C.J., Allgeier, A., Lacombe, D. and Gorlia, T. (2006) Adjuvant procarbazine lomustine, and vincristine improves progression-free survival but not overall survival in newly diagnosed anaplastic oligodendrogliomas and oligoastrocytomas: a randomized European Organisation for Research and Treatment of Cancer phase III trial. *Journal of Clinical Oncology*, **24**, 2715–2722.

4 Cairncross, G., Berkey, B., Shaw, E., Jenkins, R., Scheithauer, B., Brachman, D., Buckner, J., Fink, K., Souhami, L., Laperierre, N., Mehta, M. and Curran, W. (2006) Phase III trial of chemotherapy plus radiotherapy compared with radiotherapy alone for pure and mixed anaplastic oligodendroglioma: Intergroup Radiation Therapy Oncology Group Trial 9402. *Journal of Clinical Oncology*, **24**, 2707–2714.

5 Rasheed, B.K., Wiltshire, R.N., Bigner, S.H. and Bigner, D.D. (1999) Molecular pathogenesis of malignant gliomas. *Current Opinion in Oncology*, **11**, 162–167.

6 Collins, V.P. (1999) Progression as exemplified by human astrocytic tumors. *Seminars in Cancer Biology*, **9**, 267–276.

7 Fulci, G., Ishii, N. and Van Meir, E.G. (1998) p53 and brain tumors: from gene mutations to gene therapy. *Brain Pathology*, **8**, 599–613.

8 Reifenberger, J., Reifenberger, G., Liu, L., James, C.D., Wechsler, W. and Collins, V.P. (1994) Molecular genetic analysis of oligodendroglial tumors shows preferential allelic deletions on 19q and 1p. *The American Journal of Pathology*, **145**, 1175–1190.

9 Reifenberger, G. and Louis, D.N. (2003) Oligodendroglioma: toward molecular definitions in diagnostic neuro-oncology. *Journal of Neuropathology and Experimental Neurology*, **62**, 111–126.

10 Ueki, K., Ono, Y., Henson, J.W., Efird, J.T., von Deimling, A. and Louis, D.N. (1996) CDKN2/p16 or RB alterations occur in the majority of glioblastomas and are inversely correlated. *Cancer Research*, **56**, 150–153.

11 Ichimura, K., Schmidt, E.E., Goike, H.M. and Collins, V.P. (1996) Human glioblastomas with no alterations of the CDKN2A (p16INK4A MTS1) and CDK4 genes have frequent mutations of the retinoblastoma gene. *Oncogene*, **13**, 1065–1072.

12 Ishii, N., Maier, D., Merlo, A., Tada, M., Sawamura, Y., Diserens, A.C. and Van

Meir, E.G. (1999) Frequent co-alterations of TP53 p16/CDKN2A, p14ARF, PTEN tumor suppressor genes in human glioma cell lines. *Brain Pathology*, **9**, 469–479.

13 Riemenschneider, M.J., Buschges, R., Wolter, M., Reifenberger, J., Bostrom, J., Kraus, J.A., Schlegel, U. and Reifenberger, G. (1999) Amplification and overexpression of the MDM4 (MDMX) gene from 1q32 in a subset of malignant gliomas without TP53 mutation or MDM2 amplification. *Cancer Research*, **59**, 6091–6096.

14 Reifenberger, G., Liu, L., Ichimura, K., Schmidt, E.E. and Collins, V.P. (1993) Amplification and overexpression of the MDM2 gene in a subset of human malignant gliomas without p53 mutations. *Cancer Research*, **53**, 2736–2739.

15 Hui, A.B., Lo, K.W., Yin, X.L., Poon, W.S. and Ng, H.K. (2001) Detection of multiple gene amplifications in glioblastoma multiforme using array-based comparative genomic hybridization. *Laboratory Investigation*, **81**, 717–723.

16 Riemenschneider, M.J., Knobbe, C.B. and Reifenberger, G. (2003) Refined mapping of 1q32 amplicons in malignant gliomas confirms MDM4 as the main amplification target. *International Journal of Cancer*, **104**, 752–757.

17 Jordan, B. (2002) Historical background and anticipated developments. *Annals of the New York Academy of Sciences*, **975**, 24–32.

18 Green, E.D. and Olson, M.V. (1990) Systematic screening of yeast artificial-chromosome libraries by use of the polymerase chain reaction. *Proceedings of the National Academy of Sciences of the United States of America*, **87**, 1213–1217.

19 Schena, M., Shalon, D., Davis, R.W. and Brown, P.O. (1995) Quantitative monitoring of gene expression patterns with a complementary DNA microarray. *Science*, **270**, 467–470.

20 Wodicka, L., Dong, H., Mittmann, M., Ho, M.H. and Lockhart, D.J. (1997) Genome-wide expression monitoring in *Saccharomyces cerevisiae*. *Nature Biotechnology*, **15**, 1359–1367.

21 Gunn, S.R., Robetorye, R.S. and Mohammed, M.S. (2007) Comparative genomic hybridization arrays in clinical pathology: progress and challenges. *Molecular Diagnosis & Therapy*, **11**, 73–77.

22 Mohapatra, G., Betensky, R.A., Miller, E.R., Carey, B., Gaumont, L.D., Engler, D.A. and Louis, D.N. (2006) Glioma test array for use with formalin-fixed paraffin-embedded tissue: array comparative genomic hybridization correlates with loss of heterozygosity and fluorescence *in situ* hybridization. *The Journal of Molecular Diagnostics*, **8**, 268–276.

23 Cho, W.C. and Cheng, C.H. (2007) Oncoproteomics: current trends and future perspectives. *Expert Review of Proteomics*, **4**, 401–410.

24 Nutt, C.L., Mani, D.R., Betensky, R.A., Tamayo, P., Cairncross, J.G., Ladd, C., Pohl, U., Hartmann, C., McLaughlin, M.E., Batchelor, T.T., Black, P.M., von Deimling, A., Pomeroy, S.L., Golub, T.R. and Louis, D.N. (2003) Gene expression-based classification of malignant gliomas correlates better with survival than histological classification. *Cancer Research*, **63**, 1602–1607.

25 Freije, W.A., Castro-Vargas, F.E., Fang, Z., Horvath, S., Cloughesy, T., Liau, L.M., Mischel, P.S. and Nelson, S.F. (2004) Gene expression profiling of gliomas strongly predicts survival. *Cancer Research*, **64**, 6503–6510.

26 Kleihues, P. and Ohgaki, H. (1999) Primary and secondary glioblastomas: from concept to clinical diagnosis. *Neuro-Oncology*, **1**, 44–51.

27 Maruno, M., Ninomiya, H., Ghulam Muhammad, A.K., Hirata, M., Kato, A. and Yoshimine, T. (2000) Whole-genome analysis of human astrocytic tumors by

comparative genomic hybridization. *Brain Tumor Pathology*, **17**, 21–27.

28 Mischel, P.S., Shai, R., Shi, T., Horvath, S., Lu, K.V., Choe, G., Seligson, D., Kremen, T.J., Palotie, A., Liau, L.M., Cloughesy, T.F. and Nelson, S.F. (2003) Identification of molecular subtypes of glioblastoma by gene expression profiling. *Oncogene*, **22**, 2361–2373.

29 Tso, C.L., Freije, W.A., Day, A., Chen, Z., Merriman, B., Perlina, A., Lee, Y., Dia, E.Q., Yoshimoto, K., Mischel, P.S., Liau, L.M., Cloughesy, T.F. and Nelson, S.F. (2006) Distinct transcription profiles of primary and secondary glioblastoma subgroups. *Cancer Research*, **66**, 159–167.

30 Godard, S., Getz, G., Delorenzi, M., Farmer, P., Kobayashi, H., Desbaillets, I., Nozaki, M., Diserens, A.C., Hamou, M.F., Dietrich, P.Y., Regli, L., Janzer, R.C., Bucher, P., Stupp, R., de Tribolet, N., Domany, E. and Hegi, M.E. (2003) Classification of human astrocytic gliomas on the basis of gene expression: a correlated group of genes with angiogenic activity emerges as a strong predictor of subtypes. *Cancer Research*, **63**, 6613–6625.

31 Vertosick, F.T., Jr., Selker, R.G. and Arena, V.C. (1991) Survival of patients with well-differentiated astrocytomas diagnosed in the era of computed tomography. *Neurosurgery*, **28**, 496–501.

32 McCormack, B.M., Miller, D.C., Budzilovich, G.N., Voorhees, G.J. and Ransohoff, J. (1992) Treatment and survival of low-grade astrocytoma in adults – 1977–1988. *Neurosurgery*, **31**, 636–642 (discussion 642).

33 Reifenberger, G. and Collins, V.P. (2004) Pathology and molecular genetics of astrocytic gliomas. *Journal of Molecular Medicine*, **82**, 656–670.

34 Ohgaki, H. (2005) Genetic pathways to glioblastomas. *Neuropathology*, **25**, 1–7.

35 Ohgaki, H. and Kleihues, P. (2007) Genetic pathways to primary and secondary glioblastoma. *The American Journal of Pathology*, **170**, 1445–1453.

36 Sallinen, S.L., Sallinen, P.K., Haapasalo, H.K., Helin, H.J., Helen, P.T., Schraml, P., Kallioniemi, O.P. and Kononen, J. (2000) Identification of differentially expressed genes in human gliomas by DNA microarray and tissue chip techniques. *Cancer Research*, **60**, 6617–6622.

37 van den Boom, J., Wolter, M., Kuick, R., Misek, D.E., Youkilis, A.S., Wechsler, D.S., Sommer, C., Reifenberger, G. and Hanash, S.M. (2003) Characterization of gene expression profiles associated with glioma progression using oligonucleotide-based microarray analysis and real-time reverse transcription-polymerase chain reaction. *The American Journal of Pathology*, **163**, 1033–1043.

38 van den Boom, J., Wolter, M., Blaschke, B., Knobbe, C.B. and Reifenberger, G. (2006) Identification of novel genes associated with astrocytoma progression using suppression subtractive hybridization and real-time reverse transcription-polymerase chain reaction. *International Journal of Cancer*, **119**, 2330–2338.

39 Mueller, W., Hartmann, C., Hoffmann, A., Lanksch, W., Kiwit, J., Tonn, J., Veelken, J., Schramm, J., Weller, M., Wiestler, O.D., Louis, D.N. and von Deimling, A. (2002) Genetic signature of oligoastrocytomas correlates with tumor location and denotes distinct molecular subsets. *The American Journal of Pathology*, **161**, 313–319.

40 Sharma, M.K., Mansur, D.B., Reifenberger, G., Perry, A., Leonard, J.R., Aldape, K.D., Albin, M.G., Emnett, R.J., Loeser, S., Watson, M.A., Nagarajan, R. and Gutmann, D.H. (2007) Distinct genetic signatures among pilocytic astrocytomas relate to their brain region origin. *Cancer Research*, **67**, 890–900.

41 Modena, P., Lualdi, E., Facchinetti, F., Veltman, J., Reid, J.F., Minardi, S., Janssen, I., Giangaspero, F., Forni, M., Finocchiaro, G., Genitori, L., Giordano, F., Riccardi, R., Schoenmakers, E.F., Massimino, M. and Sozzi, G. (2006) Identification of tumor-specific molecular signatures in intracranial ependymoma and association with clinical characteristics. *Journal of Clinical Oncology*, **24**, 5223–5233.

42 Korshunov, A., Neben, K., Wrobel, G., Tews, B., Benner, A., Hahn, M., Golanov, A. and Lichter, P. (2003) Gene expression patterns in ependymomas correlate with tumor location grade, and patient age. *The American Journal of Pathology*, **163**, 1721–1727.

43 Tibshirani, R., Hastie, T., Narasimhan, B. and Chu, G. (2002) Diagnosis of multiple cancer types by shrunken centroids of gene expression. *Proceedings of the National Academy of Sciences of the United States of America*, **99**, 6567–6572.

44 Bild, A.H., Yao, G., Chang, J.T., Wang, Q., Potti, A., Chasse, D., Joshi, M.B., Harpole, D., Lancaster, J.M., Berchuck, A., Olson, J.A., Jr., Marks, J.R., Dressman, H.K., West, M. and Nevins, J.R. (2006) Oncogenic pathway signatures in human cancers as a guide to targeted therapies. *Nature*, **439**, 353–357.

45 Bild, A.H., Potti, A. and Nevins, J.R. (2006) Linking oncogenic pathways with therapeutic opportunities. *Nature Reviews. Cancer*, **6**, 735–741.

46 Choe, G., Horvath, S., Cloughesy, T.F., Crosby, K., Seligson, D., Palotie, A., Inge, L., Smith, B.L., Sawyers, C.L. and Mischel, P.S. (2003) Analysis of the phosphatidylinositol 3′-kinase signaling pathway in glioblastoma patients *in vivo*. *Cancer Research*, **63**, 2742–2746.

47 Riemenschneider, M.J., Betensky, R.A., Pasedag, S.M. and Louis, D.N. (2006) AKT activation in human glioblastomas enhances proliferation via TSC2 and S6 kinase signaling. *Cancer Research*, **66**, 5618–5623.

48 Riemenschneider, M.J., Mueller, W., Betensky, R.A., Mohapatra, G. and Louis, D.N. (2005) *in situ* analysis of integrin and growth factor receptor signaling pathways in human glioblastomas suggests overlapping relationships with focal adhesion kinase activation. *The American Journal of Pathology*, **167**, 1379–1387.

49 Dong, S., Nutt, C.L., Betensky, R.A., Stemmer-Rachamimov, A.O., Denko, N.C., Ligon, K.L., Rowitch, D.H. and Louis, D.N. (2005) Histology-based expression profiling yields novel prognostic markers in human glioblastoma. *Journal of Neuropathology and Experimental Neurology*, **64**, 948–955.

50 Brat, D.J. and Van Meir, E.G. (2004) Vaso-occlusive and prothrombotic mechanisms associated with tumor hypoxia necrosis, and accelerated growth in glioblastoma. *Laboratory Investigation*, **84**, 397–405.

51 Brat, D.J., Castellano-Sanchez, A.A., Hunter, S.B., Pecot, M., Cohen, C., Hammond, E.H., Devi, S.N., Kaur, B. and Van Meir, E.G. (2004) Pseudopalisades in glioblastoma are hypoxic express extracellular matrix proteases, and are formed by an actively migrating cell population. *Cancer Research*, **64**, 920–927.

52 Enam, S.A., Rosenblum, M.L. and Edvardsen, K. (1998) Role of extracellular matrix in tumor invasion: migration of glioma cells along fibronectin-positive mesenchymal cell processes. *Neurosurgery*, **42**, 599–607 (discussion 607–598).

53 Friedlander, D.R., Zagzag, D., Shiff, B., Cohen, H., Allen, J.C., Kelly, P.J. and Grumet, M. (1996) Migration of brain tumor cells on extracellular matrix proteins *in vitro* correlates with tumor type and grade and

involves alphaV and beta1 integrins. *Cancer Research*, **56**, 1939–1947.

54 Mahesparan, R., Tysnes, B.B., Read, T.A., Enger, P.O., Bjerkvig, R. and Lund-Johansen, M. (1999) Extracellular matrix-induced cell migration from glioblastoma biopsy specimens *in vitro*. *Acta Neuropathologica (Berlin)*, **97**, 231–239.

55 Mariani, L., Beaudry, C., McDonough, W.S., Hoelzinger, D.B., Demuth, T., Ross, K.R., Berens, T., Coons, S.W., Watts, G., Trent, J.M., Wei, J.S., Giese, A. and Berens, M.E. (2001) Glioma cell motility is associated with reduced transcription of proapoptotic and proliferation genes: a cDNA microarray analysis. *Journal of Neuro-Oncology*, **53**, 161–176.

56 Berens, M.E. and Giese, A. (1999) ''…those left behind.'' Biology and oncology of invasive glioma cells. *Neoplasia*, **1**, 208–219.

57 Hoelzinger, D.B., Mariani, L., Weis, J., Woyke, T., Berens, T.J., McDonough, W.S., Sloan, A., Coons, S.W. and Berens, M.E. (2005) Gene expression profile of glioblastoma multiforme invasive phenotype points to new therapeutic targets. *Neoplasia*, **7**, 7–16.

58 Lee, J., Kotliarova, S., Kotliarov, Y., Li, A., Su, Q., Donin, N.M., Pastorino, S., Purow, B.W., Christopher, N., Zhang, W., Park, J.K. and Fine, H.A. (2006) Tumor stem cells derived from glioblastomas cultured in bFGF and EGF more closely mirror the phenotype and genotype of primary tumors than do serum-cultured cell lines. *Cancer Cell*, **9**, 391–403.

59 Bjerkvig, R., Tysnes, B.B., Aboody, K.S., Najbauer, J. and Terzis, A.J. (2005) Opinion: the origin of the cancer stem cell: current controversies and new insights. *Nature Reviews. Cancer*, **5**, 899–904.

60 Singh, S.K., Hawkins, C., Clarke, I.D., Squire, J.A., Bayani, J., Hide, T., Henkelman, R.M., Cusimano, M.D. and Dirks, P.B. (2004) Identification of human brain tumour initiating cells. *Nature*, **432**, 396–401.

61 Vescovi, A.L., Galli, R. and Reynolds, B.A. (2006) Brain tumour stem cells. *Nature Reviews. Cancer*, **6**, 425–436.

62 Beier, D., Hau, P., Proescholdt, M., Lohmeier, A., Wischhusen, J., Oefner, P.J., Aigner, L., Brawanski, A., Bogdahn, U. and Beier, C.P. (2007) CD133(+) and CD133(−) glioblastoma-derived cancer stem cells show differential growth characteristics and molecular profiles. *Cancer Research*, **67**, 4010–4015.

63 Phillips, H.S., Kharbanda, S., Chen, R., Forrest, W.F., Soriano, R.H., Wu, T.D., Misra, A., Nigro, J.M., Colman, H., Soroceanu, L., Williams, P.M., Modrusan, Z., Feuerstein, B.G. and Aldape, K. (2006) Molecular subclasses of high-grade glioma predict prognosis delineate a pattern of disease progression, and resemble stages in neurogenesis. *Cancer Cell*, **9**, 157–173.

64 Mueller, W., Nutt, C.L., Ehrich, M., Riemenschneider, M.J., von Deimling, A., van den Boom, D. and Louis, D.N. (2007) Downregulation of RUNX3 and TES by hypermethylation in glioblastoma. *Oncogene*, **26**, 583–593.

Index

Neural Degeneration and Repair: Gene Expression Profiling, Proteomics, and Systems Biology
Edited by Hans Werner Müller
Copyright © 2008 WILEY-VCH Verlag GmbH & Co. KGaA, Weinheim
ISBN: 978-3-527-31707-3